Advanced Secure Transmission of Telemedicine-Based Bio-Medical Images

Binay Kumar Pandey
Department of Information Technology, College of Technology, Govind Balladh Pant University of Agriculture and Technology, India

A. Shaji George
TSM, Almarai Company, Saudi Arabia

Sameer Tiwari
George Mason University, USA

Salah A. Albermany
Kufa University, Iraq

Ho Sy Hung
Hong Duc University, Vietnam

IGI Global
Scientific Publishing
Publishing Tomorrow's Research Today

Vice President of Editorial Melissa Wagner
Director of Acquisitions Mikaela Felty
Director of Book Development Jocelynn Hessler
Production Manager Mike Brehm
Cover Design Jose Rosado

Published in the United States of America by
IGI Global Scientific Publishing
701 East Chocolate Avenue
Hershey, PA, 17033, USA
Tel: 717-533-8845
Fax: 717-533-7115
Website: https://www.igi-global.com E-mail: cust@igi-global.com

Library of Congress Cataloging-in-Publication Data

Names: Tiwari, Sameer, 1984- editor | Albermany, Salah A., 1971- editor | George, A. Shaji, 1971- editor | Pandey, Binay, 1983- editor | Hung, Ho Sy, 1984- editor
Title: Advanced secure transmission of telemedicine-based bio-medical images / edited by Sameer Tiwari, Salah A. Albermany, A. Shaji George, Binay Pandey, Ho Sy Hung.
Description: Hershey, PA : IGI Global Scientific Publishing, [2025] | Includes bibliographical references and index. | Summary: "This book also offers advanced steganography ways for embedding textual data on the cover image, as well as a new way for secure transmission of biological imaging, imaging with machine learning and deep learning, and 2D, 3D imaging in the field of telemedicine"-- Provided by publisher.
Identifiers: LCCN 2024060570 (print) | LCCN 2024060571 (ebook) | ISBN 9798369398210 hardcover | ISBN 9798369398227 paperback | ISBN 9798369398234 ebook
Subjects: LCSH: Medical telematics--Security measures | Image transmission | Internet in medicine--Security measures
Classification: LCC R119.95 .A375 2025 (print) | LCC R119.95 (ebook) | DDC 610.285--dc23/eng/20250331
LC record available at https://lccn.loc.gov/2024060570
LC ebook record available at https://lccn.loc.gov/2024060571
British Cataloguing in Publication Data
A Cataloguing in Publication record for this book is available from the British Library.

Table of Contents

Detailed Table of Contents

Access and convenience for both patients and providers have been significantly improved as a result of the rapid development of telemedicine, which has revolutionized the delivery of healthcare. The growing reliance on digital technologies for patient interactions, on the other hand, leads to significant concerns regarding the confidentiality and security of patient information. With a particular emphasis on a variety of privacy-protecting strategies and multi-layered security solutions, this study investigates the critical need for robust security measures in the field of telemedicine. At the same time that it discusses the fundamental security principles of confidentiality, integrity, and availability, the research highlights the vulnerabilities that are associated with the transmission and storage of sensitive medical data, such as biomedical images and pharmacy records, through an in-depth analysis.

In the field of telemedicine, the incorporation of secure image transmission technologies and workflow automation, with a particular emphasis on the impact these technologies have on service delivery. Secure image transmission, which is accomplished through encryption protocols, virtual private networks (VPNs), and cloud-based platforms, makes it possible for medical professionals to share medical images in a manner that is both secure and fast. Through the use of real-time image sharing, diagnostic accuracy can be improved, delays can be reduced, and treatment decisions can be made more quickly and effectively. The automation of workflows also helps to streamline administrative and clinical tasks, which reduces the likelihood of errors caused by humans and increases operational efficiency.

Artificial intelligence (AI) is revolutionizing the field of medical image analysis, highlighting the vital need of strong security protocols to safeguard private patient

Security cameras are typical in most systems and come in many varieties. Internet security cameras, or IP cameras, send and receive data. Free smartphone and tablet apps make live video broadcasts easy to access anytime. IP cameras can monitor a facility inside and out. Cameras can also alert guards to suspicious activity so they can investigate. Remote video monitoring using video surveillance is used for safeguarding a property or structure from intruders, theft, and dishonest personnel. CCTV cameras can monitor daily operations, speed them up, and prevent loss. Outdoor CCTV cameras are used to monitor a building. Video surveillance, roving security/protection teams, perimeter fencing, closed gates for cars and pedestrians, and intrusion detection systems can keep this region secure. For safety, CCTV camera pictures are analyzed using machine learning.

The rapid development of telemedicine has resulted in the emergence of significant challenges concerning the transmission of medical images in a secure manner. Given the growing reliance of the healthcare industry on digital platforms for diagnosis and treatment, it is of the utmost importance to protect the confidentiality and integrity of sensitive patient data. The application of machine learning (ML) in the context of improving the safety and effectiveness of telemedicine image transmission. By utilizing advanced machine learning techniques, such as dynamic encryption algorithms, real-time anomaly detection, and adaptive security protocols, healthcare providers are able to better protect themselves against cybersecurity threats while simultaneously ensuring that they have timely access to high-quality medical images.

The development of machine learning applications in the healthcare industry depends on safe medical image sharing. Protecting patient privacy is more difficult but necessary as medical imaging data grows. This paper investigates how to integrate encryption techniques and secure data-sharing methods, like blockchain, to facilitate cross-organizational collaboration while maintaining data privacy. Sensitive patient data is kept in local systems thanks to collaborative models like federated learning, which enable institutions to train machine learning algorithms on decentralized datasets. This strategy makes use of the variety of data available across healthcare facilities while protecting the privacy of medical records. The creation of machine learning models for diagnosis and treatment planning that are more reliable and accurate is made possible by the safe interchange of medical images.

The transformative potential of machine learning (ML) in disease forecasting is emphasizes how crucial secure transmission techniques are to maintaining the integrity of patient data. With the growing reliance of healthcare on sophisticated data analytics, machine learning (ML) models have become indispensable instruments for forecasting disease outbreaks and enhancing patient results. ML algorithms are able to detect patterns and trends that help with early detection and intervention in a variety of health conditions by examining large datasets that include clinical data, medical images, and environmental factors. But considering the increasing frequency of cyberattacks and data breaches in the healthcare industry, it is critical that this sensitive data be transmitted securely.

Preface

In an era of unprecedented connectivity and digital transformation, the secure transmission of biomedical and telemedicine-based images has become not only a technical challenge but a critical necessity for healthcare delivery systems worldwide. The proliferation of audiovisual content—spanning images, audio, video, and textual formats—over public networks and Internet of Things (IoT) devices brings with it enormous potential for remote diagnostics, patient care, and medical collaboration. However, it simultaneously exposes sensitive data to a host of vulnerabilities that must be addressed with advanced security frameworks.

This edited reference book, Advanced Secure Transmission of Telemedicine-Based Bio-Medical Images, explores the forefront of secure multimedia transmission in healthcare environments. It draws on a wide array of contemporary research to examine and integrate diverse approaches such as encryption, digital watermarking, cryptography, and steganography—all of which contribute to the three fundamental pillars of data security: confidentiality, integrity, and availability. These methods ensure that only authorized users can access critical information, that the information remains unaltered and trustworthy, and that it is readily accessible when needed.

Of particular emphasis is the innovative use of steganographic techniques for embedding secret data into biomedical images, as well as the application of machine learning and deep learning algorithms for secure and intelligent image processing. Chapters within this volume address the challenges of 2D and 3D medical imaging, the potential of textual image recognition, and the development of advanced methodologies for secure storage and transmission over public networks.

The contributions gathered in this volume reflect a multidisciplinary approach, bringing together insights from computer science, biomedical engineering, and healthcare technology. For researchers, practitioners, and system designers, this book offers both theoretical depth and practical guidance on developing secure, scalable, and intelligent telemedicine solutions.

As editors, our goal has been to curate a comprehensive resource that not only addresses current technological gaps but also inspires further innovation in secure healthcare data processing. We hope this volume will serve as a valuable reference for those working to enhance the reliability, safety, and efficiency of digital medical infrastructures in an increasingly interconnected world.

ORGANIZATION OF THE BOOK

In *Chapter 1*, "Ensuring Confidentiality in Telemedicine: A Comprehensive Study on Secure Transmission of Bio-Medical Images and Pharmacy Data," the authors present a compelling analysis of the vital importance of protecting patient data in telemedicine. As digital technologies increasingly facilitate remote consultations and medical services, concerns regarding confidentiality and secure data transmission intensify. This chapter delves into multi-layered security mechanisms and privacy-enhancing strategies aimed at safeguarding sensitive information, particularly bio-medical images and pharmacy records, while reinforcing the foundational security principles of confidentiality, integrity, and availability.

Chapter 2, titled "Enhancing Telemedicine Workflow Through Secure Image Transmission," explores how the integration of secure image-sharing technologies—such as encryption protocols, VPNs, and cloud infrastructures—improves diagnostic accuracy and operational efficiency. The chapter articulates how these technologies enable real-time image access, reduce delays, and enhance clinical decision-making. Furthermore, workflow automation in telemedicine minimizes human error, optimizes task execution, and creates a more streamlined, secure, and responsive healthcare delivery environment.

In *Chapter 3*, "AI Powered Secure Bio-Medical Image Analysis," the intersection of artificial intelligence and security in medical imaging is thoroughly examined. As AI reshapes diagnostics and treatment planning through powerful image analysis tools, the necessity of data protection grows proportionately. This chapter discusses advanced privacy-preserving techniques such as differential privacy, federated learning, and secure multi-party computation, all of which allow collaborative medical innovation while ensuring that sensitive patient data remains confidential and uncompromised.

Chapter 4, "Role of Secure Image Transmission in Agricultural Health Monitoring," extends the scope of image security to agriculture, showing how secure imaging technologies are crucial in monitoring the health of crops and livestock. With data sources ranging from drones to satellites, the chapter underscores the importance of encrypted transmission methods and end-to-end security protocols. By ensuring the integrity and confidentiality of agricultural data, these technologies support timely, data-driven decisions, regulatory compliance, and digital trust across the agri-tech ecosystem.

In *Chapter 5*, "Scientific Progress in Artificial Intelligence for Time-Stamped Interpretation of Camera Images in Medical Safety Systems," the use of AI-enhanced surveillance for medical and facility safety is explored. The chapter details how IP cameras, combined with real-time analytics and machine learning, contribute to the monitoring and protection of healthcare environments. From perimeter security to internal activity tracking, this chapter highlights the value of automated image analysis in boosting situational awareness and operational safety in medical settings.

Chapter 6, "Integrating Machine Learning with Secure Telemedicine Image Transmission," investigates how machine learning fortifies the transmission of medical images against cyber threats. By deploying smart encryption, real-time anomaly detection, and adaptive security models, healthcare systems can maintain the confidentiality and reliability of transmitted data. This chapter emphasizes that ML-driven image transmission not only reinforces security but also enhances the speed and precision of remote diagnosis and care delivery.

Chapter 7, "Enhancing Machine Learning Efficiency Through Secure Medical Image Sharing," discusses the growing need for privacy-preserving collaboration across healthcare institutions. With federated learning and blockchain-based sharing protocols, this chapter demonstrates how medical institutions can pool knowledge and train ML algorithms without compromising patient privacy. The secure sharing of imaging data empowers researchers and practitioners to develop more robust diagnostic models while maintaining adherence to data protection standards.

Chapter 8, "Machine Learning and Secure Image Transmission for Disease Forecasting," examines the dual role of ML and secure data handling in predicting disease trends and outbreaks. Through the analysis of large-scale clinical and environmental datasets, ML models facilitate early detection and informed intervention. However, the chapter stresses that these advancements must be underpinned by secure data transmission protocols to prevent breaches and preserve public trust in digital health systems.

Chapter 9: "IoT Driven Secure Data Sharing in Telemedicine Systems" explores the pivotal role that connected devices play in revolutionizing telemedicine. This chapter emphasizes how IoT can elevate patient care and remote health monitoring while also underlining the urgent need for robust security strategies to protect sensitive health data. As healthcare infrastructure becomes increasingly reliant on these technologies, the chapter argues for continuous innovation in securing data exchanges and adhering to evolving compliance mandates.

Chapter 10: "Telemedicine IoT Networks and Secure Image Transmission" continues this discussion by focusing on the synergy between IoT networks and the secure transmission of medical images. With accurate diagnostics heavily dependent on high-quality imaging, the chapter illustrates how IoT-enabled telemedicine must employ advanced transmission safeguards to ensure privacy and reliability while also increasing accessibility and system efficiency.

Chapter 11: "Role of IoT in Enhancing Secure Medical Image Transfers" investigates the privacy-centric transformation IoT brings to medical image handling. It details how lightweight protocols like MQTT and CoAP enable secure, real-time data sharing. This chapter contributes critical insights into how connected medical devices can securely relay sensitive visual data, ensuring faster, safer diagnoses in dynamic healthcare settings.

Chapter 12: "Securing IoT Devices for Bio-Medical Image Sharing" highlights the increasing vulnerability landscape that accompanies the proliferation of IoT in healthcare. With a strong focus on biomedical image sharing, this chapter emphasizes the necessity of end-to-end security strategies—specifically, robust authentication mechanisms, encryption models, and intelligent anomaly detection—to fortify data protection without compromising system performance.

Chapter 13: "Quantum Cryptography for Biomedical Image Security in Next-Generation Telemedicine Networks" introduces a forward-looking perspective, delving into quantum cryptography's revolutionary role in future-proofing biomedical data security. Traditional encryption is no longer sufficient against quantum computing threats; this chapter presents quantum key distribution (QKD) and advanced protocols like MDI-QKD as essential tools for safeguarding medical imaging in advanced applications such as remote surgery and teleradiology. It also addresses the practical challenges of adopting such systems at scale.

Together, these chapters reflect a unified mission: to build resilient, intelligent telemedicine ecosystems where security, accessibility, and innovation coexist. The authors contribute diverse yet complementary viewpoints, helping healthcare professionals, technologists, and researchers navigate the complexities of digital health transformation in a secure and scalable manner.

CONCLUSION

As editors of this volume, we conclude this anthology with a strong sense of urgency, possibility, and responsibility. The chapters presented throughout this book reflect the growing convergence of digital technologies—particularly IoT, AI, quantum cryptography, and secure communication protocols—with the critical domain of healthcare. Telemedicine, once considered a supplementary service, has rapidly evolved into a cornerstone of modern healthcare delivery, driven by the demand for accessibility, speed, and personalization. However, as these systems become more deeply embedded in clinical practice, the stakes around data privacy, cybersecurity, and technological integrity have never been higher.

The contributors to this work have illuminated a path forward—one that demands innovation not only in hardware and software but also in policy, design thinking, and ethical implementation. From securing biomedical image transfers to deploying quantum-resistant cryptographic systems, the chapters capture the multifaceted challenges and offer actionable insights to build resilient telemedicine infrastructures.

Ultimately, this volume serves not only as a reference for academic inquiry but as a strategic guide for practitioners, researchers, and policymakers committed to shaping a secure and equitable digital health future. As we move further into a hyperconnected era, our hope is that the knowledge curated here inspires continued research, fosters interdisciplinary collaboration, and ensures that the next wave of digital healthcare innovation is as secure as it is transformative.

Chapter 1
Ensuring Confidentiality in Telemedicine:
A Comprehensive Study on Secure Transmission of Bio-Medical Images and Pharmacy Data

Manish Kumar Thimmaraju
Department of Pharmaceutical Analysis, Balaji Institute of Pharmaceutical sciences, Warangal, India

Divya Pingili
https://orcid.org/0000-0001-5951-8910
Department of Pharmaceutical Chemistry, Sri Venkateshwara College of Pharmacy, India

Gampa Vijaya Kumar
Department of Pharmacy, KGR Institute of Technology and Management, Rampally, India

Mukundan Appadurai Paramashivan
https://orcid.org/0009-0009-5608-4788
Champions Group, Singapore

ABSTRACT

Access and convenience for both patients and providers have been significantly improved as a result of the rapid development of telemedicine, which has revolutionized the delivery of healthcare. The growing reliance on digital technologies for patient interactions, on the other hand, leads to significant concerns regarding the confidentiality and security of patient information. With a particular emphasis

DOI: 10.4018/979-8-3693-9821-0.ch001

on a variety of privacy-protecting strategies and multi-layered security solutions, this study investigates the critical need for robust security measures in the field of telemedicine. At the same time that it discusses the fundamental security principles of confidentiality, integrity, and availability, the research highlights the vulnerabilities that are associated with the transmission and storage of sensitive medical data, such as biomedical images and pharmacy records, through an in-depth analysis.

INTRODUCTION

The ability to diagnose, treat, and manage patients remotely, telemedicine has completely transformed the delivery of healthcare. In spite of this, there are significant concerns regarding the confidentiality of sensitive data, such as images of biomedical procedures and information about pharmacies. With the goal of preserving the trust of patients and adhering to ethical and legal standards, it is essential to guarantee the safe transmission of this information. In the process of being transmitted between patients and healthcare providers, biomedical images, which include X-rays, CT scans, and MRIs, contain sensitive personal health information (PHI) that must be safeguarded. Data breaches, interception by unlawful parties, and tampering are examples of common types of threats. The protection of this data is largely dependent on the utilization of encryption methods, including symmetric and asymmetric encryption, particularly. Beginning with the sender and continuing all the way through to the receiver, end-to-end encryption (E2EE) ensures that the data is protected from any unauthorized access by a third party. In addition, secure transmission protocols such as SSL/TLS offer additional layers of protection by establishing secure communication channels (Sheela, M. S. et al., 2025) between different electronic systems. Due to the fact that pharmacy data is connected to patient records, prescriptions, and medical history, it is also necessary to implement stringent security measures. Encryption, access control, and compliance with regulations such as HIPAA and GDPR are all necessary components in the process of protecting sensitive data. Through the provision of immutable records that improve data integrity and security, blockchain technology is emerging as a powerful solution for securely sharing pharmacy data. Secure application programming interfaces (APIs) guarantee that only authorized systems and personnel are able to access and share pharmacy data, thereby reducing the likelihood of data breaches (Satheesh, N. et al., 2025).

Telemedicine and its Growing Importance

The provision of medical services via digital communication technologies, known as telemedicine, allows patients and healthcare professionals to communicate remotely. It includes a broad range of services, such as follow-up care, diagnosis, treatment, and virtual consultations and remote monitoring. Telemedicine has grown in importance as a component of contemporary healthcare due to the quick development of communication technologies and healthcare systems (Kumar, M. S. et al., 2025). It addresses major issues with efficiency, cost, and accessibility. The demand for better access to healthcare, particularly in underserved or rural areas where medical facilities are frequently limited, has led to a significant increase in the importance of telemedicine. Patients no longer need to take lengthy trips to see specialists in order to receive care using telemedicine. Patients with chronic conditions who need regular monitoring and consultations will particularly benefit from this. Telemedicine eases the workload for medical facilities and expedites the process for patients and providers by enabling virtual visits. Telemedicines uptake was sped up by the COVID-19 pandemic, which highlighted its significance in preserving healthcare delivery while lowering the risk of disease transmission. Many patients found that telemedicine was their lifeline during lockdowns and restrictions, enabling them to receive care while following social distancing protocols. It also showed how useful it is for handling non-emergency scenarios, cutting down on hospital and clinic crowding, and avoiding delays in providing necessary healthcare services. Beyond ease of use and accessibility, telemedicine lowers healthcare delivery costs, which benefits the economy. In comparison to traditional in-person care, patients save on travel expenses and healthcare providers can more effectively allocate resources, providing services at a lower cost. Wearable technology and other remote monitoring tools allow for real-time tracking of patients' health conditions, which enables earlier interventions and better health outcomes. Specialized care also heavily relies on telemedicine. For example, specialists from large hospitals can visit patients in remote areas, facilitating prompt diagnosis and treatment. This is especially helpful in areas where a lot of services can be efficiently provided through telecommunication, such as radiology, dermatology, and mental health. The incorporation of cutting-edge technologies such as artificial neural network (Pandey, B. K., & Pandey, D., 2023), machine learning, and data analytics will augment the capabilities of telemedicine as it advances. These technologies can facilitate individualized treatment plans, enhance diagnostics, and offer predictive insights. Telemedicine is a vital tool in meeting the rising demand for healthcare services worldwide because of its capacity to provide healthcare more effectively, more affordably, and with greater accessibility (Yusof, M. M. et al., 2008).

Secure Transmission of Sensitive Medical Data

In telemedicine, where patients and healthcare providers exchange personal health information (PHI) like medical records, biomedical images, and pharmacy data, the safe transmission of sensitive medical data is essential. Safeguarding this data is crucial to upholding patient privacy (Pandey, B. K., & Pandey, D., 2025), fostering trust, and adhering to legal requirements as healthcare relies more and more on digital communication technologies. Since medical data is so sensitive, any compromise or illegal access may have dire repercussions. Identity theft, insurance fraud, or the unauthorized use of personal data may result from the disclosure of private information such as diagnosis, treatment plans, or prescription details. Medical data breaches have the potential to damage patient confidence in the healthcare system and discourage people from using telemedicine services, in addition to the legal and financial ramifications. The efficacy of remote care is compromised, and patients may be disinclined to divulge crucial health information, which could have an adverse effect on their course of treatment. In addition to protecting patient privacy, secure transmission is required by law. The protection of personal health data is subject to stringent regulations, including the General Data Protection Regulation (GDPR) in Europe and the Health Insurance Portability and Accountability Act (HIPAA) in the United States. Utilizing strong encryption techniques, secure transmission protocols, and access control mechanisms to prevent unwanted access, healthcare providers and telemedicine platforms must make sure that data is transferred securely. Secure data transmission relies heavily on encryption. Encryption ensures that medical data cannot be read or altered by unauthorized parties, even if it is intercepted, by encoding the data during transmission. By guaranteeing that the data can only be accessed by the intended sender and recipient, end-to-end encryption, or E2EE, further improves security. Preventing cyberattacks, phishing, and data breaches requires the use of secure communication channels like SSL/TLS protocols, multi-factor authentication (MFA), and strong password policies. Telemedicine platforms need to put these safeguards in place to guard against internal risks like employees accidentally exposing patient data and external threats like hackers (Vora, J. et al., 2018).

TELEMEDICINE DATA SECURITY REQUIREMENTS

Bio-Medical Images and Pharmacy Records

In telemedicine, the transmission of sensitive data is a primary concern, with biomedical images and pharmaceutical records being among the most critical types of information managed. These data sets encompass sensitive information regarding a patient's health, rendering confidentiality and security paramount in any telemedicine platform. Biomedical images, including X-rays, CT scans, MRIs, and ultrasound images, are essential for precise diagnosis and treatment planning. These images frequently include identifiable patient information and comprehensive visuals of a patient's condition, which must be safeguarded against unauthorized access or alteration (Konapure, C. G. et al., 2025). The substantial volume and considerable file sizes of medical images complicate their secure transmission, necessitating robust encryption techniques and secure communication channels to preserve data integrity throughout the process. In the absence of sufficient safeguards, these images may be intercepted, modified, or exploited by unauthorized individuals (Singh, S. et al., 2025), resulting in privacy infringements and possible detriment to the patient. Pharmacy records constitute a sensitive category of data within telemedicine. This documentation encompasses prescription specifics, dosage data, and a patient's pharmacological medical history. The security of pharmacy records, which are frequently linked to a patient's comprehensive treatment plan, is essential to avert misuse. Unauthorized access to these records may result in medication fraud, illicit prescription modifications, and identity theft (Sharma, M. et al., 2025). Inadequate management of pharmacy data may lead to violations of health regulations, thereby exposing healthcare providers to legal liabilities. The secure transmission of biomedical images and pharmaceutical records is essential for preserving the integrity and confidentiality of telemedicine services. Inadequate encryption, access control, and secure communication protocols elevate the risks of data breaches (Pandey, B. K. et al., 2024a), jeopardizing patient privacy and trust. As telemedicine advances, the emphasis on safeguarding sensitive data will persist as a primary concern for healthcare providers and technology developers (Mbonihankuye, S. et al., 2019).

Core Security Principles

Protecting sensitive medical data and guaranteeing safe healthcare delivery are made possible by the three main telemedicine security principles: confidentiality, integrity, and availability (Pandey, B. K. et al., 2024b). When we talk about confidentiality, we mean keeping private any sensitive medical data safe from unwanted access. This idea is crucial to the field of telemedicine because patient data, such as medical histories, biomedical images (Basha, A. J. et al., 2024), and prescription records, must be kept confidential. Strict user authentication procedures, robust access controls, and encryption are all necessary to achieve confidentiality (KVM, S. et al., 2024). Telemedicine platforms make sure that only patients and authorized healthcare providers have access to or exchange of sensitive data by putting these safeguards in place. Prioritizing confidentiality is crucial because a breach can result in serious privacy violations (Lakshmi, K. V. N. et al., 2024) and erode patient trust in telemedicine services. The goal of integrity is to keep medical data accurate and consistent during storage and transmission. Maintaining data integrity in telemedicine is essential to avoiding unauthorized changes that might lead to inaccurate diagnosis, ineffective treatments, or medication mistakes. Telemedicine platforms use digital signatures, encryption, and secure communication protocols that identify any unauthorized changes or tampering during transmission in order to protect the integrity of data (Saravanakumar, R. et al., 2024). Healthcare professionals can improve the safety and dependability of patient care by making sure the information they receive is exactly as intended. Availability guarantees that authorized users can always access medical data and telemedicine services. Continuous access to vital data is necessary for the efficient delivery of healthcare, including pharmacy data, biomedical images, and medical records. Redundancy, data backup programs, and secure cloud services all contribute to availability by reducing the effects of disruptions, cyberattacks, and system failures. High data and service availability is crucial, particularly in emergency scenarios where having instant access to patient data can save lives (Qayyum, A. et al., 2020).

SECURING BIO-MEDICAL IMAGE TRANSMISSION

Vulnerabilities During Image Transmission

Numerous vulnerabilities exist in the transmission of biomedical images during telemedicine, which may jeopardize the security and privacy of private patient information. Interception and tampering are two major threats that seriously jeopardize the accuracy of medical data (Kumarganesh, S. et al., 2024). Unauthorized access to data during transmission between locations is referred to as interception. In the context of telemedicine, this might happen when biomedical images are transferred between various healthcare systems or from a patient to a healthcare provider. Cybercriminals may obtain sensitive patient data by intercepting data packets carrying these images through the use of network security flaws (Muralidhar, L. B. et al., 2024). Identity theft, the unapproved disclosure of medical records, and serious legal and financial fallout for healthcare institutions are all possible outcomes of such breaches. It is essential to use secure communication protocols (such as SSL/TLS), strong authentication procedures, and encryption techniques to reduce the possibility of interception. Data tampering is the act of making unwanted changes to data while it is being transmitted or stored (Pandey, B. K. et al., 2024c). Modified biomedical images in telemedicine can have detrimental effects, possibly resulting in incorrect diagnosis or treatment choices. The consequences for patient care could be disastrous, for example, if a radiologist receives an image that has been altered to hide serious medical conditions. Insider threats, malicious software, and even unsafe storage techniques are some of the ways that tampering can happen. Digital signatures and checksums that confirm the integrity and validity of the transmitted images should be used by healthcare providers to reduce the possibility of tampering. These steps aid in preventing unauthorized data modifications from occurring and ensuring that any effects on patient care are avoided (Agbo, C. C. et al., 2019).

Image Storage/Retrieval Issues

The storage and retrieval of images in telemedicine pose considerable challenges, as illustrated in figure 1, owing to the substantial file sizes and the sensitive nature of medical images. Robust storage solutions are imperative to avert unauthorized access, necessitating encryption and stringent access controls. Moreover, effective retrieval systems are essential for facilitating rapid access to images by authorized healthcare professionals while maintaining security. Nonetheless, the administration of extensive databases, preservation of image quality, and assurance of data integrity during retrieval remain persistent issues. Inadequate security measures render stored images susceptible to breaches, which may result in data leaks, privacy infringements, or alterations during retrieval processes.

- *Data Security*: Biomedical images (Elarmathi, S. et al., 2024) contain sensitive patient information, rendering them prime targets for cybercriminals. Unauthorized access to these images may result in significant privacy infringements and identity theft. The potential ramifications encompass not only detriment to the individual but also considerable legal and financial consequences for the healthcare organization accountable for the data. Consequently, the implementation of robust security measures is essential. Efficient data security necessitates the implementation of sophisticated encryption techniques for both archived images and those being transmitted (Pandey, B. K. et al., 2024d). Encryption guarantees that, even if data is intercepted or accessed without permission, it remains indecipherable. Moreover, implementing stringent access controls guarantees that only authorized individuals can access or manage sensitive images. Conducting regular security audits and providing employee training on data protection practices can enhance data security measures in healthcare organizations.

- *Data Integrity*: Maintaining the integrity of biomedical images is essential, as any corruption or modification of these files can significantly impact patient care. If an image is modified due to a technical malfunction or interference, healthcare providers may rely on erroneous information for their diagnoses, which could result in unsuitable treatment plans. Ensuring data integrity requires the implementation of measures to promptly identify and correct such issues (George, W. K. et al., 2024). An effective method for ensuring data integrity is the implementation of checksums, which confirm that the data remains unaltered during transmission and storage. Regular backups are crucial, enabling healthcare organizations to restore images to their original condition in the event of corruption. Furthermore, implementing stringent data validation procedures during image upload and storage can facilitate the early detection and rectification of errors in the workflow, thereby ensuring that healthcare providers utilize precise and dependable data (Abdullahi, M. et al., 2024).
- *Scalability*: The swift expansion of telemedicine has led to a considerable rise in the quantity of biomedical images produced. Healthcare organizations must be equipped to handle the increasing data influx without sacrificing performance or accessibility. Neglecting to implement scalable storage solutions may result in system deceleration, diminished efficiency, and potential data loss, thereby adversely impacting patient care. Cloud-based storage systems present an efficient means of managing substantial data volumes, offering flexibility and scalability (Kumar, B. et al., 2024). These systems can adapt dynamically to the evolving storage requirements of healthcare organizations, facilitating seamless expansion as necessary. Cloud storage generally incorporates inherent redundancy, guaranteeing the preservation of images despite hardware malfunctions or other interruptions. By utilizing cloud technologies, healthcare providers can adequately address escalating data requirements.
- *Efficiency of Retrieval*: Immediate access to biomedical images is essential for healthcare providers, especially in critical situations where prompt diagnoses can influence patient outcomes. Prolonged retrieval of medical images can obstruct clinical workflows, resulting in increased patient wait times and potentially jeopardizing care quality (Khadka, M. et al., 2025). Consequently, enhancing retrieval efficiency is crucial for effective telemedicine practices. One method to improve retrieval efficiency is the implementation of sophisticated indexing protocols that classify and arrange images according to diverse parameters, such as patient demographics or medical conditions.

Intuitive interfaces can markedly enhance the search experience for healthcare professionals, enabling them to swiftly and effortlessly locate essential images. Investing in high-performance storage solutions can expedite retrieval times, guaranteeing that healthcare professionals have prompt access to essential patient information (Pandey, D. et al., 2024).

- *Compliance with Regulations*: Adherence to legal and ethical standards concerning data privacy and security is a critical issue for healthcare organizations. The storage and retrieval of biomedical images must comply with regulations such as HIPAA in the United States and GDPR in Europe, which impose stringent guidelines for safeguarding sensitive health information. Non-compliance may result in significant legal repercussions, including substantial fines and harm to the organizations reputation. Healthcare organizations must formulate and execute thorough policies and procedures for the management of biomedical images to ensure compliance (Shahul, A. et al., 2024). Consistent training for personnel on compliance mandates and optimal data management practices is imperative. Performing regular audits to evaluate compliance with regulatory standards enables organizations to detect potential vulnerabilities and implement corrective measures. By emphasizing compliance, healthcare providers can preserve patient trust and sustain the integrity of their telemedicine services.

Figure 1. Image storage/retrieval issues

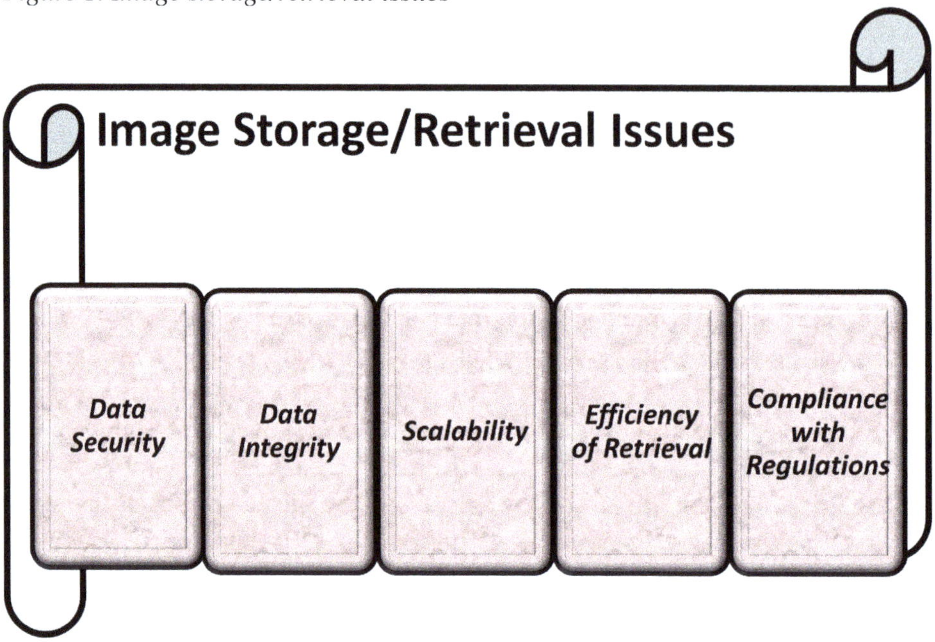

PHARMACY DATA CONFIDENTIALITY CONCERNS

Transmission Risks to Pharmacies

Modern healthcare, especially telemedicine, relies on pharmacy data transmission to pharmacies and healthcare providers. This process may compromise patient data confidentiality, integrity, and availability (Muniandi, B. et al., 2024). These risks must be understood to develop effective pharmacy data transmission security measures. Interception of pharmacy data is a major risk. Man-in-the-middle attacks and packet sniffing are used by cybercriminals to steal data from unsecured networks. When healthcare providers send prescription details and patient identifiers to pharmacies, this can happen. Data intercepted can be used for identity theft or unauthorized medication dispensing. Healthcare organisations must encrypt all data transmissions to reduce this risk. Data intercepted by unauthorized parties is unreadable with encryption. VPNs and TLS can improve data in transit security. Regular network security audits and employee threat awareness training help prevent interception (Singh, S. et al., 2025). Tampering with pharmacy data is another concern. Unauthorized individuals may change prescriptions, dosages, or patient identifiers, posing risks. Changing a prescription to increase dosage or medication can pose serious health risks. Tampering data can also lead to misdiagnosis and inappropriate treatment plans, endangering patients. Healthcare organisations should use digital signatures and checksums to prevent tampering. Digital signatures verify data authenticity and integrity, preventing change in transit. Monitoring data logs can help identify transmission discrepancies for quick investigation and correction. Another pharmacy data transmission risk is inadequate access controls. Failure to enforce access controls can compromise patient confidentiality by allowing unauthorized access to sensitive information. In healthcare data sharing environments, this risk increases the risk of unintentional exposure or malicious access. This risk must be reduced by strong access control. RBAC restrict data access to authorized users based on their roles (Vinodhini, V. et al., 2022). To prevent unauthorized access, review and update access permissions regularly. MFA adds another layer of security by requiring users to verify their identity through multiple methods before accessing sensitive data. The pharmacy data transmission infrastructure can add risk. Cybercriminals exploit network hardware or software vulnerabilities to steal data during transmission. Attacks can exploit outdated software or unpatched systems. Public Wi-Fi networks lack security, making them vulnerable. Healthcare organizations need regular system updates and patches to mitigate these vulnerabilities. Network vulnerabilities can be found and fixed by regular vulnerability assessments. Secure, private networks are essential for transmitting pharmacy data to reduce outside threats. Another pharmacy data transmission risk is human error. Healthcare providers who enter incorrect patient or prescription information can harm patient care. Miscommunication between healthcare providers can also complicate patient treatment. Healthcare organisations should standardise data entry and transmission to reduce human error (Rai, P. K. et al., 2024). Data handling best practices training for healthcare staff can reduce errors. User-friendly interfaces and error-checking in software systems can improve data transmission accuracy. Pharmacy data transmission must comply with US regulations like HIPAA. Healthcare organizations can suffer legal and financial penalties for noncompliance. Regulatory violations can damage patient trust and the organization's reputation. Staying current on regulations and best practices helps healthcare organizations comply. Staff training on compliance requirements and regulatory-compliant policies and procedures are essential. Audits of compliance can help organizations improve and comply with laws. Pharmacy data transmitted across multiple systems or platforms can fragment, causing inconsistencies and gaps in information. Communication between healthcare providers and pharmacies can be hampered by fragmentation, causing medication delays or treatment errors. Interoperable systems that enable cross-platform data sharing can help healthcare organizations reduce data fragmentation. Creating data transmission standards can also improve stakeholder communication and reduce inconsistencies (Kumar Pandey, B. et al., 2021).

Impacts of Data Leaks on Patient Privacy

Data leaks can severely impact patient privacy, affecting individuals, healthcare organizations, and the healthcare system. Understanding these consequences emphasizes the need for strong data protection for providers and patients. Patient confidentiality is immediately affected by data leaks. Patients lose privacy when medical histories, prescriptions, and personal identifiers are exposed. Vulnerable people may suffer significant emotional distress and anxiety from this breach. Patients worry about how their data will be used, who has access to it, and whether it will be misused, which can damage trust in healthcare providers. Trust fosters open communication and honesty about medical conditions, which is crucial for patient-provider relationships. Patient safety can also be compromised by data leaks. Criminals can use exposed data to commit identity theft or fraud. Example: Personal health information can be used to forge prescriptions and dispense unauthorized medications. This can harm the healthcare system and patients, especially those with chronic conditions who need accurate prescriptions and medical histories for treatment. Patients may avoid medical care out of concern for data misuse. Data leaks can harm healthcare organizations as well as patients. Organizations may face legal and financial consequences from data breaches. Patient lawsuits for breach damages may result in costly legal battles and settlements. For violating data protection laws like HIPAA in the US, regulators may fine companies. Financial strain can detract from patient care and lower service quality. Data breaches make patients wary of seeking care from firms that may compromise their personal data. This decline in patient trust can reduce patient retention and business, threatening the organization's finances. In an age of word-of-mouth and online reviews, a single breach can damage a healthcare providers reputation. Clinical research and studies use patient data to improve healthcare. Patients may fear privacy breaches and be less willing to share their data for research after data leaks. This reluctance can stifle medical progress and new treatment development, lowering patient care.

IMAGE COMPRESSION AND ENCRYPTION TECHNIQUES

Image Encryption for Secure Storage and Transmission

Image encryption is essential for digital image storage and transmission, especially in healthcare, finance, and personal privacy. Encrypting images prevents data breaches by preventing unauthorized users from viewing or manipulating them. Data confidentiality is one of image encryption's main goals. Telemedicine images often contain patient identifiers, medical history, and diagnostic images. Intercepted transmission or unsecured storage of these images can lead to identity theft, fraudulent claims, and privacy violations. By using strong encryption, organizations can restrict access to sensitive data and images to intended recipients. Images are encrypted during storage and transmission using various methods. Most people use symmetric key encryption, which uses the same key for encryption and decryption. Fast encryption and decryption of large image files is possible with this method. High-security and efficient algorithms like AES are widely used. AES can meet different security needs by supporting key lengths. In contrast, asymmetric key encryption uses two keys—public and private. This method eliminates the need to share the decryption key, making it ideal for secure transmission. Common asymmetric encryption algorithms are RSA and ECC. Although slower than symmetric encryption, these methods offer better security for exchanging encryption keys or signing images to verify their authenticity. To accommodate image data's unique structure, specialized image encryption methods have been developed. Block-based encryption and pixel shuffling make it difficult for unauthorised users to reconstruct the original image without the key. These image-specific methods can improve security without affecting image quality. A comprehensive security strategy must include encryption and other data protection measures. Encryption with TLS or SSL secures images during network transmission. Data in transit is encrypted by these protocols to prevent interception and unauthorized access. Encryption key management is essential for security. Organizations need regular key rotation, secure key storage, and strict access controls. This protects encryption keys from unauthorized access, ensuring encryption integrity.

Methods for Balancing Compression and Security

Achieving equilibrium between image compression and security is vital in telemedicine applications, where it is imperative to maintain data integrity and confidentiality while enhancing storage and transmission efficiency. Several methods exist to attain this equilibrium. Attaining equilibrium between compression and security in image management necessitates a comprehensive strategy that prioritizes data integrity and confidentiality. Organizations can improve the efficiency of image storage and transmission, while ensuring strong data protection, by utilizing methods such as selective compression, hybrid techniques, adaptive algorithms, and user-controlled settings. This equilibrium is particularly crucial in fields such as telemedicine, where the privacy and precision of patient data are essential. In telemedicine, striking a balance between image compression and security requires the application of cutting-edge methods that give equal weight to data protection and efficiency. One method is to use lossy compression to reduce file size in less important areas of an image and lossless compression for sensitive areas of the image to ensure no detail is lost. Security is largely dependent on encryption, and contemporary algorithms make sure that even compressed images are safe for transmission and storage. New hybrid models that simultaneously combine encryption and compression are starting to appear. These models allow for real-time processing without sacrificing the security or integrity of the image.

- *Targeted Compression Methods*: The utilization of selective compression techniques makes it possible to compress specific regions of an image in accordance with the significance of those regions. When it comes to critical domains that require high fidelity, such as diagnostic information in medical imaging, it is possible to compress them in a less aggressive manner or to preserve them in lossless formats. On the other hand, regions that are not as significant may undergo more intense lossy compression, which maintains the functionality of the image as a whole while simultaneously improving the efficiency of the file size.
- *Hybrid Encryption Methods*: There is the potential to achieve a successful equilibrium through the utilization of a hybrid approach that incorporates both compression and encryption strategies. By first compressing images and then encrypting the data that has been compressed, businesses are able to reduce the amount of information that needs to be encrypted, which in turn improves the speed at which they process information. On the other hand, encrypting data before compressing it can be inefficient because encryption can produce data that is less amenable to compression.
- *Adaptive Compression Algorithms*: Image content and transmission context are taken into consideration by adaptive compression algorithms, which then dynamically adjust compression levels accordingly. It is possible for these algorithms to improve compression ratios while simultaneously protecting sensitive information. This is accomplished by analyzing the significance of various image attributes. This method makes it possible to manage file sizes more effectively without compromising the information that is essential to the image.

- *Error-Correction Protocols*: The utilization of error-correction mechanisms can make it easier to retrieve data that was lost during the compression process, particularly when lossy compression techniques are utilized. It is possible for organizations to ensure that the fundamental content will be preserved even in the event that certain parts of the image are lost or compromised if they integrate redundant information. In circumstances where image precision is of the utmost importance, this is of extremely great significance.
- *Secure Compression Protocols*: With the implementation of secure compression protocols that incorporate encryption during the compression process, it is possible to ensure the safety of data while simultaneously facilitating efficient compression. Establishing a secure channel for the transmission of compressed images is made possible by protocols such as Secure Sockets Layer (SSL), which protects data from being intercepted while it is being transmitted.
- *Assessment and Appraisal*: The identification of potential vulnerabilities and the evaluation of the effectiveness of the techniques that are being utilized are both made easier through the consistent testing and evaluation of compression and security methodologies. The results of trials can shed light on the effects that different compression levels have on data security, which offers businesses the opportunity to improve their strategies in order to achieve the highest possible level of performance.

Figure 2. Methods for balancing compression and security

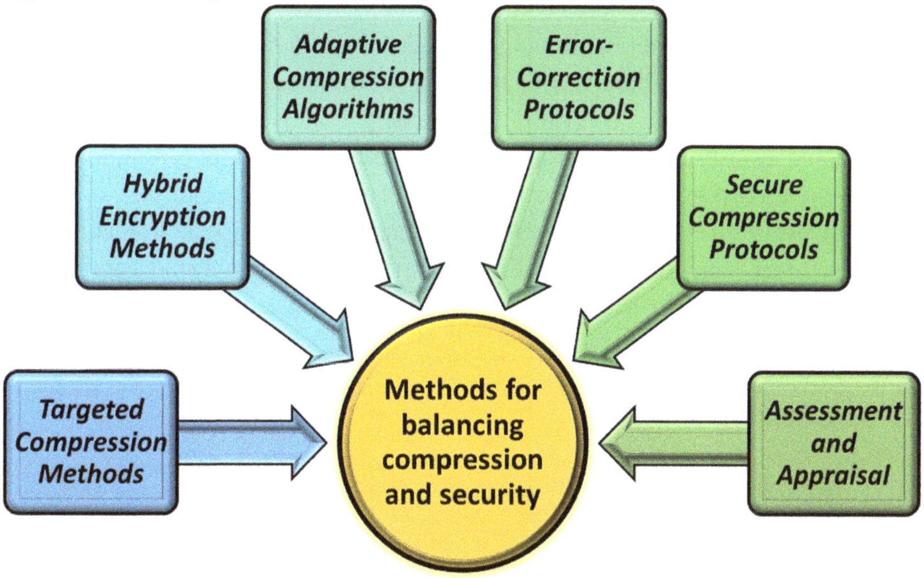

MULTI-LAYER SECURITY IMPLEMENTATION

Today's digital landscape requires multi-layered security solutions, especially for sensitive sectors like healthcare, finance, and government. Defense in depth, or a multi-layered approach, combines multiple security measures to mitigate risks and protect against diverse threats. If one layer is compromised, other layers protect critical assets, improving security. Multi-layered security often starts with perimeter defenses like firewalls and IDS. Firewalls monitor and control incoming and outgoing traffic based on security rules to separate trusted internal and external networks. Intrusion detection systems monitor network traffic for threats and suspicious activity. These perimeter defenses protect against unauthorized access and cyberattacks as the first line of defense. After perimeter security, endpoint security comes next. Computers, smartphones, and servers that access the network must be secured. Endpoint protection solutions like antivirus, anti-malware, and EDR tools help identify and eliminate device threats. Protecting all endpoints prevents malware spread and reduces attacker vulnerabilities. Data protection is another important part of multi-layered security. Confidential data is encrypted at rest and in transit to prevent unauthorized access. DLP solutions can also monitor and control data transfers to prevent sensitive information from being shared or leaked. Organizations can reduce data breaches and comply with data protection laws by securing data throughout its lifecycle. Protecting sensitive data and systems requires user authentication and access control. Multi-factor authentication (MFA) improves security by requiring users to verify their identity multiple times. RBAC reduces insider threats by restricting access to data and systems to roles. To meet changing staff and organizational needs, access controls must be reviewed and updated regularly. Employee security awareness training is another important step. Human error is a leading cause of security breaches, so staff must be trained to recognize phishing and social engineering attacks. Staff training can help employees make informed data handling and security decisions, fostering a security-conscious culture. A multi-layered security solution needs continuous monitoring and incident response. Companies should invest in SIEM systems to collect and analyze security data in real time for proactive threat detection and response. Organizations can quickly mitigate security incidents and resume normal operations with a well-defined incident response plan.

CONCLUSION

The security and confidentiality of patient data in telemedicine are essential, particularly as the healthcare sector progressively adopts digital solutions. Our investigation into privacy-preserving techniques, multi-layered security strategies, and the particular vulnerabilities linked to telemedicine underscores the urgent necessity for stringent measures to safeguard sensitive information. The findings highlight that although telemedicine provides considerable benefits in accessibility and convenience, it also poses distinct challenges that require resolution through robust security measures. Anticipating the future, numerous trends are poised to influence the domain of telemedicine security. A significant trend is the implementation of artificial intelligence (AI) powered security measures, which can improve threat detection and response efficacy. Artificial Intelligence can evaluate extensive datasets in real time, detecting patterns and anomalies that may signify potential security breaches. The advancement of quantum encryption offers the potential to greatly improve data security, delivering unparalleled protection through the principles of quantum mechanics. As these technologies advance, they possess the capacity to transform security protocols in telemedicine, facilitating more secure and efficient patient care. To guarantee data confidentiality in telemedicine, healthcare providers must adopt several essential recommendations. Organizations should implement a multi-faceted security strategy that integrates encryption, access controls, and ongoing monitoring. Investing in user education and training is crucial for enhancing awareness of potential threats and optimal data protection practices. Moreover, adherence to pertinent regulatory standards, including HIPAA and GDPR, must be prioritized to guarantee the responsible management of patient data. By proactively mitigating security issues and adopting emerging technologies, healthcare providers can enhance the protection of patient information, thereby cultivating trust and facilitating the ongoing expansion of telemedicine.

REFERENCES

Abdullahi, M., Ahmad, A., Pandey, B. K., & Pandey, D. (2024). Digital Currency Adoption: A Comparative Analysis of Global Trends and the Nigerian eNaira Digital Currency. *SN Computer Science*, *5*(5), 1–11. DOI: 10.1007/s42979-024-02882-6

Agbo, C. C., Mahmoud, Q. H., & Eklund, J. M. (2019, April). Blockchain technology in healthcare: A systematic review. [). MDPI.]. *Health Care*, *7*(2), 56. PMID: 30987333

Basha, A. J., Maheshwari, R. U., Pandey, B. K., & Pandey, D. (2024). Ultra-sensitive photonic crystal fiber–based SPR sensor for cancer detection utilizing hybrid nanocomposite layers. *Plasmonics*, •••, 1–15. DOI: 10.1007/s11468-024-02584-y

Elarmathi, S., Rishabavarthani, P., Sindhuja, M., Elayaraja, P., & Malathi Murugesan, S. (2024). Novel manufacturing systems for cancer diagnosis using ultra-sensitive photonic crystal fiber biosensor with dual-functionalized aptamer-nanocavity. *Microsystem Technologies*, •••, 1–20. DOI: 10.1007/s00542-024-05820-x

George, W. K., Silas, E. I., Pandey, D., & Pandey, B. K. (2024). Utilization of Industry 4.0 Technologies in Nigerian Technical and Vocational Education: A Conundrum for Educators. In *Examining the Rapid Advance of Digital Technology in Africa* (pp. 270–293). IGI Global. DOI: 10.4018/978-1-6684-9962-7.ch014

Khadka, M., Sah, M., Chaudhary, R., Sahani, S. K., Sahani, K., Pandey, B. K., & Pandey, D. (2025). Spectroscopic, quantum chemical, and topological calculations of the phenylephrine molecule using density functional theory. *Scientific Reports*, *15*(1), 208. DOI: 10.1038/s41598-024-81633-2 PMID: 39747169

. Konapure, C. G., Pandey, D., Shete, H., Thakar, C. M., Pandey, B. K., & George, A. S. (2025). Artificial Intelligence in Automated Concrete Mix Design Using Computerized Grading Curves. Interdisciplinary Approaches to AI, Internet of Everything, and Machine Learning, 567-586.

. Kumar, B., Pandey, D., Pandey, B. K., & George, A. S. (2024). Higher Education in the Last Four Decades: A Review of Paradigm Shifts in Policy Frameworks. Design and Implementation of Higher Education Learners' Learning Outcomes (HELLO), 333-348.

Kumar, M. S., Prasanna, P. L., Lalitha, M., Joy, M., Jha, S. S., & Pandey, B. K. (2025). Utilizing the Internet of Everything and Artificial Intelligence for Real-Time Workforce Management. In Role of Internet of Everything (IOE), VLSI Architecture, and AI in Real-Time Systems (pp. 153-168). IGI Global Scientific Publishing.

Kumar Pandey, B., Pandey, D., Nassa, V. K., Ahmad, T., Singh, C., George, A. S., & Wakchaure, M. A. (2021). Encryption and steganography-based text extraction in IoT using the EWCTS optimizer. *Imaging Science Journal*, *69*(1-4), 38–56. DOI: 10.1080/13682199.2022.2146885

Kumarganesh, S., & Malathi Murugesan, C. (2024). Hybrid plasmonic biosensors with deep learning for colorectal cancer detection. *Plasmonics*, •••, 1–15. DOI: 10.1007/s11468-024-02568-y

KVM, S., Pandey, B. K., & Pandey, D. (2024). Design of Surface Plasmon Resonance (SPR) Sensors for Highly Sensitive Biomolecular Detection in Cancer Diagnostics. *Plasmonics*, •••, 1–13.

Lakshmi, K. V. N., Rajan, R., Pandey, D., & Pandey, B. K. (2024). Circular economy: A catalyst for economic growth-an empirical study. *Circular Economy and Sustainability*, •••, 1–22.

Mbonihankuye, S., Nkunzimana, A., & Ndagijimana, A. (2019). Healthcare data security technology: HIPAA compliance. *Wireless Communications and Mobile Computing*, *2019*(1), 1927495.

Muniandi, B., Nassa, V. K., Pandey, D., Pandey, B. K., Dadheech, P., & George, A. S. (2024). Pattern Analysis for Feature Extraction in Complex Images. In Using Machine Learning to Detect Emotions and Predict Human Psychology (pp. 145-167). IGI Global. DOI: 10.4018/979-8-3693-1910-9.ch007

Muralidhar, L. B., Lakshmi, K. V. N., Swapna, H. R., Rupani, J., Nethravathi, K., Pandey, B. K., & Pandey, D. (2024). Impact of Organizational Culture on The Level of Corporate Social Responsibility Investments: An Exploratory Study. *Circular Economy and Sustainability*, *4*(3), 1–19. DOI: 10.1007/s43615-024-00371-9

Pandey, B. K., Nassa, V. K., Mukundan, A. P., Mahajan, D. A., Pandey, D., George, A. S., & Dadheech, P. (2024c). An Industry-Focused Traffic System Utilising Internet of Things. In *Emerging Engineering Technologies and Industrial Applications* (pp. 200–213). IGI Global. DOI: 10.4018/979-8-3693-1335-0.ch009

Pandey, B. K., & Pandey, D. (2023). Parametric optimization and prediction of enhanced thermoelectric performance in co-doped CaMnO3 using response surface methodology and neural network. *Journal of Materials Science Materials in Electronics*, *34*(21), 1589. DOI: 10.1007/s10854-023-10954-1

Pandey, B. K., & Pandey, D. (2025). Securing healthcare medical image information using advance morphological component analysis, information hiding systems, and hybrid convolutional neural networks on IoMT. *Computers in Biology and Medicine*, *185*, 109499. DOI: 10.1016/j.compbiomed.2024.109499 PMID: 39642698

Pandey, B. K., Pandey, D., & Lelisho, M. E. (2024a). Face mask identification with enhanced cuckoo optimization and deep learning-based faster regional neural network. *Scientific Reports*, *14*(1), 29719. DOI: 10.1038/s41598-024-78746-z PMID: 39613761

Pandey, B. K., Pandey, D., & Sahani, S. K. (2024b). Autopilot control unmanned aerial vehicle system for sewage defect detection using deep learning. *Engineering Reports*, •••, 12852.

Pandey, B. K., Paramashivan, M. A., Pandey, D., George, A. S., Agarwal, A., Mahajan, D. A., . . . Pramanik, S. (2024d). Future Directions of Digital Twin Architectures for 6G Communication Networks. In Security Issues and Solutions in 6G Communications and Beyond (pp. 197-211). IGI Global.

Pandey, D., Nassa, V. K., Pandey, B. K., Mahajan, D. A., Patidar, P. K., Dadheech, P., & George, A. S. (2024). An Analysis of Internet-of-Things-Based Fire Detection and Alert Systems. In *Emerging Engineering Technologies and Industrial Applications* (pp. 295–304). IGI Global. DOI: 10.4018/979-8-3693-1335-0.ch014

Qayyum, A., Qadir, J., Bilal, M., & Al-Fuqaha, A. (2020). Secure and robust machine learning for healthcare: A survey. *IEEE Reviews in Biomedical Engineering*, *14*, 156–180. DOI: 10.1109/RBME.2020.3013489 PMID: 32746371

Rai, P. K., Pandey, D., & Pandey, B. K. (2024). The future of enterprise and innovation is compute as a commodity, or CaaC. *Partners Universal International Research Journal*, *3*(2), 89–94.

Saravanakumar, R., TamilSelvi, T., Pandey, D., Pandey, B. K., Mahajan, D. A., & Lelisho, M. E. (2024). Big data processing using hybrid Gaussian mixture model with salp swarm algorithm. *Journal of Big Data*, *11*(1), 167. DOI: 10.1186/s40537-024-01015-3

Satheesh, N., Gopisankar, N., Kumarganesh, S., Anthoniraj, S., Saravanakumar, S., & Martin Sagayam, K. (2025). Advanced AI-driven emergency response systems for enhanced vehicle and human safety. *Iran Journal of Computer Science*, •••, 1–16. DOI: 10.1007/s42044-025-00228-w

Shahul, A., Muniandi, B., Paramashivan, M. A., Pandey, D., Pandey, B. K., Dadheech, P., & George, H. (2024). An Analysis of Algorithms and Methods Based on Image Processing for Medical Applications. In *Emerging Engineering Technologies and Industrial Applications* (pp. 173–186). IGI Global. DOI: 10.4018/979-8-3693-1335-0.ch007

Sharma, M., Talwar, R., Nassa, V. K., Binay, K., & Pandey, D. (2025). Design and performance analysis of a multiband vivaldi antenna for wireless broadband communication in 3-5.6 GHz spectrum. In *Artificial Intelligence and Information Technologies* (pp. 86–91). CRC Press.

Sheela, M. S., Kumarganesh, S., Pandey, B. K., & Lelisho, M. E. (2025). Integration of silver nanostructures in wireless sensor networks for enhanced biochemical sensing. *Discover Nano*, *20*(1), 7. DOI: 10.1186/s11671-024-04159-6 PMID: 39804434

Singh, S., Madaan, G., Swapna, H. R., Singh, A., Pandey, D., George, A. S., & Pandey, B. K. (2025). Empowering Connectivity: Exploring the Internet of Things. In Interdisciplinary Approaches to AI, Internet of Everything, and Machine Learning (pp. 89-116). IGI Global Scientific Publishing.

Vinodhini, V., Kumar, M. S., Sankar, S., Pandey, D., Pandey, B. K., & Nassa, V. K. (2022). IoT-based early forest fire detection using MLP and AROC method. *International Journal of Global Warming*, *27*(1), 55–70. DOI: 10.1504/IJGW.2022.122794

Vora, J., Italiya, P., Tanwar, S., Tyagi, S., Kumar, N., Obaidat, M. S., & Hsiao, K. F. (2018, July). Ensuring privacy and security in e-health records. In *2018 International conference on computer, information and telecommunication systems (CITS)* (pp. 1-5). IEEE. DOI: 10.1109/CITS.2018.8440164

Yusof, M. M., Papazafeiropoulou, A., Paul, R. J., & Stergioulas, L. K. (2008). Investigating evaluation frameworks for health information systems. *International Journal of Medical Informatics*, *77*(6), 377–385. DOI: 10.1016/j.ijmedinf.2007.08.004 PMID: 17904898

Chapter 2
Enhancing Telemedicine Workflow Through Secure Image Transmission

Niladri Maiti
https://orcid.org/0009-0000-6030-7424
School of Dentistry, Central Asian University, Tashkent, Uzbekistan

Riddhi Chawla
School of Dentistry, Central Asian University, Tashkent, Uzbekistan

T. Illakiya
https://orcid.org/0000-0001-5890-529X
Faculty of Engineering and Technology, SRM Institute of Science and Technology, Chennai, India

Chinnem Rama Mohan
Department of Computer Science and Engineering, Narayana Engineering College, Nellore, India

S. Meena
https://orcid.org/0000-0001-9979-8689
Department of Chemistry, Dayanandasagar College of Engineering, Bangalore, India

Souvik Sen
Health and Family Welfare Department, Government of West Bengal, India

A. Shaji George
https://orcid.org/0000-0002-8677-3682
Almarai Company, Saudi Arabia

ABSTRACT

In the field of telemedicine, the incorporation of secure image transmission technologies and workflow automation, with a particular emphasis on the impact these technologies have on service delivery. Secure image transmission, which is accomplished through encryption protocols, virtual private networks (VPNs), and cloud-based platforms, makes it possible for medical professionals to share medical images in a manner that is both secure and fast. Through the use of real-time

DOI: 10.4018/979-8-3693-9821-0.ch002

image sharing, diagnostic accuracy can be improved, delays can be reduced, and treatment decisions can be made more quickly and effectively. The automation of workflows also helps to streamline administrative and clinical tasks, which reduces the likelihood of errors caused by humans and increases operational efficiency.

INTRODUCTION

Professionals can diagnose, assess, and treat patients from a distance with the help of telemedicine, which is the practice of providing medical services remotely using digital communication tools. Technology such as messaging apps, mobile platforms, phone calls, and video conferencing are used in this approach (Pandey, B. K. et al., 2024a). Improving access to care is the main goal, especially for those who live in underserved or remote areas with limited access to facilities or experts. Real-time interactions, store-and-forward techniques, and continuous monitoring are the three ways that remote consultations can be conducted. Instant assessments, symptom evaluations, and prescription advice are all possible during real-time consultations via video or live chat, which mimic in-person meetings. When medical data, like images (Shahul, A. et al., 2024) or medical records, are sent so experts can review them later, this is referred to as store-and-forward. Get second opinions on MRI scans and X-rays, for example, is a non-urgent situation where this method works well. Typically used for long-term condition management, remote monitoring entails tracking a patients vital signs or health metrics via wearables or sensors (Pandey, D. et al., 2024). Enhancing service accessibility is among the many notable benefits. There is no need to travel for consultations for those who live in remote areas or have restricted mobility. Managing chronic conditions such as diabetes or heart disease requires careful attention to detail (Pandey, B. K. et al., 2024b). Furthermore, by optimizing resource utilization and reducing in-person visits, digital approaches ease the burden on healthcare facilities. The other two major advantages are convenience and cost savings. Individuals save money and time on travel, and healthcare systems save money on maintaining physical facilities and scheduling in-person visits. Regular patient interaction helps identify health problems early and allows for prompt intervention. Notwithstanding, certain obstacles persist, including safeguarding information transfer, upholding confidentiality, and surmounting technological constraints in areas with inadequate internet connectivity.

Secure Image Transfer's Significance

Secure medical image transmission is essential to telemedicine in order to guarantee patient privacy and high-quality care. Imaging tests, like MRIs, CT scans, ultrasounds, and X-rays, are essential for both diagnosing and tracking a wide range of medical conditions. In order to facilitate prompt and precise medical interventions, these images must be securely and quickly transmitted between patients, healthcare providers, and specialists. However, security throughout the transmission process is crucial because medical data is sensitive. Patient privacy protection is the main justification for secure image transfer. Personal identifiers are frequently included in medical images along with health-related information. There may be data breaches, identity theft, or fraud if these are intercepted or accessed by unauthorized parties. Secure transmission techniques protect this data by rendering it unreadable by unauthorized parties, such as AES (Advanced Encryption Standard) or RSA (Rivest-Shamir-Adleman) encryption protocols. There are stringent guidelines regarding the storage and transmission of medical data, including images, enforced by healthcare regulations such as the GDPR (General Data Protection Regulation) in Europe and the HIPAA (Health Insurance Portability and Accountability Act) in the United States. Not only is adherence to these laws required by law, but it also fosters confidence between healthcare providers and their patients. Breaking these rules could have serious legal and financial repercussions, such as large fines or reputational damage. Ensuring image quality during transmission is just as important as security. Inadequate transmission protocols have the potential to compress data too much, which lowers the clarity or resolution of medical images and jeopardizes the accuracy of diagnosis. Modern image transmission technologies guarantee that high-quality images travel to their destination undamaged by providing options like error correction and lossless compression. More streamlined telemedicine workflows are facilitated by the safe and effective transfer of medical images. Healthcare providers can provide prompt consultations and treatment plans with the help of fast and dependable access to diagnostic images, which improves patient outcomes and boosts the effectiveness of telemedicine services overall (Puvvadi, U. L. et al., 2015).

CURRENT TELEMEDICINE WORKFLOW

Steps in Telemedicine Consultations

Telemedicine consultations ensure secure and efficient remote healthcare. Typical telemedicine consultation steps are listed here are shown in the figure 1. Telemedicine consults mimic the efficiency and effectiveness of in-person visits while being more convenient. Remote healthcare services can provide personalized, comprehensive medical care without physical contact by following structured steps from appointment scheduling to follow-up.

- *Scheduling Appointments*: Telemedicine consultations begin with scheduling. The healthcare provider's online portal, mobile app, or clinic phone number can be used for this. Many telemedicine systems have simple interfaces where patients can choose a time, doctor, and reason for the visit. Some systems let patients choose between video, phone, or secure messaging consultations. Patients can upload medical records, lab reports, and prescriptions during this phase to give the provider preliminary information. Most appointment scheduling systems are integrated with patient management platforms, giving providers access to vital information (Swapna, H. R. et al., 2024a). This step improves convenience and lets doctors assess the patient's condition before the consultation, focusing the discussion. This step eliminates travel and wait times for remote or disabled patients. The provider and patient are well-prepared before the consultation, reducing administrative time.
- *Pre-Consultation Setup*: Patients may receive detailed instructions on how to access the video conferencing platform or telemedicine app before the virtual meeting. In this phase, patients and healthcare providers need the right technology (Pandey, B. K. et al., 2024d). Providers test their equipment to ensure stable video and audio connections, while patients may be asked to check their internet connection, camera, and microphone, and find a quiet, private space for the consultation. Patients unfamiliar with video calls can get troubleshooting help on some platforms. Patients are also advised to upload relevant medical documents, imaging results, and medical history into a secure portal beforehand (Pandey, B. K. et al., 2024e). This pre-consultation phase helps the doctor understand the patient's condition. In more complex cases, patients may be asked to pre-provide vital signs like blood pressure, temperature, and glucose using at-home medical devices. Smoothly completing this step improves consultation efficiency and prevents interruptions (Pandey, B. K. et al., 2024f).
- *Virtual Consultation*: Telemedicine visits revolve around a video conferencing or secure messaging session. The provider reviews symptoms, asks detailed questions, and asks about medical history after connecting with the patient. The provider may ask the patient to check for swelling or redness or perform basic movement tests to assess muscle or joint function on camera, depending on the condition (Swapna, H. R. et al., 2024b). The provider evaluates the information and may take notes in the patient's EHR. If uploaded, medical images or lab results can be shared in real time during virtual consul-

tations to help the provider assess the patient's condition. The provider may instruct the patient on how to use at-home monitoring tools like a pulse oximeter or blood pressure cuff and provide immediate feedback. This interactive virtual consultation keeps remote care comprehensive and personalized (Filonenko, A., & Jo, K. H., 2016).

- *Diagnosis and treatment plan*: If necessary, the provider diagnoses or refers the patient for further testing after the virtual consultation. The doctor will usually explain the diagnosis and next steps. Prescriptions, lifestyle changes, and follow-up consultations may be recommended. The provider may order local lab tests or imaging in serious cases. These test results are usually sent to the provider electronically for review. The provider discusses the treatment plan with the patient and sends prescriptions electronically to the patient's preferred pharmacy. Telemedicine platforms integrate prescription services, simplifying this process. Medication, physical therapy, and other treatment instructions are also given to patients. For more continuous care, providers may use remote monitoring devices to track patient progress between visits.
- *Prescription and Documentation*: After agreeing on a treatment plan, the provider must document the consultation. This includes documenting the diagnosis, treatment plan, and session advice in the patient's EMR. Legally and medically, documentation ensures continuity of care for future visits. Most providers use digital health records that other doctors can access if the patient needs a specialist. The provider sends an electronic prescription to the patient's preferred pharmacy for pickup or delivery. This method reduces handwritten prescription errors and saves time. Some telemedicine systems let patients track their prescriptions, set reminders, and request refills via the app. Clear documentation simplifies insurance claims for patients and providers (Kim, B. et al., 2017).
- *Follow-up*: Telemedicine consultations, especially for chronic conditions or ongoing treatments, require follow-up. Depending on the illness, the provider may schedule a virtual follow-up to monitor progress. Another video call, phone check-in, or in-person visit may be needed for this follow-up. For patients using remote monitoring devices, the provider may review data (Swapna, H. R. et al., 2024c) to assess treatment response. To ensure treatment is effective and make adjustments, follow-ups are necessary. The provider may recommend additional diagnostic tests or refer the patient to specialists. Virtual follow-ups allow patients to ask questions and provide updates on their condition without in-person visits (Bhatt, D. et al., 2024). This method improves long-term outcomes for patients with chronic diseases or complex health conditions by providing continuous care.

Figure 1. Key steps in telemedicine consultations

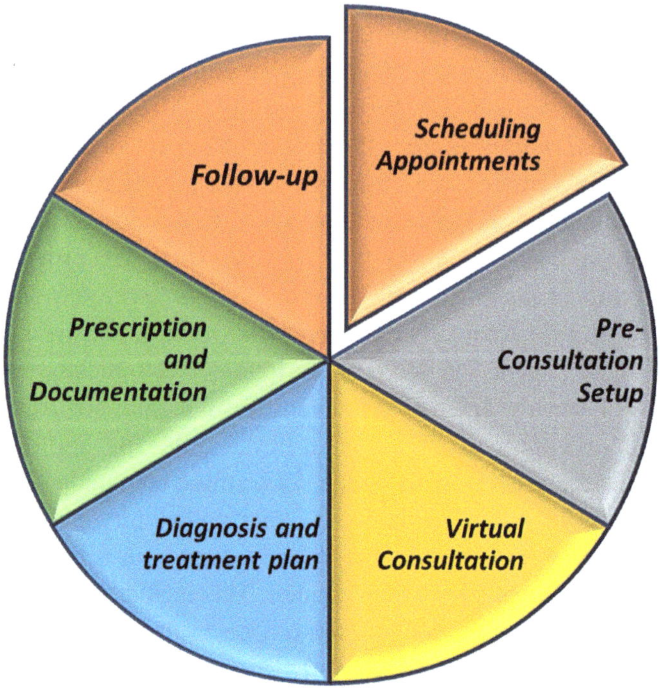

Medical Imaging in Remote Diagnosis

The utilization of medical imaging for the purpose of facilitating accurate diagnoses during telemedicine consultations is of utmost importance. X-rays, magnetic resonance imaging (MRI), computed tomography (CT) scans, and ultrasounds are examples of technologies that enable medical professionals to evaluate internal structures and conditions that are not visible to the naked eye. It is not necessary for the patient to be physically present in order for these images to be transmitted digitally to specialists or primary care providers during remote consultations. These providers are able to analyze the images and make appropriate diagnostic decisions based on their findings. It is absolutely necessary for accurate remote diagnosis to have the capability to share medical images in a secure and efficient manner (Pandey, B. K. et al., 2023). When it comes to diagnosing a wide variety of conditions, including fractures, tumors, organ dysfunctions, and infections, high-quality images provide essential details that are helpful in making diagnostic decisions. Especially when dealing with serious or complicated health problems, these images are frequently used as the basis upon which treatment plans are constructed. Furthermore, the store-and-forward model of telemedicine enables patients to upload their imaging results in advance, providing physicians with ample time to review the data before the consultation begins. This results in an improvement in the quality of care that is provided remotely (Maheshwari, R. Uma. et al., 2024). The elimination of geographical barriers is another benefit of medical imaging in remote healthcare, in addition to the improvement of diagnostic accuracy. The ability to receive high-quality care without having to travel is available to patients who live in underserved or rural areas, who might otherwise have difficulty gaining access to advanced diagnostic tools. For the purpose of providing second opinions or guiding local healthcare providers in the delivery of more precise treatment, specialists are able to interpret images from a geographical distance. This shortens the amount of time it takes to diagnose conditions and begin treatment, which, in some instances, can mean the difference between life and death. Additionally, the rapid sharing of images helps streamline workflows in telemedicine, which ultimately results in care that is both more efficient and more effective (Lin, Z. et al., 2016).

IMAGE QUALITY IN TELEMEDICINE

High-Resolution Images in Accurate Diagnosis

In the field of medical diagnostics, high-resolution images are essential because they greatly improve the precision and dependability of assessments made by medical professionals. With the help of imaging technologies like digital X-rays, CT scans, and MRIs, doctors can more accurately detect abnormalities because they offer detailed views of the body's internal structures. High-resolution images can provide detailed information that is essential for diagnosing a range of conditions, including organ abnormalities, soft tissue injuries, tumors, and fractures. An important advantage of high-resolution imaging is that it can increase diagnostic confidence (Abdulkarim, Yadgar I. et al., 2024). Improved clarity makes it possible for specialists and radiologists to identify minute alterations in organs and tissues that could go undetected in lower-quality pictures. For example, in oncology, the ability to see small tumors can have a big influence on treatment choices and results. In the fight against cancer and other serious diseases, high-resolution images are crucial because early detection frequently results in a better prognosis (Revathi, T. K. et al., 2022). High-resolution photos also help healthcare providers communicate with each other more effectively. Experts can work together more productively on complicated cases, exchange ideas, and come to a consensus on possible treatments when they have access to detailed images. This is especially crucial for telemedicine, where digital image transmission is used for remote assessment. By guaranteeing that all parties have access to the same degree of detail, high-resolution imaging lowers the possibility of misunderstandings and raises the standard of care overall. The significance of high-resolution images only increases with the advancement of medical imaging technology. With the increasing prevalence of innovations like 3D imaging and sophisticated visualization software, providers can now analyze data in previously unfeasible ways. To summarise, high-resolution images play a crucial role in precise diagnosis, early detection, improved teamwork, and ultimately better patient outcomes (Kokkonis, G. et al., 2017).

Poor Image Quality on Clinical Decisions

When it comes to clinical decisions, the effects of low-quality images are considered. The accuracy of diagnoses and the efficacy of treatment plans can be called into question when the image quality is poor, which can have a significant impact on clinical decisions. X-rays, magnetic resonance imaging (MRI), and computed tomography (CT) scans are examples of medical images that can be distorted or obscured if they have a low resolution or are captured less accurately. It is possible for healthcare providers to misinterpret as a result of this, which may lead to incorrect diagnoses or the failure to recognize abnormalities that ought to be addressed immediately. The potential for a delay in patient care is one of the most significant dangers that are associated with images of poor quality (Khan, B. et al., 2021). It is possible that additional imaging will be necessary in the event that a radiologist is unable to accurately evaluate an image due to its poor quality. This will cause the diagnostic process to take longer. For patients who are suffering from serious conditions, such as cancers or acute injuries, where prompt intervention is essential, this delay can be especially detrimental. Therefore, the likelihood of complications or the progression of the disease to a more advanced stage may increase, which will have a negative impact on the outcomes for the patient. There is a correlation between poor image quality and a reduction in the level of trust and communication that exists between patients and providers (Devasenapathy, D. et al., 2023). To make decisions that are based on accurate assessments, patients rely on their healthcare professionals to provide them with accurate information. It is possible for confusion and dissatisfaction to result when diagnoses are made based on images that are not clear. Patients may have doubts about the dependability of their healthcare provider, which can put a strain on the relationship between the provider and the patient and result in a reduction in the patient's behavior in accordance with the recommendations for treatment. Clinical decision-making is significantly hampered by low-quality medical images, which can lead to the possibility of incorrect diagnoses, delays in treatment, and a reduction in patient trust. Obtaining images that are of a high resolution and have been captured correctly is absolutely necessary for efficient medical evaluation and the best possible outcomes for patients (Stergiou, C. et al., 2017).

NEED FOR SECURE IMAGE TRANSMISSION

Sensitivity of Medical Data

The term "medical data" refers to a wide range of information, including but not limited to medical histories, test results, treatment plans, and demographic details. Due to the highly personal nature of this information, it is of the utmost importance to maintain both its confidentiality and its integrity (Saxena, A. et al., 2021). Because it includes not only a patient's personal health information but also identifiable details that can have an impact on the patient's privacy, security (Dhanasekar, S. et al., 2023), and overall wellbeing, the sensitivity of medical data is a significant concern in the healthcare industry. The potential for medical data to be misused is the source of its sensitivity. Theft of identity, insurance fraud, and discrimination against individuals based on their health status are all potential outcomes that can result from unauthorized access to health records. For instance, if a person's mental health history is disclosed without their consent, it may have a detrimental effect on their employment opportunities or their relationships with other people. Therefore, healthcare providers are required to implement stringent measures in order to protect this data from being breached or accessed by unauthorized parties (Kim, I. C. et al., 2022). Regulations in the United States, such as the Health Insurance Portability and Accountability Act (HIPAA), impose stringent guidelines on the manner in which medical data should be handled. Encryption, access controls, and regular audits are some of the specific protocols that healthcare organizations are required to implement in order to comply with these regulations and protect patient information. Compliance with these laws not only protects patients, but it also protects healthcare organizations from the potential legal and financial repercussions that are associated with data breaches. In this day and age of digital health technologies, the sensitivity (Pandey, B. K. et al., 2022) of medical data is further amplified by the growing reliance on telemedicine and electronic health records of patients. The risk of cyberattacks and data breaches increases in tandem with the growing amount of patient information that is stored and transmitted electronically. The protection of patients' medical information is not only a legal requirement, but also an ethical obligation that healthcare providers must make a priority in order to preserve the trust and confidence of patients in the healthcare system (Yang, X. et al., 2015).

Data Breaches and Unauthorized Access

Patients and healthcare organizations are at serious risk from data breaches and illegal access to medical records. Serious repercussions from these incidents may include financial losses, patient privacy violations, and harm to healthcare providers' reputations. Due to its sensitive nature, medical data is especially prone to cyber-attacks of all kinds, with potentially devastating long-term effects. The disclosure of personal health information (PHI) is among the most pressing risks connected to data breaches. Unauthorized access to medical records can provide hackers with comprehensive details about a patient's diagnosis, course of treatment, medical history, and even financial information. A patient's financial situation and credit score may be negatively impacted by identity theft using this information (Tareke, S. A. et al., 2022), which can result in fraudulent activities. Unexpected financial burdens could arise, for instance, if someone uses their insurance information to get prescription drugs or medical services without their knowledge. Violations may have a big impact on patient confidence. Patients' trust in the healthcare system may be damaged when organizations fail to protect sensitive data.

Patients may be reluctant to provide essential information to their providers out of concern that their information won't be kept private. This resistance can impede clear diagnosis, treatment planning, and communication (Pandey, B. K. et al., 2024g), ultimately jeopardizing patient care. A healthcare organization's ability to attract new patients and retain existing ones may also be hampered if it has a reputation for experiencing frequent data breaches. Another important outcome of data breaches is financial losses. Costs associated with breach detection, investigation, and remediation can be very high for healthcare organizations. Studies show that when legal fees, regulatory fines, and customer compensation are taken into account, the typical cost of a data breach in the healthcare industry can reach the millions of dollars. Entities may encounter legal actions from impacted patients or regulatory agencies, resulting in further financial burden. When discussing the risks associated with data breaches, compliance with regulations like the Health Insurance Portability and Accountability Act (HIPAA) is also relevant. Businesses that violate HIPAA regulations risk severe consequences, which may include high fines and other sanctions. The necessity of upholding strong data security procedures to safeguard sensitive information is highlighted by this regulatory scrutiny (Plageras, A. P. et al., 2016).

TECHNOLOGIES FOR SECURE IMAGE TRANSMISSION

Protecting sensitive medical data during telemedicine and healthcare operations requires the use of secure image transmission technologies (Pandey, B. K. et al., 2024h). Some important techniques are cloud storage services with strong security features. In order to protect patient privacy and adhere to data protection laws, these technologies make sure that medical images are transmitted securely and are only accessible by recognized healthcare professionals. These technologies that are shown in the Figure 2, can help healthcare organizations secure medical image transmission, protecting patient data and meeting regulatory requirements. The use of technologies that allow for secure image transmission is absolutely necessary in order to safeguard patient information during the process of exchanging medical images in telemedicine. Data (Kumar Pandey, B. et al., 2021) is protected by sophisticated encryption methods such as AES and RSA, which ensure that only authorized personnel are able to access the data it contains (Stergiou, C. et al., 2018). The transmission of images between healthcare providers can be accomplished through the use of encrypted channels that are created by secure communication methods such as TLS. In addition, secure cloud platforms provide solutions for both storage and transmission, which guarantees that images are stored securely while still being accessible for clinical use. In addition to ensuring compliance with regulations and fostering trust in digital healthcare systems, these technologies (Sahani, K. et al., 2024b) contribute to the preservation of data integrity and preserving privacy.

1. *Encryption Protocols*: The use of encryption protocols like AES and RSA is essential for securing medical images during transmission. For large datasets like medical images, AES is efficient because it uses symmetric encryption, where the same key is used for encryption and decryption. An asymmetric encryption algorithm like RSA uses public and private keys to secure data exchange. This dual approach protects sensitive data from unauthorized users without the right decryption keys. End-to-end encryption protects images during transmission.
2. *Virtual Private Networks* (VPNs): VPNs encrypt data sent between devices made up of semiconductor materials (Du John, H. V. et al., 2022) over the internet, allowing healthcare professionals to securely access and share medical images. VPNs hide users' IP addresses, making data theft harder. Telemedicine and remote consultations benefit from VPNs, which allow healthcare providers to securely access images on remote servers or cloud services. Organizations can also enforce VPN policies to ensure secure remote connections.
3. *Image Compression Methods*: Lossless compression algorithms like PNG or JPEG2000 can reduce medical image file sizes without compromising quality, speeding up transmission. Telemedicine and remote diagnostics require

efficient image compression to speed up uploads and downloads and conserve bandwidth. Compression must be combined with security measures to preserve image integrity during transfer. Optimized compression keeps high-resolution images accessible without overloading network resources.

4. *Two-Factor Authentication* (2FA): User authentication with two forms of identification before accessing medical images increases security. This usually requires a password and a smartphone app that generates a verification code. By using 2FA, healthcare organizations can reduce the risk of unauthorized access and restrict sensitive medical image viewing to verified personnel. Regular security audits and staff training can strengthen 2FA.
5. *Blockchain Technology*: A secure and decentralized method for storing and transmitting medical images. A tamper-proof ledger records each data transaction or transfer, ensuring data integrity and image access by authorized parties. Blockchain allows real-time tracking of image access and modification, providing an audit trail that improves accountability. Smart contracts can also automate medical image sharing to enforce permissions based on predefined criteria.
6. *Cloud Storage Solutions*: Highly secure cloud storage solutions efficiently store and transmit medical images. Cloud platforms can encrypt and restrict access to images for authorized users. Multiple-factor authentication, data redundancy, and automated backups improve data security and availability. Cloud services also meet HIPAA requirements, allowing healthcare organizations to store and share sensitive medical data without compromising patient privacy.
7. *Secure File Transfer Protocols* (SFTP): SFTP, a secure version of FTP, encrypts data during transmission, making medical image transmission secure. Unlike traditional FTP, SFTP encrypts command and data channels to protect sensitive data. SFTP supports public key authentication for added security. Many healthcare organizations transfer large image files using SFTP to ensure data security and compliance.
8. *End-to-End Encryption*: This method encrypts data on the sender's device and decrypts it on the recipient's, preventing intermediaries from accessing it during transmission. To protect privacy, end-to-end encryption restricts medical image viewing to intended recipients. Telemedicine, where patient confidentiality is paramount, requires this. End-to-end encryption requires strong key management to protect encryption keys and medical data throughout its lifecycle.

Figure 2. Secure image transmission technologies

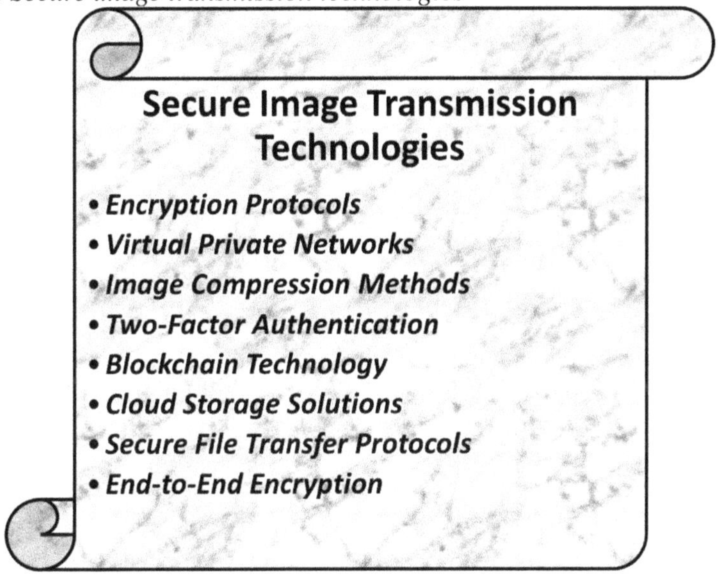

PROPOSED WORKFLOW ENHANCEMENT

Real-Time Healthcare Professional Image Sharing

Real-time image sharing has transformed Healthcare professionals collaboration and patient care decisions. Modern healthcare delivery relies on instantaneous medical image transmission due to advances in telemedicine and digital imaging. This capability improves diagnosis and treatment speed and patient care quality. Patient and provider wait times are reduced by real-time image sharing. In the past, a patient would undergo imaging, then wait days or weeks for the images to be reviewed and interpreted before receiving feedback. Specialists and primary care physicians can instantly receive X-rays, MRIs, and CT scans via real-time sharing. Rapid diagnosis and treatment can be crucial in emergencies. Healthcare professionals can collaborate remotely using real-time image sharing. Specialists can analyze images simultaneously and provide quick feedback. In complex cases where multidisciplinary teams must reach a consensus, this collaborative approach is beneficial. Radiologist, oncologist, and surgeon can share imaging data (Kennedy, G. W. et al., 2024) and discuss findings and treatment options in real time. This collective input improves decision-making and patient care strategies. Real-time medical image sharing has improved with cloud-based platforms and secure communication technologies. These platforms provide secure, centralized storage for healthcare professionals to access images from any internet accessible device. HIPAA-compliant cloud solutions protect patient data with strong encryption and security. Health professionals can annotate images, comment, and collaborate directly on the platform, streamlining communication and reducing misinterpretation. Sharing health information in real time empowers patients. Patients can access their medical images and reports through patient portals, improving their healthcare experience. Participation in care improves health outcomes by encouraging patients to follow treatment plans and follow-up appointments. Real-time image sharing has drawbacks despite its many benefits. System outages, slow internet connections, and software compatibility issues can hinder sharing. For real-time sharing to work, healthcare organizations need reliable infrastructure and staff training. Due to its sensitivity, medical data requires strong security to prevent breaches. Imaging system and healthcare platform interoperability is a concern. Sharing images can be difficult for professionals using different systems due to inconsistent formats and standards. Standards like DICOM (Digital Imaging and Communications in Medicine) can help make images universally accessible and interpretable.

Workflow Automation for Efficiency

There has been a significant rise in the importance of workflow automation as a tool for improving clinical efficiency. Optimising their operations can ultimately lead to improved patient care and satisfaction. This can be accomplished by streamlining processes, automating routine tasks, and reducing the number of manual interventions that are performed. Artificial neural network (Pandey, B. K., & Pandey, D., 2023) based technologies can be utilized in a variety of departments within the healthcare industry, ranging from administrative tasks to clinical workflows, thereby facilitating operations that are both more efficient and more streamlined. One of the most significant benefits of workflow automation is its capacity to reduce the amount of errors that are caused by human intervention. Automated systems have the potential to significantly reduce the errors that are associated with manual data entry, scheduling, and other repetitive tasks in the healthcare industry, which places a high premium on precision (Pandey, B. K., & Pandey, D., 2025). Automatic scheduling systems, for example, are able to manage appointment bookings, cancellations, and reminders in an effective manner. This allows administrative staff to focus on more complex tasks while also ensuring that patients receive timely notifications. The patient experience is improved as a result of this, as wait times and scheduling conflicts are reduced. This not only improves operational efficiency but also improves patient satisfaction. Automation of workflows also improves data management and accessibility respectively (Saravanakumar, R. et al., 2024). For the purpose of providing healthcare professionals with prompt access to vital information, automated systems make it possible to store patient information in a secure manner, organize it, and retrieve it in real time (Kumarganesh, S. et al., 2024). Through the facilitation of informed decision-making and the promotion of collaboration among healthcare teams, this seamless access to information contributes to an improvement in the quality of care that is provided to people.

PROVISION OF HEALTHCARE

The implementation of cutting-edge technologies in the healthcare industry, in particular with regard to the sharing of images in real time and the automation of workflows, has greatly altered the delivery of healthcare (Basha, A. J. et al., 2024). A better patient outcome, increased cost savings, and improved operational efficiency have all resulted from these advancements, which have also led to improved diagnosis accuracy and speed. One of the most notable effects of these technological advancements is an increase in how quickly and accurately diagnoses can be made. Healthcare professionals are able to gain access to high-quality medical images almost instantly thanks to real-time image sharing (Lakshmi, K. V. N. et al., 2024), which enables them to make interpretations that are both more accurate and more quickly. By allowing clinicians to make decisions in a timely manner, this rapid access to diagnostic information helps to reduce the amount of time that passes between the initial consultation and the diagnosis. The ability of multiple specialists to work together in real time, reviewing images and exchanging insights (Rai, P. K. et al., 2024), helps to reduce the likelihood of making an incorrect diagnosis, which in turn improves the accuracy of diagnoses even further. There is a direct correlation between these enhancements and improved patient effects. By making diagnoses more quickly and accurately, it is possible to begin treatment earlier, which is especially important for conditions such as cancer or injuries that are more severe. An early intervention program has the potential to significantly improve recovery rates, enhance quality of life, and even save lives altogether. In addition, increased collaboration among healthcare professionals supports the development of a more holistic approach to patient care. This approach ensures that all aspects of a patient's health are taken into consideration and addressed. The adoption of these technologies results in cost savings and increased operational efficiency, which are both benefits that arise. Healthcare organizations are able to reduce their administrative overhead and more effectively allocate resources if they focus on streamlining workflows and reducing the number of manual processes. By way of illustration, automated scheduling and patient management systems have the potential to reduce the number of patients who do not show up and optimize staff allocation, which ultimately results in lower operational costs. This combination of faster diagnosis, improved patient outcomes, and increased operational efficiency (Sahani, S. K. et al., 2024a) contributes to a more sustainable healthcare system. It enables organizations to provide high-quality care while effectively managing expenses, which is a significant benefit by itself.

CONCLUSION

The combination of technologies that allow for the transmission of images in a secure manner and the automation of workflow has completely transformed the delivery of healthcare. The implementation of these advancements has resulted in the speedier and more precise diagnosis of patients, the enhancement of collaboration among healthcare professionals, the improvement of patient outcomes, and the realization of significant cost savings through increased operational efficiency. While healthcare organizations ensure the privacy and security of patient information by encrypting sensitive medical data, using virtual private networks (VPNs), and utilizing secure platforms, real-time image sharing improves the decision-making and treatment processes available to patients. The security of telemedicine will involve additional innovations to address new cyber threats. This is something that can be expected. The implementation of more advanced blockchain solutions, the assurance of system interoperability, and the improvement of data encryption methods will be among the most important priorities. Further protection of patient information can be achieved through the development of robust security systems that are driven by artificial intelligence and can detect and prevent breaches. To ensure the long-term viability of telemedicine and its ability to successfully provide high-quality healthcare that is easily accessible, it will be essential to keep a strong focus on security as it continues to develop.

REFERENCES

Abdulkarim, Y. I., Awl, H. N., Muhammadsharif, F. F., Saeed, S. R., Sidiq, K. R., Khasraw, S. S., Dong, J., Pandey, B. K., & Pandey, D. (2024). Metamaterial-based sensors loaded corona-shaped resonator for COVID-19 detection by using microwave techniques. *Plasmonics*, *19*(2), 595–610. DOI: 10.1007/s11468-023-02007-4

Basha, A. J., Maheshwari, R. U., Pandey, B. K., & Pandey, D. (2024). Ultra-Sensitive Photonic Crystal Fiber–Based SPR Sensor for Cancer Detection Utilizing Hybrid Nanocomposite Layers. *Plasmonics*, •••, 1–15. DOI: 10.1007/s11468-024-02584-y

Bhatt, D., Swapna, H. R., Madaan, G., Gayathri, D. K., Mahajan, D. A., Mahajan, R. D., & Paramashivan, M. A. (2024). From Theory to Practice: The Evolution of Artificial Intelligence in Business. In Utilization of AI Technology in Supply Chain Management (pp. 1-14). IGI Global.

Devasenapathy, D., Madhumathy, P., Umamaheshwari, R., Pandey, B. K., & Pandey, D. (2023). Transmission-efficient grid-based synchronized model for routing in wireless sensor networks using Bayesian compressive sensing. *SN Computer Science*, *5*(1), 128. DOI: 10.1007/s42979-023-02410-y

Dhanasekar, S., Martin Sagayam, K., Pandey, B. K., & Pandey, D. (2023). Refractive index sensing using metamaterial absorbing augmentation in elliptical graphene arrays. *Plasmonics*, •••, 1–11.

Du John, H. V., Jose, T., Jone, A. A. A., Sagayam, K. M., Pandey, B. K., & Pandey, D. (2022). Polarization insensitive circular ring resonator based perfect metamaterial absorber design and simulation on a silicon substrate. *Silicon*, *14*(14), 9009–9020. DOI: 10.1007/s12633-021-01645-9

Filonenko, A., & Jo, K. H. (2016). Unattended object identification for intelligent surveillance systems using sequence of dual background difference. *IEEE Transactions on Industrial Informatics*, *12*(6), 2247–2255. DOI: 10.1109/TII.2016.2605582

Kennedy, G. W., Sunday, S. E., Pandey, D., Kabari, A. D., Pandey, B. K., George, A. S., & Dadheech, P. (2024). Building Information Modeling: Harnessing Innovations for Professional Proficiency. In *Emerging Engineering Technologies and Industrial Applications* (pp. 305-331). IGI Global.

Khan, B., Hasan, A., Pandey, D., Ventayen, R. J. M., Pandey, B. K., & Gowwrii, G. (2021). Fusion of datamining and artificial intelligence in prediction of hazardous road accidents. In *Machine learning and iot for intelligent systems and smart applications* (pp. 201–223). CRC Press. DOI: 10.1201/9781003194415-12

Kim, B., Psannis, K., & Bhaskar, H. (2017). Special section on emerging multimedia technology for smart surveillance system with IoT environment. *The Journal of Supercomputing*, *73*(3), 923–925. DOI: 10.1007/s11227-016-1939-9

Kim, I. C., Kim, Y. J., & Chin, S. Y. (2022). Sound localization framework for construction site monitoring. *Applied Sciences (Basel, Switzerland)*, *12*(21), 10783. DOI: 10.3390/app122110783

Kokkonis, G., Psannis, K. E., Roumeliotis, M., & Schonfeld, D. (2017). Real-time wireless multisensory smart surveillance with 3D-HEVC streams for internet-of-things (IoT). *The Journal of Supercomputing*, *73*(3), 1044–1062. DOI: 10.1007/s11227-016-1769-9

Kumar Pandey, B., Pandey, D., Nassa, V. K., Ahmad, T., Singh, C., George, A. S., & Wakchaure, M. A. (2021). Encryption and steganography-based text extraction in IoT using the EWCTS optimizer. *Imaging Science Journal*, *69*(1-4), 38–56. DOI: 10.1080/13682199.2022.2146885

Kumarganesh, S., & Malathi Murugesan, C. (2024). Hybrid Plasmonic Biosensors with Deep Learning for Colorectal Cancer Detection. *Plasmonics*, •••, 1–15. DOI: 10.1007/s11468-024-02568-y

Lakshmi, K. V. N., Rajan, R., Pandey, D., & Pandey, B. K. (2024). Circular Economy: A Catalyst for Economic Growth-An Empirical Study. *Circular Economy and Sustainability*, •••, 1–22.

Lin, Z., Ding, G., Han, J., & Wang, J. (2016). Cross-view retrieval via probability-based semantics-preserving hashing. *IEEE Transactions on Cybernetics*, *47*(12), 4342–4355. DOI: 10.1109/TCYB.2016.2608906 PMID: 28113531

Maheshwari, R., Kumarganesh, S., K v M, S., Gopalakrishnan, A., Selvi, K., Paulchamy, B., Rishabavarthani, P., Sagayam, K. M., Pandey, B. K., & Pandey, D. (2024). Advanced plasmonic resonance-enhanced biosensor for comprehensive real-time detection and analysis of deepfake content. *Plasmonics*, •••, 1–18. DOI: 10.1007/s11468-024-02407-0

Pandey, B. K., Mukundan, A. P., Nassa, V. K., Pandey, D., George, A. S., Hameed, A. S., & Dadheech, P. (2024f). Deployment of Load Balancing in Cloud Computing: Industrial Application and Benefits. In Emerging Engineering Technologies and Industrial Applications (pp. 342-354). IGI Global.

Pandey, B. K., Nassa, V. K., Mukundan, A. P., Mahajan, D. A., Pandey, D., George, A. S., & Dadheech, P. (2024d). An Industry-Focused Traffic System Utilising Internet of Things. In *Emerging Engineering Technologies and Industrial Applications* (pp. 200–213). IGI Global. DOI: 10.4018/979-8-3693-1335-0.ch009

Pandey, B. K., & Pandey, D. (2023). Parametric optimization and prediction of enhanced thermoelectric performance in co-doped CaMnO3 using response surface methodology and neural network. *Journal of Materials Science Materials in Electronics*, *34*(21), 1589. DOI: 10.1007/s10854-023-10954-1

Pandey, B. K., & Pandey, D. (2025). Securing healthcare medical image information using advance morphological component analysis, information hiding systems, and hybrid convolutional neural networks on IoMT. *Computers in Biology and Medicine*, *185*, 109499. DOI: 10.1016/j.compbiomed.2024.109499 PMID: 39642698

Pandey, B. K., Pandey, D., & Agarwal, A. (2022). Encrypted information transmission by enhanced steganography and image transformation. [IJDAI]. *International Journal of Distributed Artificial Intelligence*, *14*(1), 1–14. DOI: 10.4018/IJDAI.297110

Pandey, B. K., Pandey, D., Dadheech, P., Mahajan, D. A., George, A. S., & Hameed, A. S. (2023). Review on Smart Sewage Cleaning UAV Assistance for Sustainable Development. In *Handbook of Research on Safe Disposal Methods of Municipal Solid Wastes for a Sustainable Environment* (pp. 69–79). IGI Global. DOI: 10.4018/978-1-6684-8117-2.ch005

Pandey, B. K., Paramashivan, M. A., Hasan, A., Pramanik, S., Dadheech, P., Manaktala, S. S., & George, A. S. (2024a). Social Psychological Obstacles to the Implementation of Artificial Intelligence in Supply Chain Management. In AI and Machine Learning Impacts in Intelligent Supply Chain (pp. 17-24). IGI Global. DOI: 10.4018/979-8-3693-1347-3.ch002

Pandey, B. K., Paramashivan, M. A., Kanike, U. K., Mahajan, D. A., Mahajan, R., George, A. S., & Hameed, A. S. H. (2024b). Impacts of Artificial Intelligence and Machine Learning on Intelligent Supply Chains. In *AI and Machine Learning Impacts in Intelligent Supply Chain* (pp. 57–73). IGI Global. DOI: 10.4018/979-8-3693-1347-3.ch005

Pandey, B. K., Paramashivan, M. A., Mahajan, R., Mahajan, D. A., Behare, N., Gowwrii, G., & Pramanik, S. (2024c). Applications of Artificial Intelligence and Machine Learning in Supply Chain Management: An In-Depth Investigation. In *AI and Machine Learning Impacts in Intelligent Supply Chain* (pp. 74–90). IGI Global. DOI: 10.4018/979-8-3693-1347-3.ch006

Pandey, B. K., Paramashivan, M. A., Nassa, V. K., Mahajan, D. A., Dadheech, P., George, A. H., & George, A. S. (2024h). Blockchain's Potential Effect on the Healthcare Industry. In Emerging Engineering Technologies and Industrial Applications (pp. 214-232). IGI Global. DOI: 10.4018/979-8-3693-1335-0.ch010

. Pandey, B. K., Paramashivan, M. A., Pandey, D., George, A. S., Agarwal, A., Dadheech, P., & Mahajan, D. A. (2024g). A Recent Survey on 6G Vehicular Technology: Applications and Challenges. 6G Security Education and Multidisciplinary Implementation, 337-350.

Pandey, B. K., Paramashivan, M. A., Pandey, D., George, A. S., Agarwal, A., Mahajan, D. A., . . . Pramanik, S. (2024e). Future Directions of Digital Twin Architectures for 6G Communication Networks. In Security Issues and Solutions in 6G Communications and Beyond (pp. 197-211). IGI Global.

Pandey, D., Pandey, B. K., Paramashivan, M. A., Mahajan, D. A., Dadheech, P. D., George, A. S., & Hameed, A. S. (2024). Advanced Digital Data Processing Using Cloud Cryptography: Industrial Applications. In Emerging Engineering Technologies and Industrial Applications (pp. 255-268). IGI Global.

Plageras, A. P., Psannis, K. E., Ishibashi, Y., & Kim, B. G. (2016, October). IoT-based surveillance system for ubiquitous healthcare. In *IECON 2016-42nd Annual Conference of the IEEE Industrial Electronics Society* (pp. 6226-6230). IEEE. DOI: 10.1109/IECON.2016.7793281

Puvvadi, U. L., Di Benedetto, K., Patil, A., Kang, K. D., & Park, Y. (2015). Cost-effective security support in real-time video surveillance. *IEEE Transactions on Industrial Informatics*, *11*(6), 1457–1465. DOI: 10.1109/TII.2015.2491259

Rai, P. K., Pandey, D., & Pandey, B. K. (2024). The future of enterprise and innovation is compute as a commodity, or CaaC. *Partners Universal International Research Journal*, *3*(2), 89–94.

Revathi, T. K., Sathiyabhama, B., Sankar, S., Pandey, D., Pandey, B. K., & Dadeech, P. (2022). An intelligent model for coronary heart disease diagnosis. In *Networking Technologies in Smart Healthcare* (pp. 309–327). CRC Press. DOI: 10.1201/9781003239888-15

Sahani, K., Khadka, S. S., Sahani, S. K., Pandey, B. K., & Pandey, D. (2024b). A possible underground roadway for transportation facilities in Kathmandu Valley: A racking deformation of underground rectangular structures. *Engineering Reports*, *6*(8), e12821. DOI: 10.1002/eng2.12821

Sahani, S. K., Pandey, B. K., & Pandey, D. (2024a). *Single-valued Signals, Multi-valued Signals and Fixed-Point of Contractive Signals*. Mathematics Open. DOI: 10.1142/S2811007224500020

Saravanakumar, R., TamilSelvi, T., Pandey, D., Pandey, B. K., Mahajan, D. A., & Lelisho, M. E. (2024). Big data processing using hybrid Gaussian mixture model with salp swarm algorithm. *Journal of Big Data, 11*(1), 1–29. DOI: 10.1186/s40537-024-01015-3

Saxena, A., Sharma, N. K., Pandey, D., & Pandey, B. K. (2021). Influence of tourists satisfaction on future behavioral intentions with special reference to desert triangle of Rajasthan. *Augmented Human Research, 6*(1), 13. DOI: 10.1007/s41133-021-00052-4

Shahul, A., Muniandi, B., Paramashivan, M. A., Pandey, D., Pandey, B. K., Dadheech, P., & George, H. (2024). An Analysis of Algorithms and Methods Based on Image Processing for Medical Applications. In *Emerging Engineering Technologies and Industrial Applications* (pp. 173–186). IGI Global. DOI: 10.4018/979-8-3693-1335-0.ch007

Stergiou, C., Psannis, K. E., Kim, B. G., & Gupta, B. (2018). Secure integration of IoT and cloud computing. *Future Generation Computer Systems, 78*, 964–975. DOI: 10.1016/j.future.2016.11.031

Stergiou, C., Psannis, K. E., Plageras, A. P., Kokkonis, G., & Ishibashi, Y. (2017, June). Architecture for security monitoring in IoT environments. In *2017 IEEE 26th international symposium on industrial electronics (ISIE)* (pp. 1382-1385). IEEE. DOI: 10.1109/ISIE.2017.8001447

Swapna, H. R., Bigirimana, E., Geetha, R., Paramashivan, M. A., George, A. S., Dadheech, P., & Vyas, V. (2024c). New Insights Into Strategic Consumer Behavior From the Field of Operations Management. In Utilization of AI Technology in Supply Chain Management (pp. 289-298). IGI Global. DOI: 10.4018/979-8-3693-3593-2.ch019

Swapna, H. R., Geetanjali, S., Lakshmi, K. V. N., Paramashivan, M. A., Nikhil, M. S., Dadheech, P., & Vyas, V. (2024b). Navigating the Transformative Journey: AI's Progression in Business Applications. In Utilization of AI Technology in Supply Chain Management (pp. 15-25). IGI Global.

Swapna, H. R., Hukkeri, S. V., Pandey, D., & Paramashivan, M. A. (2024a). Cosmopolitan living during the COVID-19 Era: Navigating Challenges and Uniting Communities-An Impact Analysis. In Impact of Climate Change on Mental Health and Well-Being (pp. 1-10). IGI Global.

Tareke, S. A., Lelisho, M. E., Hassen, S. S., Seid, A. A., Jemal, S. S., Teshale, B. M., & Pandey, B. K. (2022). The prevalence and predictors of depressive, anxiety, and stress symptoms among Tepi town residents during the COVID-19 pandemic lockdown in Ethiopia. *Journal of Racial and Ethnic Health Disparities*, •••, 1–13. PMID: 35028903

Yang, X., Qian, X., & Mei, T. (2015). Learning salient visual word for scalable mobile image retrieval. *Pattern Recognition*, *48*(10), 3093–3101. DOI: 10.1016/j.patcog.2014.12.017

Chapter 3
AI-Powered Secure Bio-Medical Image Analysis

Shaik Balkhis Banu
https://orcid.org/0000-0001-8014-0342
Department of Physiotherapy, Fatima College of Health Sciences, Al Ain, UAE

Geetha Kathirvelu
Independent Researcher, Oman

S. Meena
https://orcid.org/0000-0001-9979-8689
Department of Chemistry, Dayanandasagar College of Engineering, Bangalore, India

Devanga Dharani Lakshmi
https://orcid.org/0009-0008-3812-8663
Department of Computer Science and AI, Central University of Andhra Pradesh, Ananthapuramu, India

T. Keerthika
https://orcid.org/0000-0002-1911-1785
School of Artificial Intelligence, Amrita Vishwa Vidyapeetham, Coimbatore, India

Anantha Murthy
https://orcid.org/0000-0002-9009-7541
NMAM, Institute of Technology, Nitte University, India

A. S. Hovan George
Tbilisi State Medical University, Georgia

ABSTRACT

Artificial intelligence (AI) is revolutionizing the field of medical image analysis, highlighting the vital need of strong security protocols to safeguard private patient information. The use of cutting-edge analytical tools improves the precision and effectiveness of medical imaging, enabling earlier diagnoses and better treatment outcomes as healthcare increasingly uses AI-driven technologies. But using a lot of patient data creates serious privacy issues, so data protection needs to be prioritized.

DOI: 10.4018/979-8-3693-9821-0.ch003

Differential privacy, federated learning, and secure multi-party computation are three important approaches that are covered. These techniques enable collaborative analysis without disclosing raw data.

INTRODUCTION

Healthcare is changing as a result of faster and more accurate medical imaging made possible by AI-powered biomedical image analysis (Pandey, B. K., & Pandey, D., 2025). Modern machine learning algorithms are able to identify subtle patterns in images, such as MRIs and X-rays, and can frequently spot abnormalities earlier than more conventional techniques. For illnesses like cancer, heart disease, and neurological disorders, this has resulted in better diagnosis and more individualized treatment regimens. But there are issues with data security and privacy as digital image processing becomes more and more common (Satheesh, N. et al., 2025). Sensitive information is frequently contained in medical images, making it susceptible to cyberattacks during storage, transmission, and analysis. Advanced encryption techniques are employed to protect this data at every stage of its lifecycle, guaranteeing that even in the event of access, the data cannot be read by unauthorized parties. When data is transferred between imaging systems and healthcare providers, secure transmission protocols like VPNs further safeguard it (Sheela, M. S. et al., 2025). Apart from encryption, real-time monitoring systems assist in identifying questionable activities related to the access or usage of data. These systems are able to identify possible breaches before they have a major negative impact. Collaborative analysis of medical data is made possible by privacy-preserving techniques that prevent external systems from seeing the actual images (Kumar, M. S. et al., 2025). This keeps privacy violations less likely while allowing for thorough analysis.

Landscape of Biomedical Imaging

The field of biomedical imaging is currently characterized by rapid technological advancements that have significantly improved the accuracy, speed, and resolution of medical images. These advancements have had a significant impact on the field. In clinical settings (Khadka, M. et al., 2025), diagnostic procedures such as magnetic resonance imaging (MRI), computed tomography (CT) scans, X-rays, and ultrasound are frequently utilized for the purpose of diagnosing, monitoring, and treating a wide variety of medical conditions. Clinicians are able to visualize the internal structures of the body through the use of these imaging modalities (Konapure, C. G. et al., 2025), which assists in the diagnosis of diseases such as cancer, cardiovascular disorders, and neurological issues. In recent years, the incorporation of digital technology has resulted in an improvement in image quality and has made it possible to conduct more in-depth analyses (Singh, S. et al., 2025a). Imaging techniques such as high-resolution imaging, three-dimensional reconstruction, and functional imaging are now able to provide more in-depth insights into the anatomical and physiological changes that occur within the body. As a result of this progress, it is now possible to detect diseases at earlier stages, to personalize treatment plans, and to improve the outcomes for patients.

The increasing application of artificial intelligence and machine learning in the field of biomedical imaging is causing a transformation in the way that images are analysed (Singh, S. et al., 2025b). The ability of automated systems to assist radiologists in the detection of abnormalities, thereby reducing the likelihood of human error and increasing diagnostic precision, is now available. Despite these advancements, there are still challenges to be faced, particularly with regard to the management of large volumes of imaging data and the protection of patient information in terms of both privacy and security. As imaging technology continues to advance, the future of biomedical imaging will be shaped by the emphasis placed on making it more accessible, accurate, and secure (Bajwa, J. et al., 2021).

AI Integration for Efficiency

The application of artificial intelligence (AI) to biomedical imaging has resulted in a significant improvement in both the accuracy and efficiency of image analysis (Pandey, B. K. et al., 2024a). When it comes to interpreting medical images, traditional methods frequently rely on human expertise, which can be error-prone and time-consuming, especially when dealing with findings that are complex or subtle. The ability to analyse vast amounts of imaging data in a short amount of time and with a high degree of accuracy is a capability of artificial intelligence systems, particularly those that are based on machine learning and deep learning (Pandey, B. K. et al., 2024b). Human diagnosticians are often outperformed by these systems in certain tasks because they are able to recognize patterns, recognize anomalies, and classify medical conditions with remarkable accuracy. Artificial intelligence tools (Maheshwari, R. U. et al., 2024) have the ability to automate routine tasks such as image segmentation, tumor detection, and organ delineation, which significantly reduces the amount of time required for analysis that is required. Consequently, this not only expedites the workflows involved in diagnostic procedures, but it also guarantees more consistent results across a wider range of patients. AI systems are able to detect minute changes in tissue or structures that may be difficult for the human eye to notice. This enables earlier diagnosis and intervention in cases such as the detection of neurological disorders or instances of cancer. AI-driven models are constantly getting better as they are presented with more data. As they process more information (Maheshwari, R. Uma. et al., 2024), they become more adept at dealing with a variety of cases and learning from the results of previous cases. Both the speed and the quality of medical diagnoses are ultimately improved as a result of the efficiency gained from the integration of AI (Saxena, A. et al., 2024). This efficiency frees up clinicians to focus on more complex decision-making and patient care. Medical imaging solutions that are quicker, more accurate, and more cost-effective are being developed as a result of this shift, which is reshaping the healthcare industry (Al Kuwaiti, A. et al., 2023).

Security and Privacy in Sensitive Medical Data

The significance of security and privacy in managing sensitive medical data is paramount, especially regarding biomedical imaging. Medical images frequently encompass intricate and confidential patient information, rendering them exceptionally sensitive and valuable. Unauthorized access to this data may result in significant privacy breaches (Rai, P. K. et al., 2024), identity theft, or the improper use of medical information. Healthcare institutions are often targeted by cyberattacks because of the significant value of patient data in black markets (Lakshmi, K. V. N. et al., 2024). Securing medical images is essential for preserving patient trust and adhering to regulatory standards such as HIPAA and GDPR. These regulations mandate healthcare providers to safeguard patient data by ensuring it is encrypted, anonymized, and securely stored. Security breaches may result in legal liabilities, substantial penalties, and reputational harm to healthcare organizations.

AI-driven systems utilized in biomedical imaging present heightened security challenges due to the processing and storage of substantial data volumes across networks and cloud infrastructures. Secure transmission protocols, strong encryption methods, and access controls are vital to safeguard this data from unauthorized access and manipulation (Saravanakumar, R. et al., 2024). Privacy-preserving technologies, including federated learning, enable the training of AI models on decentralized datasets without the need to centralize sensitive patient data, thereby mitigating the risk of exposure (Mohammed, M. A. et al., 2022).

AI AND ITS ROLE IN BIOMEDICAL IMAGING

Image analysis accuracy and efficiency are crucial to biomedical imaging with artificial neural network (Pandey, B. K., & Pandey, D., 2023). Deep learning algorithms excel at image segmentation, classification, and anomaly detection, enabling early detection of cancer and diabetic retinopathy. Training on large datasets helps these algorithms learn complex patterns and improve. By automating labour-intensive processes, AI frees up healthcare professionals to make important decisions (Kumarganesh, S. et al., 2024). AI in biomedical imaging improves diagnostic precision, improving patient outcomes and healthcare delivery. AI significantly transforms biomedical imaging by augmenting diagnostic capabilities, optimizing workflow efficiency (Muralidhar, L. B. et al., 2024), and enhancing patient outcomes, while simultaneously tackling challenges within the healthcare sector. The Impact of Artificial Intelligence on Biomedical Imaging are as shown in the figure 1.

Figure 1. Impact of AI on biomedical imaging

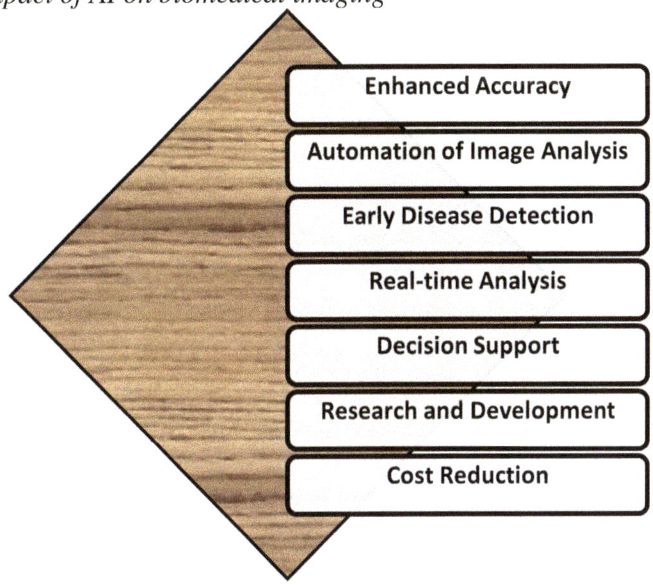

- *Enhanced Accuracy*: AI algorithms can evaluate medical images with exceptional accuracy, frequently detecting anomalies that human radiologists might miss. Deep learning models have demonstrated significant efficacy in identifying conditions such as lung cancer in chest X-rays and diabetic retinopathy in retinal images. These models are trained on comprehensive datasets, enabling them to comprehend the intricacies of diverse pathologies and apply this understanding uniformly across various cases. Machine learning models enhance diagnostic precision by perpetually learning from extensive datasets. As additional images are input into these systems, they adjust and optimize their algorithms, thereby improving their performance over time. This iterative learning process enables AI to remain up-to-date with emerging medical knowledge and evolving disease patterns, rendering it an invaluable asset in the dynamic healthcare landscape.

- *Automation of Image Analysis*: Artificial Intelligence streamlines labor-intensive processes including image segmentation, feature extraction, and classification. By optimizing these processes, AI alleviates the workload of healthcare professionals, enabling them to focus on advanced decision-making. In MRI scans, AI can rapidly delineate structures such as tumors, blood vessels, or organs, thereby enabling expedited and more precise evaluations. This automation alleviates the burden on radiologists, enabling them to concentrate on intricate cases and patient care. By removing redundant tasks, AI systems allow radiologists to dedicate more time to patient interaction and collaboration with other healthcare professionals. This not only improves care quality but also fosters increased job satisfaction among healthcare professionals.
- *Early Disease Detection*: AI systems are capable of identifying diseases at earlier stages, thereby enhancing treatment outcomes, particularly for ailments such as cancer. AI algorithms can examine mammograms to detect early indicators of breast cancer, potentially facilitating earlier interventions and improved prognoses. Timely identification is essential for effective treatment, rendering AI a vital partner in preventive medicine. Algorithms are developed to identify nuanced patterns and alterations in imaging data that signify the existence of disease. By concentrating on these preliminary indicators, AI can detect conditions that may be overlooked during standard assessments. This proactive strategy allows healthcare providers to adopt preventive measures, thereby diminishing the burden of advanced disease and related healthcare expenses (Hurkmans, C. W. et al., 2001).
- *Real-time Analysis*: AI-driven tools are capable of processing and analyzing images instantaneously, offering immediate feedback and assistance to clinicians during procedures. This ability is especially significant in interventional radiology, where rapid decisions are frequently required based on real-time imaging data. AI can identify areas of concern or assist clinicians in navigating intricate anatomical structures, thereby improving procedural safety and efficacy. This ability improves decision-making and enables prompt interventions. Real-time insights enable healthcare professionals to respond more rapidly to complications or unforeseen findings, resulting in enhanced patient outcomes. This responsiveness is particularly vital in emergency medicine, where each second is critical for preserving lives.
- *Decision Support*: AI offers decision support tools that aid radiologists in analyzing intricate images, emphasizing areas of interest and proposing potential diagnoses. These tools provide supplementary support, assisting clini-

cians in validating their interpretations and improving diagnostic precision. AI enhances confidence in clinical decision-making by offering evidence-based recommendations. These instruments improve the diagnostic procedure and diminish the likelihood of misdiagnosis. The utilization of AI in image interpretation reduces the probability of errors, resulting in enhanced patient care. This partnership between AI and human expertise fosters a synergistic relationship that enhances outcomes while preserving a human element in healthcare.

- *Research and Development*: Artificial Intelligence is employed in research to create novel imaging techniques and improve existing ones, fostering innovation in the discipline. Researchers are investigating AI's capabilities in sophisticated imaging techniques, including functional MRI and molecular imaging. Utilizing AI, researchers can identify innovative methods that enhance imaging resolution and offer fresh perspectives on disease mechanisms. Collaborative initiatives among researchers and healthcare practitioners are enhancing diagnostic capabilities. These collaborations facilitate the conversion of research outcomes into clinical applications, thereby enhancing patient care. As artificial intelligence advances, its impact on research is expected to produce substantial innovations in medical imaging and healthcare.
- *Cost Reduction*: Enhancing accuracy and efficiency through AI may lead to a decrease in healthcare expenses linked to misdiagnosis and postponed treatments. Prompt and precise identification of diseases can facilitate timely interventions, thereby diminishing the necessity for costly and invasive procedures in the future. This proactive strategy can substantially reduce total healthcare expenditures. Optimized workflows result in reduced operational expenses for healthcare institutions. AI improves the efficiency of imaging departments by automating routine tasks and optimizing resource allocation. The cost savings can be reinvested in patient care initiatives, thereby enhancing the quality of services offered to patients.

DATA SECURITY IN BIOMEDICAL IMAGE ANALYSIS

Handling Large-Scale, Sensitive Patient Data

A crucial component of contemporary healthcare is managing sensitive patient data on a large scale, especially in light of the growing reliance on digital technologies and data-driven strategies. The need for effective data management and protection has never been greater as healthcare systems produce enormous volumes of data from numerous sources, including genetic data, medical imaging, and electronic health records (EHRs). Sensitive information about patients is inherent; it contains personal information that, in the wrong hands, can result in identity theft, privacy violations, and serious personal injury. Healthcare organizations need to put strong data governance frameworks in place in order to manage large amounts of patient data. For data collection, storage, sharing, and disposal, this entails creating explicit policies and procedures. Data governance guarantees the ethical and responsible handling of sensitive information in compliance with legal mandates such as the General Data Protection Regulation (GDPR) in Europe and the Health Insurance Portability and Accountability Act (HIPAA) in the United States. Strict protocols for data access are mandated by these regulations, necessitating the implementation of safeguards like encryption, access controls, and periodic audits by organizations to ensure patient information is protected. There are advantages and disadvantages to managing sensitive data when AI and machine learning technologies are integrated in the healthcare industry. Large datasets can be processed and analyzed by AI effectively, improving patient outcomes and diagnostics. But there are also security and privacy issues with using AI. It is essential to make sure AI systems are created with privacy in mind. Methods like federated learning can assist in training algorithms without disclosing private patient information. Models can learn from distributed datasets using this method while protecting the privacy of the data. Building a data security culture among medical staff members is another essential component of managing massive patient data sets. To teach employees the value of data privacy and the best practices for safeguarding sensitive information, ongoing training and awareness campaigns are crucial. Human error is still the main cause of data breaches, but healthcare organizations can reduce this risk by fostering a security-first mentality (Vinod, S. K. et al., 2016).

Cyberattack Risks in Healthcare

Data breaches from healthcare cyberattacks are a major concern. Medical records contain sensitive patient information like names, addresses, medical histories, and finances. Cybercriminals can steal identities, commit fraud, or sell this data on the dark web. This violates privacy and damages patient trust in healthcare providers. Hospitals and clinics can lose patient confidence and face regulatory fines due to data breaches. Healthcare is facing more ransomware attacks. Hackers demand ransom to decrypt critical healthcare data. These attacks can disrupt hospital operations, making patient records, diagnostics, and critical care services difficult to access. Some hospitals have had to divert patients or delay critical treatments, endangering lives. Healthcare providers often pay ransoms, recover, and lose revenue from downtime, which causes significant financial damage. Healthcare operations disruption is another major risk. Hospitals and clinics can lose all workflow when cyberattacks cripple IT systems. EHRs and imaging systems may be lost, preventing healthcare providers from providing timely and accurate care. This can cause missed diagnoses, delayed treatments, and poor patient outcomes, especially in emergencies where seconds matter. With more connected medical devices like pacemakers and insulin pumps, cyberattacks could endanger patients. Hackers could tamper with these devices, causing malfunctions or incorrect treatments. This endangers patients and the healthcare system. Cybercriminals thrive on unsecured devices and vulnerable network infrastructure (Pandey, B. K. et al., 2024c). Healthcare organizations suffer significant legal and financial consequences from cyberattacks. Healthcare providers must notify patients after breaches and face costly lawsuits and regulatory fines. Rebuilding patient and stakeholder trust can take years, especially in smaller healthcare organizations that lack the resources to recover quickly. Thus, healthcare organizations must prioritize cybersecurity measures like continuous monitoring, threat detection, and rapid response. Insufficient cybersecurity infrastructure plagues many healthcare systems. Budget constraints and outdated technology make them attackable. Cyber incidents are also caused by human error, such as phishing attacks and improper data handling. Accidental or malicious insider threats complicate security, requiring regular staff training and strict access controls (Wang, S. et al., 2021).

TECHNOLOGIES FOR SECURING BIOMEDICAL DATA

Encryption Techniques in Biomedical Imaging

Encryption methods are crucial for protecting biomedical imaging data from unauthorized access and breaches (Pandey, B. K. et al., 2024d). These methods guarantee the protection of sensitive patient information, including MRI scans and X-rays, during both storage and transmission. Symmetric encryption employs a singular key for both encryption and decryption, providing rapidity and efficiency, thus rendering it appropriate for extensive datasets. Conversely, asymmetric encryption employs a key pair, augmenting security while necessitating greater processing power. Techniques such as Advanced Encryption Standard (AES) and RSA are frequently utilized in biomedical imaging. By employing the encryption techniques illustrated in Figure 2, healthcare organizations can preserve patient confidentiality and adhere to data protection regulations. Encryption methods are essential for protecting sensitive biomedical imaging data from unauthorized access and breaches. Healthcare organizations (Elarmathi, S. et al., 2024) can effectively safeguard patient information and promote collaboration and research in the medical field by utilizing a combination of symmetric and asymmetric encryption, homomorphic techniques, and specialized image encryption algorithms.

1. *Symmetric Encryption*: Symmetric encryption employs a singular key for both encryption and decryption, rendering it efficient for processing extensive datasets, such as those produced in biomedical imaging. Algorithms such as Advanced Encryption Standard (AES) are frequently employed for their efficiency and security. In biomedical imaging, symmetric encryption safeguards sensitive data during storage and transmission, ensuring that only authorized individuals can access patient images and related metadata. The difficulty resides in the secure distribution and management of encryption keys among authorized individuals.
2. *Asymmetric Encryption*: Asymmetric encryption utilizes a key pair: a public key for encryption and a private key for decryption. This approach improves security by removing the necessity for key exchange, allowing the public key to be disseminated openly while the private key remains secure. Asymmetric encryption can be utilized in biomedical imaging to protect communication between devices, including imaging machines and healthcare databases. It facilitates the secure transmission of images across networks, guaranteeing that only the designated recipient can decrypt and access the confidential information.
3. *Homomorphic Encryption*: Homomorphic encryption enables the execution of computations on encrypted data without prior decryption. This method is especially significant in biomedical imaging, where data confidentiality is crucial. Researchers can examine encrypted imaging data to derive significant insights while safeguarding sensitive patient information. This method facilitates collaborative research while ensuring adherence to privacy regulations, as the foundational data remains safeguarded during the analytical process.
4. *Image Encryption Algorithms*: Numerous specialized algorithms are specifically developed for the encryption of image data. Block-based encryption and chaotic encryption are effective techniques for securing biomedical images. Block-based encryption segments images into smaller blocks, encrypting each individually, thereby improving security and efficiency. Chaotic encryption employs chaotic systems to generate intricate encryption keys, rendering it exceedingly challenging for unauthorized individuals to decode the encrypted images. These algorithms guarantee that, even if an assailant acquires encrypted images, they cannot extract valuable information without the decryption key.
5. *Data Masking*: Data masking is a method employed to conceal particular data elements within a dataset while preserving the overall structure and functionality. In biomedical imaging, data masking safeguards sensitive information, such as patient identifiers, by substituting them with fictitious values. This method is especially advantageous in situations where imaging data must be disseminated for research or educational objectives. Although not a conventional encryption technique, data masking functions as a supplementary security measure, safeguarding sensitive patient information from exposure during analysis.

6. *Quantum Encryption*: Quantum encryption, grounded in the principles of quantum mechanics, presents a potentially transformative method for securing biomedical imaging data. Quantum Key Distribution (QKD) enables two parties to produce and exchange encryption keys in a manner that is theoretically impervious to interception. The application of quantum encryption in biomedical imaging, though primarily experimental, shows potential for attaining exceptional data security as quantum computing progresses.

Figure 2. Encryption methods for biomedical imaging

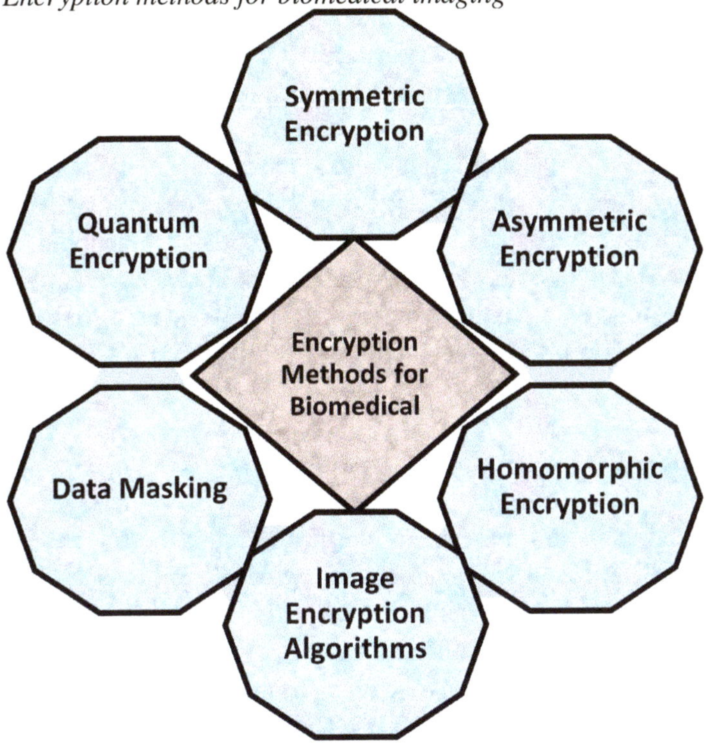

Secure Transmission Protocols

Sensitive medical image sharing between imaging facilities, patients, and health-care providers requires the use of secure transmission protocols. Considering the sensitive nature of biomedical data, strong protocols must be used to guarantee availability, confidentiality, and integrity. Secure Socket Layer (SSL) is one popular protocol that creates an encrypted connection between the client and server. This technique protects data on the network from interception and unauthorized access. By ensuring the secure transmission of images and related data, SSL deters malevolent actors from intercepting sensitive content. The replacement for SSL, Transport Layer Security (TLS), is another significant standard. TLS provides enhanced security features, including stronger encryption methods and increased defense against different types of attacks. Healthcare organizations can guarantee the confidentiality of medical images while they are being transmitted over internal networks or the internet by putting TLS into place. File transfers can be done securely with the help of Secure File Transfer Protocol (SFTP). By encrypting data and commands, SFTP offers a safe channel for exchanging medical images. Ensuring the protection of sensitive information during the transfer of large datasets is made possible by this protocol. An extension of HTTP, Hypertext Transfer Protocol Secure (HTTPS) uses TLS to encrypt web traffic. Applications in the healthcare industry that share images via web-based platforms frequently depend on HTTPS to encrypt data transfers between browsers and servers. This protocol makes sure that patient photos are kept private and gives authorized users easy access. Virtual Private Networks (VPNs) can also be used to add an additional degree of security. Healthcare practitioners can safely share images over public networks by using virtual private networks (VPNs) to create a secure tunnel for data transmission. By limiting access to the data to only those who are authorized, this method improves privacy.

AI-DRIVEN SECURITY APPROACHES

The protection of sensitive data in industries such as healthcare, finance, and critical infrastructure is being revolutionized by security approaches that are driven by artificial intelligence (AI). Traditional security measures are improved by these approaches, which also provide more robust defenses against evolving threats (Pandey, B. K. et al., 2024e). These approaches make use of advanced machine learning algorithms and data analytics. Having the capacity to perform real-time analysis on massive amounts of data is one of the most significant benefits that intelligent systems bring to the field of security. The detection of anomalous behavior, which may be an indication of a security breach or cyberattack, is being made possible by this capability. As an illustration, these systems are able to monitor access patterns to electronic health records (EHRs) in the healthcare industry and identify unusual attempts to gain access, such as multiple failed logins or access from strange locations. Organizations are able to speedily respond to potential threats and reduce the likelihood of data breaches if they are able to identify these anomalies.

To add insult to injury, intelligent systems are able to improve their predictive capabilities by learning from historical data. In order to train machine learning models to recognize the signs of potential future attacks, it is necessary to first analyze previous incidents and the patterns that are associated with them (JayaLakshmi, G. et al., 2024). Because of this proactive approach, organizations are able to enhance their defenses and anticipate potential threats before an attack takes place. When it comes to systems, for example, predictive analytics can identify vulnerabilities, which enables timely patching and updates to be implemented. Intelligent security solutions have the capability to automate responses to security incidents, which is another important aspect of these capabilities. Predefined responses can be triggered by these systems whenever a threat is identified. These responses may include isolating the systems that are affected, notifying security teams, or putting countermeasures into place to eliminate the threat. Not only does this automation lessen the workload of human security personnel, but it also shortens the amount of time it takes for them to respond to incidents. This frees them up to concentrate on more difficult tasks that require human judgment and expertise. Intelligent solutions improve the collection of threat intelligence (George, W. K. et al., 2024). These systems are able to provide organizations with valuable insights into emerging threats and vulnerabilities by continuously analysing data from a variety of sources, such as threat reports, conversations on social media, and activities on the dark web. With this information, security teams are able to take preventative measures against potential threats and put in place the necessary defenses. It is essential to acknowledge that intelligent security is not a silver bullet, despite the large number of advantages it offers. Despite the fact that these systems are susceptible to adversarial attacks that aim to take advantage of their weaknesses, their effectiveness is directly proportional to the data that they are trained on. Therefore, it is imperative that organizations implement a multi-layered security strategy that incorporates both cutting-edge tools and more conventional security measures, as well as human expertise and ongoing monitoring.

PRIVACY-PRESERVING AI TECHNIQUES

Differential Privacy for Anonymization

Differential privacy protects privacy while allowing large datasets, especially in artificial intelligence models (Abdullahi, M. et al., 2024). It anonymizes data mathematically, so including or excluding any individual's data doesn't affect analysis.

Organizations that want to use sensitive data without compromising privacy will benefit from this feature. Disparate privacy adds noise to data or algorithm output to make it hard to infer specific information about individuals in the dataset. Privacy and data utility are balanced by calibrating this noise. By adjusting noise, organizations can maintain data analysis while reducing the risk of identifying individuals. This flexibility allows businesses to comply with GDPR and HIPAA while using their datasets for insights. AI models use input and output perturbation to implement differential privacy (Kumar, B. et al., 2024). Noise is added to data before feeding it to the model to teach it from distorted data. Noise makes it harder to directly attribute data points to individuals, anonymizing contributions. Output perturbation injects noise into the model's predictions or outputs to ensure privacy without changing the training data. Both approaches can be tailored to an organization's needs and data sensitivity (Pandey, D. et al., 2024a). With differential privacy, organizations can analyze data and learn without re-identifying people. Healthcare researchers can use differential privacy to analyze patient records for trends and correlations while protecting patient identities. While maintaining privacy, researchers can gain valuable insights by preventing data points from being linked to individuals. Diverse privacy has benefits but also drawbacks. The mathematical principles and context of this approach must be understood before applying it. To maintain data utility and privacy, organizations must balance noise (Pandey, D. et al., 2024b). Transparency in differential privacy implementation is needed so stakeholders understand the implications of the privacy guarantees.

Federated Learning for Decentralized Training

Federated learning is a cutting-edge method of training AI models that puts data security and privacy first, especially in delicate industries like healthcare. Sensitive patient data does not need to be centralized in one place for several parties to work together to train a shared model thanks to this decentralized approach. Rather, the data stays on the servers or devices from which it was originally obtained, lowering the possibility of data breaches (Kennedy, G. W. et al., 2024) and guaranteeing adherence to privacy laws. Conventional machine learning involves gathering and centrally storing data for analysis. This method has a number of drawbacks, including the possibility of illegal access to private patient data and challenges in adhering to legal obligations like GDPR and HIPAA. By keeping the data local, federated learning reduces these risks and allows healthcare organizations to take part in the training process without disclosing patient information to outside parties. A central server coordinates the training of a global model in federated learning, with local servers or individual devices training their own versions of the model on their own datasets. The model updates are sent to the central server after every local training round, not the raw data (Shahul, A. et al., 2024). This server builds a fresh, enhanced global model by combining the updates from all involved parties. Iteratively going forward, this procedure protects patient confidentiality by letting the model learn from a variety of datasets. This method not only increases data privacy but also boosts the efficiency of the model. Federated learning has the potential to generate models that are more effective in real-world applications by utilizing data from multiple sources and improving their generalization across various populations. In the healthcare industry, for instance, federated learning-trained models are better able to accommodate the varied features of patient populations across various hospitals, resulting in more precise diagnosis and treatment recommendations. Federated learning has certain drawbacks despite its benefits (Pandey, D. et al., 2024c). Communication efficiency is a concern because, particularly when working with large models or datasets, transmitting model updates can demand a substantial amount of bandwidth. Furthermore, it is critical to guarantee secure aggregation and accurate training of local models. To further improve security and safeguard patient data, federated learning can incorporate strategies like differential privacy.

Secure Multi-Party Computation for Collaboration

Secure multi-party computation (SMPC) allows multiple parties to analyze data while protecting their datasets. This method works well in healthcare, finance, and research, where sensitive data is involved. SMPC meets the growing need for privacy-preserving collaboration by letting organizations compute functions on their data without revealing it (Pandey, D., & Pandey, B. K., 2022). In a typical SMPC scenario, each participant has their own dataset and wants to compute with everyone. Participants encrypt their data instead of sharing it. A protocol lets the parties compute the desired function on the encrypted inputs. After the computation, participants receive the result without access to the datasets. This protects sensitive data like patient records and financial data during analysis. The versatility of SMPC is a major benefit. It can be used for statistical analyses, machine learning model training, and data mining. For instance, hospitals can share patient data to identify treatment outcomes trends without disclosing sensitive patient information. Researchers can use SMPC to perform joint analyses that improve insights while complying with patient privacy laws. SMPC implementation is difficult despite its benefits. Encrypting data and performing secure computations increases processing time and resource consumption. This overhead can be significant for large datasets or complex algorithms. SMPC protocols are becoming more efficient due to cryptographic and optimization advances. The trustworthiness of participating parties and the robustness of the protocols also make SMPC effective. If one party is malicious or misbehaves, the results may be compromised. Thus, careful protocol design and strong security are necessary to build trust in the collaborative process.

CONCLUSION

Medical image analysis is changing as a result of the collaboration between artificial intelligence and security, which is putting patient privacy and data protection first while opening up possibilities for improved diagnostic capabilities. Healthcare organizations can increase the accuracy of medical imaging procedures while guaranteeing the security of sensitive patient data by combining sophisticated algorithms with strong security measures. This dual emphasis on privacy and performance is essential in a time when the need for effective healthcare solutions is rising quickly. Through cutting-edge methods like deep learning, artificial intelligence (AI) greatly improves the accuracy of medical image analysis, enabling more accurate diagnosis and classification of a range of medical conditions. With the use of these technologies, imaging data anomalies can be more easily detected, which can result in earlier diagnosis and better treatment outcomes. Meanwhile, patient data handling is guaranteed by the use of secure multi-party computation, differential privacy, and secure transmission protocols. The amalgamation of improved precision and strengthened security signifies a holistic approach to healthcare that places equal emphasis on patient well-being and data integrity. As artificial intelligence (AI) technologies advance, there will be more chances to create models that prioritize data privacy ethics in addition to performance. Building trust between patients and healthcare professionals will require ongoing research and investments in security measures, which will eventually increase the acceptance of AI-driven solutions in clinical practice. The healthcare industry may greatly enhance patient outcomes while protecting sensitive data by establishing a cooperative atmosphere that values both innovation and security.

REFERENCES

Abdullahi, M., Ahmad, A., Pandey, B. K., & Pandey, D. (2024). Digital Currency Adoption: A Comparative Analysis of Global Trends and the Nigerian eNaira Digital Currency. *SN Computer Science*, *5*(5), 1–11. DOI: 10.1007/s42979-024-02882-6

Al Kuwaiti, A., Nazer, K., Al-Reedy, A., Al-Shehri, S., Al-Muhanna, A., Subbarayalu, A. V., Al Muhanna, D., & Al-Muhanna, F. A. (2023). A review of the role of artificial intelligence in healthcare. *Journal of Personalized Medicine*, *13*(6), 951. DOI: 10.3390/jpm13060951 PMID: 37373940

Bajwa, J., Munir, U., Nori, A., & Williams, B. (2021). Artificial intelligence in healthcare: Transforming the practice of medicine. *Future Healthcare Journal*, *8*(2), e188–e194. DOI: 10.7861/fhj.2021-0095 PMID: 34286183

Elarmathi, S., Rishabavarthani, P., Sindhuja, M., Elayaraja, P., & Malathi Murugesan, S. (2024). Novel manufacturing systems for cancer diagnosis using ultra-sensitive photonic crystal fiber biosensor with dual-functionalized aptamer-nanocavity. *Microsystem Technologies*, •••, 1–20. DOI: 10.1007/s00542-024-05820-x

George, W. K., Silas, E. I., Pandey, D., & Pandey, B. K. (2024). Utilization of Industry 4.0 Technologies in Nigerian Technical and Vocational Education: A Conundrum for Educators. In *Examining the Rapid Advance of Digital Technology in Africa* (pp. 270–293). IGI Global. DOI: 10.4018/978-1-6684-9962-7.ch014

. Hurkmans, C. W., Borger, J. H., Pieters, B. R., Russell, N. S., Jansen, E. P., & Mijnheer, B. J. (2001). Variability in target volume delineation on CT scans of the breast. International Journal of Radiation Oncology* Biology* Physics, 50(5), 1366-1372.

JayaLakshmi. G., Pandey, D., Pandey, B. K., Kaur, P., Mahajan, D. A., & Dari, S. S. (2024). Smart big data collection for intelligent supply chain improvement. In AI and Machine Learning Impacts in Intelligent Supply Chain (pp. 180-195). IGI Global Scientific Publishing.

Kennedy, G. W., Sunday, S. E., Pandey, D., Kabari, A. D., Pandey, B. K., George, A. S., & Dadheech, P. (2024). Building Information Modeling: Harnessing Innovations for Professional Proficiency. In Emerging Engineering Technologies and Industrial Applications (pp. 305-331). IGI Global.

Khadka, M., Sah, M., Chaudhary, R., Sahani, S. K., Sahani, K., Pandey, B. K., & Pandey, D. (2025). Spectroscopic, quantum chemical, and topological calculations of the phenylephrine molecule using density functional theory. *Scientific Reports*, *15*(1), 208. DOI: 10.1038/s41598-024-81633-2 PMID: 39747169

. Konapure, C. G., Pandey, D., Shete, H., Thakar, C. M., Pandey, B. K., & George, A. S. (2025). Artificial Intelligence in Automated Concrete Mix Design Using Computerized Grading Curves. Interdisciplinary Approaches to AI, Internet of Everything, and Machine Learning, 567-586.

. Kumar, B., Pandey, D., Pandey, B. K., & George, A. S. (2024). Higher Education in the Last Four Decades: A Review of Paradigm Shifts in Policy Frameworks. Design and Implementation of Higher Education Learners' Learning Outcomes (HELLO), 333-348.

Kumar, M. S., Prasanna, P. L., Lalitha, M., Joy, M., Jha, S. S., & Pandey, B. K. (2025). Utilizing the Internet of Everything and Artificial Intelligence for Real-Time Workforce Management. In Role of Internet of Everything (IOE), VLSI Architecture, and AI in Real-Time Systems (pp. 153-168). IGI Global Scientific Publishing.

Kumarganesh, S., & Malathi Murugesan, C. (2024). Hybrid plasmonic biosensors with deep learning for colorectal cancer detection. *Plasmonics*, •••, 1–15. DOI: 10.1007/s11468-024-02568-y

Lakshmi, K. V. N., Rajan, R., Pandey, D., & Pandey, B. K. (2024). Circular economy: A catalyst for economic growth-an empirical study. *Circular Economy and Sustainability*, •••, 1–22.

Maheshwari, R., Kumarganesh, S., K v M, S., Gopalakrishnan, A., Selvi, K., Paulchamy, B., Rishabavarthani, P., Sagayam, K. M., Pandey, B. K., & Pandey, D. (2024). Advanced plasmonic resonance-enhanced biosensor for comprehensive real-time detection and analysis of deepfake content. *Plasmonics*, •••, 1–18. DOI: 10.1007/s11468-024-02407-0

Maheshwari, R. U., Paulchamy, B., Pandey, B. K., & Pandey, D. (2024). Enhancing sensing and imaging capabilities through surface plasmon resonance for deepfake image detection. *Plasmonics*, •••, 1–20. DOI: 10.1007/s11468-024-02492-1

Mohammed, M. A., Mohammed, V. A., & Mohammed, V. A. (2022). Impact of Artificial Intelligence on the Automation of Digital Health System. [IJSEA]. *International Journal of Software Engineering and Its Applications*, •••, 13.

Muralidhar, L. B., Lakshmi, K. V. N., Swapna, H. R., Rupani, J., Nethravathi, K., Pandey, B. K., & Pandey, D. (2024). Impact of Organizational Culture on The Level of Corporate Social Responsibility Investments: An Exploratory Study. *Circular Economy and Sustainability*, *4*(3), 1–19. DOI: 10.1007/s43615-024-00371-9

Pandey, B. K., Kanike, U. K., George, A. S., & Pandey, D. (Eds.). (2024d). *AI and machine learning impacts in intelligent supply chain*. IGI Global. DOI: 10.4018/979-8-3693-1347-3

Pandey, B. K., Nassa, V. K., Mukundan, A. P., Mahajan, D. A., Pandey, D., George, A. S., & Dadheech, P. (2024c). An Industry-Focused Traffic System Utilising Internet of Things. In *Emerging Engineering Technologies and Industrial Applications* (pp. 200–213). IGI Global. DOI: 10.4018/979-8-3693-1335-0.ch009

Pandey, B. K., & Pandey, D. (2023). Parametric optimization and prediction of enhanced thermoelectric performance in co-doped CaMnO3 using response surface methodology and neural network. *Journal of Materials Science Materials in Electronics*, *34*(21), 1589. DOI: 10.1007/s10854-023-10954-1

Pandey, B. K., & Pandey, D. (2025). Securing healthcare medical image information using advance morphological component analysis, information hiding systems, and hybrid convolutional neural networks on IoMT. *Computers in Biology and Medicine*, *185*, 109499. DOI: 10.1016/j.compbiomed.2024.109499 PMID: 39642698

Pandey, B. K., Pandey, D., & Lelisho, M. E. (2024a). Face mask identification with enhanced cuckoo optimization and deep learning-based faster regional neural network. *Scientific Reports*, *14*(1), 29719. DOI: 10.1038/s41598-024-78746-z PMID: 39613761

Pandey, B. K., Pandey, D., & Sahani, S. K. (2024b). Autopilot control unmanned aerial vehicle system for sewage defect detection using deep learning. *Engineering Reports*, •••, 12852.

Pandey, B. K., Paramashivan, M. A., Pandey, D., George, A. S., Agarwal, A., Mahajan, D. A., . . . Pramanik, S. (2024e). Future Directions of Digital Twin Architectures for 6G Communication Networks. In Security Issues and Solutions in 6G Communications and Beyond (pp. 197-211). IGI Global.

Pandey, D., Nassa, V. K., Pandey, B. K., Thankachan, B., Dadheech, P., Mahajan, D. A., & George, A. S. (2024a). Artificial Intelligence and Machine Learning and Its Application in the Field of Computational Visual Analysis. In Emerging Engineering Technologies and Industrial Applications (pp. 36-57). IGI Global. DOI: 10.4018/979-8-3693-1335-0.ch003

Pandey, D., & Pandey, B. K. (2022). An efficient deep neural network with adaptive galactic swarm optimization for complex image text extraction. In *Process Mining Techniques for Pattern Recognition* (pp. 121–137). CRC Press. DOI: 10.1201/9781003169550-10

Pandey, D., Pandey, B. K., Nassa, V. K., Mahajan, D. A., George, A. S., & Dadheech, P. (2024c). Optimized Throughput-Based Broadcasting for Next Generation Wireless Networks. In Emerging Engineering Technologies and Industrial Applications (pp. 355-368). IGI Global. DOI: 10.4018/979-8-3693-1335-0.ch018

Pandey, D., Pandey, B. K., Paramashivan, M. A., Mahajan, D. A., Dadheech, P. D., George, A. S., & Hameed, A. S. (2024b). Advanced Digital Data Processing Using Cloud Cryptography: Industrial Applications. In Emerging Engineering Technologies and Industrial Applications (pp. 255-268). IGI Global.

Rai, P. K., Pandey, D., & Pandey, B. K. (2024). The future of enterprise and innovation is compute as a commodity, or CaaC. *Partners Universal International Research Journal*, *3*(2), 89–94.

Saravanakumar, R., TamilSelvi, T., Pandey, D., Pandey, B. K., Mahajan, D. A., & Lelisho, M. E. (2024). Big data processing using hybrid Gaussian mixture model with salp swarm algorithm. *Journal of Big Data*, *11*(1), 167. DOI: 10.1186/s40537-024-01015-3

Satheesh, N., Gopisankar, N., Kumarganesh, S., Anthoniraj, S., Saravanakumar, S., & Martin Sagayam, K. (2025). Advanced AI-driven emergency response systems for enhanced vehicle and human safety. *Iran Journal of Computer Science*, •••, 1–16. DOI: 10.1007/s42044-025-00228-w

Saxena, A., Agarwal, A., Pandey, B. K., & Pandey, D. (2024). Examination of the Criticality of Customer Segmentation Using Unsupervised Learning Methods. *Circular Economy and Sustainability*, *4*(2), 1–14. DOI: 10.1007/s43615-023-00336-4

Shahul, A., Muniandi, B., Paramashivan, M. A., Pandey, D., Pandey, B. K., Dadheech, P., & George, H. (2024). An Analysis of Algorithms and Methods Based on Image Processing for Medical Applications. In *Emerging Engineering Technologies and Industrial Applications* (pp. 173–186). IGI Global. DOI: 10.4018/979-8-3693-1335-0.ch007

Sheela, M. S., Kumarganesh, S., Pandey, B. K., & Lelisho, M. E. (2025). Integration of silver nanostructures in wireless sensor networks for enhanced biochemical sensing. *Discover Nano*, *20*(1), 7. DOI: 10.1186/s11671-024-04159-6 PMID: 39804434

Singh, S., Madaan, G., Swapna, H. R., Singh, A., Pandey, B. K., George, A. S., & Pandey, D. (2025b). Unleashing the Power of AI and Data Analysis: Transforming Insights into Action. In Interdisciplinary Approaches to AI, Internet of Everything, and Machine Learning (pp. 1-24). IGI Global Scientific Publishing.

Singh, S., Madaan, G., Swapna, H. R., Singh, A., Pandey, D., George, A. S., & Pandey, B. K. (2025a). Empowering Connectivity: Exploring the Internet of Things. In Interdisciplinary Approaches to AI, Internet of Everything, and Machine Learning (pp. 89-116). IGI Global Scientific Publishing.

Vinod, S. K., Jameson, M. G., Min, M., & Holloway, L. C. (2016). Uncertainties in volume delineation in radiation oncology: A systematic review and recommendations for future studies. *Radiotherapy and Oncology : Journal of the European Society for Therapeutic Radiology and Oncology*, *121*(2), 169–179. DOI: 10.1016/j.radonc.2016.09.009 PMID: 27729166

Wang, S., Cao, G., Wang, Y., Liao, S., Wang, Q., Shi, J., Li, C., & Shen, D. (2021). Review and prospect: Artificial intelligence in advanced medical imaging. *Frontiers in Radiology*, *1*, 781868. DOI: 10.3389/fradi.2021.781868 PMID: 37492170

Chapter 4
Role of Secure Image Transmission in Agricultural Health Monitoring

Daneshwari A Noola
https://orcid.org/0009-0000-6030-7424
Department of Information Science, BLDEA's VP Dr. PG Halakatti College of Engineering and Technology, India

Chinnem Rama Mohan
Department of Computer Science and Engineering, Narayana Engineering College, Nellore, India

Shailendra M. Pardeshi
https://orcid.org/0000-0001-6297-6074
RC Patel Institute of Technology, Shirpur, India

Krishna Murthy Inumula
https://orcid.org/0000-0002-4556-549X
Symbiosis International University, Pune, India

P. Asha
Computer Science and Engineering, Sathyabama Institute of Science and Technology, Chennai, India

Bhawna Janghel Rajput
https://orcid.org/0009-0006-8062-0462
Department of Computer Science and Engineering, Rungta College of Engineering and Technology, Bhilai, India

ABSTRACT

Digital technology adoption for health monitoring has become essential in the quickly changing agricultural landscape. In order to protect sensitive data that is gathered from a variety of sources, including drones, sensors, and satellites, this chapter examines the crucial role that secure image transmission plays in agricultural health monitoring. In order to preserve data integrity and guarantee that agricultural stakeholders receive timely and accurate information for efficient decision-making,

DOI: 10.4018/979-8-3693-9821-0.ch004

secure transmission techniques such as encryption and end-to-end protocols are crucial. This chapter outlines the many advantages of secure image transmission, such as improved data integrity, prompt decision-making, heightened stakeholder trust, and defense against cyberattacks. Strong security measures are also required for compliance with data privacy regulations and efficient resource management as agricultural data becomes more digitalized.

INTRODUCTION

Real-time data collection and monitoring are essential in today's agriculture to maximize crop yields and farm operations. In order for farmers, agronomists, and other agricultural stakeholders to gather visual data from a variety of sources, including drones, satellites, and sensors, image transmission (Pandey, B. K., & Pandey, D., 2025) is essential. In the age of precision agriculture, the ability to precisely and effectively manage crops, livestock, and environmental conditions is made possible by these images.Real-time monitoring of crops and fields is one of the main applications of image transmission in agriculture. Drones with high-resolution cameras and sensors are able to take precise pictures of the farmland, which can be used to learn important information about possible pest infestations, crop health, and soil moisture levels. On the other hand, a larger-scale perspective provided by satellite imagery makes it possible to monitor a large area of agricultural land. Farmers can identify trends, monitor different stages of growth, and evaluate the effects of weather-related events like droughts and floods with the use of these photos. Farmers are better able to react proactively to new issues because they have instant access to visual data, which facilitates faster and more informed decision-making.

The use of image transmission in precision agricultureis a significant additional benefit. In precision agriculture, inputs like pesticides, fertilizers, and water are applied selectively to different parts of a field according to their individual needs (Khadka, M. et al., 2025). Farmers can identify stress areas in their crops, such as nutrient deficiencies or pest infestations, by analysing the transmitted images and applying treatments only as needed. Because it avoids using excessive amounts of chemicals and water, this minimizes waste, lowers production costs, and has a minimal negative impact on the environment. By guaranteeing that resources are used effectively, precision agriculture raises overall productivity and produces healthier and higher-yielding crops.Image transmission is useful for evaluating livestock health in addition to crop monitoring. Farmers can identify early signs of illness or injury by using real-time images and videos of animals captured by livestock monitoring systems fitted with cameras and sensors. Artificial intelligence (AI) (Satheesh, N. et al., 2025) can be integrated with these systems to analyze the images and notify farmers automatically of any anomalies, such as odd behavior or changes in the animals' physical characteristics (Sheela, M. S. et al., 2025). By lowering the possibility of disease outbreaks and boosting farm productivity overall, this proactive approach assists farmers in maintaining the health and wellbeing of their livestock. But as agriculture depends more and more on digital technologies (Kumar, M. S. et al.,2025), security concernsabout the transfer of private information, including images, are rising. Critical data regarding a farms operations, such as crop yields, land use patterns, and resource management tactics, are frequently contained in the photos taken by drones, satellites, and sensors. This data could result in large financial losses, competitive disadvantages, or even threats to food security if it is intercepted or tampered with while it is being transmitted (Konapure, C. G. et al.,2025). For example, an image transmission breach may reveal a farm's susceptibility to environmental conditions or pests, which competitors or bad actors may take advantage of secure image transmission protocols are crucial to addressing these issues (Singh, S. et al.,2025a). The data can be protected during transmission by using encryption techniques like Advanced Encryption Standard (AES), which guarantees that only authorized users can access the information. Furthermore, end-to-end encryption ensures that the data is safe all the way from its source—drones and sensorsto its destinationfarm management systems or cloud storage (Singh, S. et al., 2025b). In addition to improving data security, blockchain technology offers potential solutions by generating a decentralized, tamper-proof record of image transmission (Pandey, B. K. et al., 2024a).

Agricultural Health Monitoring

Agricultural health monitoring is a crucial practice in contemporary farming that emphasizes the ongoing evaluation of crops, soil, and livestock to guarantee their optimal health and productivity (Pandey, B. K. et al., 2024b). This monitoring process enables farmers to identify problems promptly, including diseases, pests, or nutrient deficiencies, facilitating timely corrective actions. This not only increases yield and minimizes crop losses but also improves the overall sustainability of agricultural practices (Maheshwari, R. U. et al.,2024). The emergence of precision agriculture and advanced technologies has enhanced the efficiency (Maheshwari, R. Uma. et al.,2024), accuracy, and effectiveness of monitoring agricultural health, thereby addressing challenges in both small and large-scale farming.A crucial element of agricultural health monitoring is the assessment of crop vitality. Through crop monitoring, farmers can identify indicators of stress resulting from pests, diseases, or unfavourable weather conditions. Prompt identification facilitates timely interventions, such as pesticide application or irrigation adjustments, which can prevent substantial crop damage.

Historically, this monitoring was conducted manually; however, drones, satellite imagery, and remote sensors now offer real-time data on crop conditions. These technologies allow farmers to evaluate the condition of their fields remotely and respond promptly to emerging issues, thereby averting minor problems from developing into significant threats that could diminish yield.Soil is equally vital in the monitoring of agricultural health. Nutritious soil is the cornerstone of efficient agriculture, supplying the vital nutrients and moisture required for crop growth. Assessing soil health entails evaluating multiple factors including moisture levels, pH balance, nutrient composition, and organic matter content. Advanced soil sensors and monitoring systems provide farmers with real-time data on these parameters, facilitating precise management of irrigation, fertilization, and other soil treatments. Preserving optimal soil health is essential for enhancing crop yields and ensuring long-term sustainability. Healthy soils diminish the necessity for chemical inputs, decrease agricultural expenses, and assist in alleviating climate change impacts by improving the soil's ability to sequester carbon and retain moisture.In livestock farming, the surveillance of animal health is equally essential (Zarei, M. et al., 2016). Livestock health monitoring systems, utilizing cameras, sensors, and wearable devices, continuously track vital signs, movements, and behavioural patterns of animals.

Timely identification of diseases, injuries, or nutritional deficiencies in livestock can markedly enhance animal welfare and productivity. If sensors identify anomalous body temperatures or irregular movement patterns in livestock, farmers can promptly intervene by isolating affected animals or modifying their feeding or care protocols. This proactive measure mitigates the risk of disease outbreaks, enhances animal welfare, and boosts overall farm efficiency by sustaining healthier livestock.Agricultural health monitoring is essential for enhancing productivity, sustainability, and profitability in contemporary farming. The utilization of drones for crop health assessment, sensors for soil monitoring, and wearable technology for livestock enables farmers to consistently monitor and manage these essential components, thereby optimizing their operations. Utilizing real-time data and advanced technology enables farmers to more effectively address environmental challenges, resource limitations, and potential threats, resulting in healthier ecosystems and more sustainable agricultural practices (Ray, P. P., 2018).

TECHNOLOGIES INVOLVED IN IMAGE TRANSMISSION

Drones and IoT Devices

Modern farmers use drones and IoT devices to collect real-time images (Saxena, A. et al., 2024) and environmental data to better manage their fields and livestock. These technologies have transformed farming by providing accurate, up-to-date data on crop health, soil conditions, and livestock well-being.High-resolution cameras and sensors on drones capture aerial images of fields, giving a bird's-eye view. These images can show crop health, pests, water stress, and soil variations. Drones allow farmers to inspect their crops without time-consuming physical inspections by flying over large areas quickly. This real-time data lets farmers quickly identify field issues and apply water or nutrients only where needed, reducing waste and improving efficiency.Multispectral and thermal sensors on drones can measure crop heat and light absorption in addition to imagery. Farmers use this data to assess plant health, growth, and even detect early disease signs. Airborne drones can locate and assess livestock health and movement patterns in large-scale livestock operations.IoT devices provide continuous environmental data through a network of farm sensors to complement drones. To measure soil moisture, temperature, humidity, and animal health, these devices are embedded in soil, attached to plants, or worn by livestock. Soil sensors can measure moisture and nutrient levels in different fields, giving farmers detailed information about their land. Precision farming requires this data to optimize irrigation, fertilization, and planting schedules based on real-time conditions (Rai, P. K. et al., 2024), improving resource efficiency and crop yields.IoT devices also impact livestock monitoring. Wearable sensors on animals can track their health, activity, and location, alerting them to abnormal behavior like illness or distress. This real-time monitoring helps farmers address issues quickly, improving animal welfare and reducing disease outbreaks.Drones and IoT devices give modern farmers real-time insights into their farms. These technologies help farmers make informed decisions, boost productivity, and improve sustainability by using resources more efficiently (Lakshmi, K. V. N. et al., 2024).

Satellite Imaging

The provision of high-resolution images that provide a broad and comprehensive view of large farming areas is one of the most important contributions that satellite imaging makes to the field of conventional agriculture. Satellite imagery covers vast regions, allowing farmers and agricultural experts to observe entire fields or landscapes at the same time. This is in contrast to ground-based monitoring, which can be time-consuming (Saravanakumar, R. et al.,2024) and limited in scope. As a result of its ability to assist in evaluating crop health, monitoring environmental conditions, and making decisions based on data in order to maximize agricultural productivity, this technology has evolved into an indispensable instrument for large-scale farming operations.One of the most significant benefits of satellite imaging is that it can quickly and accurately evaluate large areas with just a single image capture.

In order to monitor their land without having to physically inspect every area, satellite images offer a method that is both cost-effective and efficient (Kumarganesh, S. et al., 2024). This is especially useful for farmers who are responsible for managing expansive fields or agricultural companies that oversee vast regions. These high-resolution images make it possible to identify patterns and trends across the landscape. They provide insights into the health of the soil, the growth of crops, the distribution of water, and the impact of environmental factors such as droughts and floods.The use of satellite imagery is also highly important for monitoring the health of crops. Through the utilization of various spectral bands, such as visible, near-infrared, and thermal, satellites are able to capture a more comprehensive picture of crops than just a visual representation (Muralidhar, L. B. et al., 2024). The use of these sensors allows for the detection of variations in plant vitality, water stress, and even early signs of disease or pest infestations that may not be visible to the naked eye to the average person. For instance, the Normalized Difference Vegetation Index (NDVI) is a common tool that is derived from satellite data and measures the health of plants based on the amount of light that is absorbed by the vegetation. NDVI provides farmers with the ability to understand which crops are flourishing and which require intervention. This enables farmers to apply targeted treatments and reduces the amount of resources that are wasted.The monitoring of soil and the environment is another important application for satellite imaging, in addition to crop health measurements. The ability of satellites to monitor changes in soil moisture, temperature, and topography over time provides crucial information for the management of water resources and the preservation of soil content (Asghari, P. et al., 2019).

This information assists farmers in optimizing irrigation practices, which allows them to reduce water consumption in regions where moisture levels are adequate and increase water consumption in regions that are exhibiting signs of dryness. In addition, satellite data can assist in the identification of soil erosion and degradation, which enables preventative measures to be taken in order to preserve the long-term fertility of the soil.Satellite imaging has the capability of monitoring changes in climate and the environment, which is another significant advantage of this technology. Satellite imagery allows for the collection of vital information regarding weather patterns, such as temperature, precipitation, and wind conditions, all of which have an impact on agricultural productivity. Farmers are able to make adjustments to planting schedules, forecast potential risks such as droughts or storms, and plan harvests in a more efficient manner for their crops when they analyze this data.This is accomplished by providing an overall view of their land and providing detailed insights into the health of their crops, the conditions of their soil, and the environmental factors that are at play. The capability of continuously monitoring these variables ensures that farmers are able to take timely and precise actions to maintain the health of their crops and land, which ultimately results in increased yields, decreased resource consumption, and more sustainable farming practices (Jensen, M. H., & Malter, A. J., 1995).

Edge Computing

In the field of agricultural health monitoring, edge computing is becoming increasingly utilized to perform preliminary processing on images and data prior to their transmission to central servers or cloud-based systems. With edge computing, images are pre-processed before being transmitted, which results in reduced latency. When large amounts of raw data are transmitted over networks, edge computing significantly reduces the amount of latency that is involved (Pandey, B. K. et al., 2024c). This is accomplished by performing computations closer to the source of the data, such as on drones, sensors, or local devices. For precision agriculture, this ensures that decisions are made more quickly and that responses are provided in real time (Pandey, B. K. et al., 2024d).Having the capability to handle image pre-processing locally is one of the most significant advantages of edge computing. Transmission to a remote server can be time-consuming and bandwidth-intensive due to the fact that high-resolution images captured by drones or Internet of Things sensors in the field can be very large. The data can be analysed and filtered at the source by edge computing devices, which allows them to extract only the most pertinent information for transmission rather than sending raw images. In the case of crop health, for instance, algorithms are able to identify anomalies, such as signs of disease or water stress, and then send only those portions of the image that require attention, rather than sending the entire data set (Elarmathi, S. et al., 2024). By reducing the load on networks, this selective transmission speeds up the delivery of insights that can be put into action.One of the most important aspects of time-sensitive agricultural operations is the reduction of latency, which can be accomplished by minimizing the need to transfer large data sets to a central location. When farmers use edge computing, they are able to receive alerts almost instantly, which enables them to take prompt action, such as applying pesticides or adjusting irrigation at the appropriate time. Edge computing enhances data security by limiting the amount of sensitive information (Pandey, B. K. et al.,2024e) that needs to be transmitted over potentially insecure networks. At the time of transmission, there is less risk of being exposed to cyber threats because the majority of data processing takes place locally (Mekala, M. S. & Viswanathan, P., 2017). When dealing with potentially confidential farming data or other sensitive information, such as satellite images or yield predictions, this is of utmost importance.Edge computing also plays a role in efficient resource management, which is another advantage of this technology. The use of this is especially beneficial in farming areas that are located in rural or remote areas, where internet connectivity may be limited or unreliable (JayaLakshmi, G. et al., 2024). Through the utilization of edge computing, even in regions that have a limited bandwidth, it is possible to process and act upon vital data without the need for continuous access to a high-speed internet connection (George, W. K. et al., 2024).

SECURE IMAGE TRANSMISSION'S OBSTACLES

The use of secure image transmission in agriculture is hampered by a number of serious issues, as illustrated in figure 1. Strong security measures are required because sensitive information is at risk from data breaches and cybersecurity threats. Older network infrastructure can also result in vulnerabilities and make a system more vulnerable to attacks, especially in rural areas. While latency and transmission delays can impede timely decision-making (Abdullahi, M. et al., 2024), high bandwidth requirements for transmitting large images can strain connectivity. Because manipulation can affect the accuracy of transmitted images, data integrity must be ensured. Implementing robust security measures is made more difficult by the limited processing power of IoT devices, and data privacy regulations add yet another level of complexity (Kumar, B.et al.,2024).

- *Data Breach and Cybersecurity Threats*: Data breaches are a risk for the agricultural industry since it depends more and more on digital technology. It is possible for sensitive data to be intercepted during transmission, including farm plans and crop health. Cyberattacks can result in large financial losses, disruptions to operations, and loss of competitive advantage. These include phishing, ransomware, and malware. For sensitive data to be shielded from malicious actors, strong cybersecurity measures are necessary. A single breach can also jeopardize financial information and supply chains, among other components of a farming operation, due to the interconnectedness of contemporary agricultural systems. This underlines the necessity of all-encompassing cybersecurity strategies that include incident response plans, frequent security audits, staff training, and data encryption (Pandey, D. et al., 2024a).
- *Network Vulnerabilities*: It is common for network infrastructure to be antiquated or unstable in agricultural settings, particularly in rural regions. A

man-in-the-middle attack, in which an attacker intercepts and modifies communication between two parties, is one of the many cyberthreats that can befall data transmitted over weak wireless connections (Pandey, D. et al., 2024b). These flaws have the potential to corrupt data transmission integrity, which could result in inaccurate information and bad decisions. Agricultural activities also frequently employ a variety of tools and technologies (Kennedy, G. W. et al., 2024), each with varying degrees of security. It is crucial to implement standardized security protocols across all field-used devices because this heterogeneity can lead to security holes that hackers could take advantage of it (Shahul, A. et al.,2024).

- *High Bandwidth Requirements*:When it comes to areas with poor internet connectivity, transmitting high-resolution images from drones, sensors, and satellites can be very difficult due to the required large bandwidth. Slow transmission rates, higher latency, and even possible data loss can be caused by insufficient bandwidth (Pandey, D. et al., 2024c). Precision agriculture techniques may be less effective as a result of this limitation, which can impede real-time monitoring capabilities. Farmers may need to investigate alternate options, like satellite-based internet or 5G networks, which offer greater bandwidth and lower latency, as the amount of data produced by agricultural technologies keeps increasing. Advanced agricultural practices can be seamlessly integrated by investing in such technologies, which can improve data transmission capabilities.
- *Latency and Transmission Delays*: In agricultural settings, where prompt action can minimize crop losses and boost yield, real-time monitoring systems are indispensable. Making decisions slowly, however, can be a result of network congestion or poor infrastructure causing delays in data transmission. Elevated latency can compromise the efficacy of critical crop health interventions like pest management and irrigation modifications. Instantaneous communication is especially necessary as agricultural systems become more automated and dependent on real-time data. Addressing latency issues in secure image transmission is crucial because farmers may encounter difficulties when implementing automated systems that need instantaneous data inputs (Kamilaris, A., &Prenafeta-Boldú, F. X., 2018).
- *Data Integrity and Tampering*: To make trustworthy decisions, it is essential to ensure the integrity of transmitted images. Farming practices may suffer from distorted information resulting from images that have been manipulated or altered during transmission (Pandey, D., & Pandey, B. K., 2022). To guarantee that data is preserved and unaltered during the transmission process, robust encryption protocols and verification techniques must be implemented. Organisations should also take into account the possibility of enhancing data

integrity by implementing blockchain technology. Blockchain can assist in the establishment of a transparent and verifiable chain of custody, guaranteeing that any alterations to the images can be promptly identified and corrected, by generating a decentralized and tamper-proof record of all transmitted data.

- *Limited Processing Capability*: Given their low processing power, many drones and Internet of Things (IoT) devices used in agriculture make it difficult to deploy strong encryption and security measures without sacrificing efficiency. Weaker security measures may be used to maintain speed and efficiency, which can result in vulnerabilities in data transmission. More advanced processing capabilities on edge devices will also be required as the agricultural sector adopts smart technologies (Pandey, B. K., & Pandey, D., 2023).) at a faster rate. In order to ensure that data stays secure and to enable timely and efficient monitoring, farmers may need to invest in more sophisticated hardware that can support improved encryption algorithms and security measures without sacrificing performance.
- *Compliance with Data Privacy Regulations*: Secure image transmission may become more difficult in the agricultural industry due to the mandatory compliance with multiple data privacy laws and regulations. Strict data protection measures must be implemented by organizations in order to comply with regulations, such as the General Data Protection Regulation (GDPR) in Europe. There may be fines, legal ramifications, and reputational harm if compliance is not maintained. Ensuring that staff members comprehend the significance of data protection and adhere to legal requirements may also be necessary for managing these regulations. Encouraging a culture of data privacy and security will be crucial as agricultural operations continue to incorporate digital technologies in order to safeguard the company and the sensitive data it manages.

Figure 1. Challenges of secure image transmission

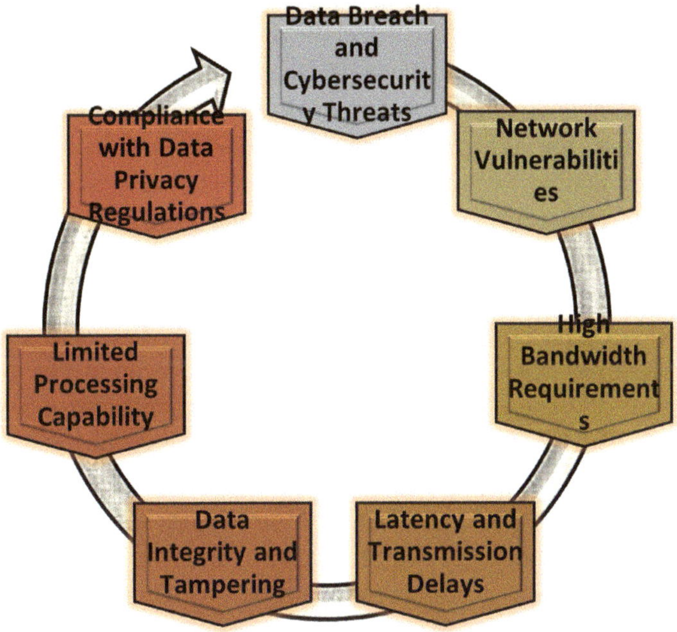

ENCRYPTION TECHNIQUES FOR SECURE IMAGE TRANSMISSION

AES (Advanced Encryption Standard)

The Advanced Encryption Standard, also known as AES, is a symmetric encryption algorithm that is widely considered to be among the most secure methods for encrypting sensitive data, including images. Since its inception in 2001 by the National Institute of Standards and Technology (NIST) of the United States of America, Advanced Encryption Standard (AES) has evolved into the encryption standard that is utilized worldwide in a variety of fields, including agriculture, government, and finance. Its robust security features make it particularly suitable for applications that require the protection of sensitive information while it is being transmitted. One example of such an application is agricultural health monitoring, which requires image data collected from drones or sensors to be protected against unauthorized access.The use of a symmetric key, which means that the same key is used for both encryption and decryption, is what gives Advanced Encryption Standard (AES) its strength. The Advanced Encryption Standard (AES) allows for key lengths of 128, 192, or 256 bits, with longer keys providing higher levels of security. Because of this versatility, organizations are able to select the appropriate key length based on the specific security requirements and threat landscape that they face. In order to achieve a high level of complexity, the algorithm works on blocks of data, processing 128 bits at a time. It uses a series of transformation rounds, which include substitution, permutation, and mixing, in order to accomplish this. Because of this, even if an adversary makes an attempt to decipher the encrypted image data, the amount of computational effort that is required to break the encryption is prohibitively high. This makes AES a formidable barrier against unauthorized access.In addition to its security features, Advanced Encryption Standard (AES) is well-known for its efficiency and speed, which enables encryption and decryption processes to take place in real time. It is especially useful for agricultural applications, where having timely access to data is essential for making effective decisions, because this characteristic is particularly advantageous (Wolfert et al., 2017). Through the utilization of Advanced Encryption Standard (AES) for the purpose of securing image data, farmers are able to guarantee the confidentiality of sensitive information concerning the health of their crops and the weather conditions. This enables them to react quickly to challenges while simultaneously safeguarding their competitive advantage.

End-to-End Encryption

A communication method known as end-to-end encryption (E2EE) ensures that data is encrypted on the device that is sending it and is only decrypted on the device that is receiving it. This prevents unauthorized access to the data while it is being transmitted. Agricultural health monitoring is an area in which sensitive data, such as images collected from drones or sensors, must be protected from potential dangers. This approach is especially important in this context. Farmers and agricultural organizations are able to protect the confidentiality and integrity of their data from the moment it is captured until it reaches its final destination if they do so through the implementation of E2EE.The ability of end-to-end encryption to provide a high level of data integrity is one of the most significant advantages of this type of encryption that is used. Any unauthorized attempts to intercept or alter the information while it is being transmitted can be easily pinpointed due to the fact that the data remains encrypted throughout its journey. If the data that has been encrypted is altered in any way, it will become unreadable to the person who is supposed to receive it. This will cause alerts to be triggered and will enable prompt action to be taken in order to address any potential security breaches. Because timely and accurate information is essential for effective decision-making in agriculture, this quality is especially important in the agricultural sector. An example of this would be if an image that indicates the health of a crop is altered while it is being transmitted. This could result in actions that are not intended and could put the yield at risk.

The parties involved in the data exchange are more likely to trust one another when end-to-end encryption is used. In the absence of any potential exposure to third parties, such as service providers or hackers, farmers can have the peace of mind that their sensitive information will be kept private and secure. Because it encourages the sharing of valuable data, which can lead to increased productivity and improved agricultural practices, this trust is the most important factor in the adoption of digital technologies in agriculture. In addition, E2EE ensures compliance with a variety of data privacy regulations by restricting access to sensitive information and safeguarding the rights of individuals who are participants in agricultural operations. When it comes to secure image transmission, end-to-end encryption is an essential component that offers robust protection for critical data throughout its entire lifecycle.

Blockchain-Based Solutions

Blockchain technology has emerged as a transformative force in securing image storage and transmission, especially in sectors such as agriculture, where data integrity and security are critical. Blockchain is fundamentally a distributed ledger technology (DLT) that documents transactions across numerous computers, ensuring that recorded transactions cannot be modified retroactively. The intrinsic immutability of blockchain renders it a formidable instrument for guaranteeing the authenticity and security of image data acquired from diverse sources, including drones and sensors utilized in agricultural health monitoring.A principal advantage of utilizing blockchain for image storage is its capacity to establish a verifiable and immutable recordof all image transactions. Every image uploaded to the blockchain is paired with a distinct cryptographic hash, functioning as a digital fingerprint. This hash is connected to the preceding block in the chain, establishing an unbroken sequence of data that is exceedingly difficult to modify without detection. In agriculture, this implies that farmers can securely archive images of their crops or soil conditions while preserving a comprehensive record of alterations or access attempts.

This transparency is essential for building trust among stakeholders, such as farmers, suppliers, and consumers. Blockchain enables secure image transmission by encrypting data at its origin prior to its entry into the distributed ledger. This encryption guarantees that only authorized individuals can access the images, safeguarding sensitive agricultural data from unauthorized access or breaches during transmission. Smart contractsself-executing agreements encoded with the terms of the contractenable farmers to automate processes like data sharing and payment settlements through image verification. This not only optimizes operations but also improves accountability and traceability in agricultural supply chains.The decentralized nature of blockchain diminishes dependence on single points of failure, thereby enhancing the system's resilience to cyberattacks. Blockchain mitigates the risks inherent in centralized data storage by dispersing data across multiple nodes, preventing a single breach from jeopardizing the entire system. In an agricultural context, this signifies that even if a single node is compromised, the integrity of the overall data is preserved, protecting essential information regarding crop health and environmental conditions.

IMPACT OF SECURE IMAGE TRANSMISSION ON AGRICULTURAL HEALTH

- *Enhanced Data Integrity*: Agriculture data like crop health and environmental conditions are protected during secure image transmission. Farmers can address issues with accurate monitoring and decision-making thanks to this integrity. Data corruption can lead to misguided interventions that lower crop yields and farm productivity. A farmer may apply fertilizers ineffectively if a field image shows nutrient deficiency but is altered during transmission. This wastes resources and may pollute nearby waterways during runoff. By using encryption and digital signatures, farmers can trust the data they receive. Trusting data leads to better decisions, healthier crops, better soil, and more sustainable farming. For supply chain traceability, data integrity helps farmers document their practices and results. Meet regulatory requirements and ensure accountability with this documentation, promoting agricultural transparency.

Figure 2. Impact of secure image transmission on agricultural health

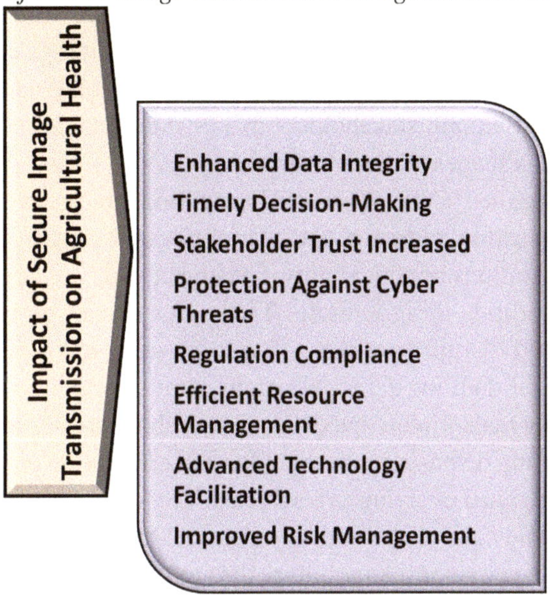

- *Timely Decision-Making*: Secure transmission lets farmers quickly access real-time data. This allows for immediate irrigation and pesticide adjustments, improving crop yields and minimizing losses. Timing matters in agriculture. Early image transmission can help farmers control pests before they cause significant damage. Secure transmission also ensures that farmers receive this vital information quickly, allowing them to make quick decisions. Quick action can save a crop or destroy it, which has serious financial consequences. Farmers can also adjust their strategies with real-time data as climate change makes weather unpredictable. Access to secure data can help farmers manage risks and seize opportunities when adjusting planting schedules, water conservation, or emergency pest management. This proactive approach boosts crop health and agricultural system resilience.
- *Stakeholder Trust Increased*: When sensitive agricultural data is transmitted securely, farmers, suppliers, and consumers trust each other. This trust encourages data sharing and collaboration, improving agricultural supply chain practices and transparency. The ability to ensure data security and reliability fosters collaboration in an industry where stakeholders depend on accurate data for decision-making. Suppliers can tailor fertilizer and pest control recommendations based on farmers' accurate crop health data. Additionally, consumers want food production transparency. Farmers develop credibility

and customer loyalty by sharing secure images of their practices, such as organic certification or sustainable farming. Trust can lead to larger industry partnerships like cooperatives and research. Partnerships can promote innovation and best practices, resulting in more sustainable agriculture and food security. Trust among stakeholders makes the agricultural ecosystem more resilient to challenges and opportunities.

- *Protection Against Cyber Threats*: Encrypting images reduces cyberattack risk. By protecting sensitive data, farmers can maintain their competitive edge and operations confidentiality. Cybercriminals are targeting digital system vulnerabilities in agriculture. These attacks can cost money, compromise data, and disrupt operations. Ransomware could prevent farmers from accessing vital data for daily operations, threatening crop health and yield. Cryptography makes intercepted data unreadable, making secure image transmission a strong defense. Security audits and encryption protocol updates can also protect against evolving cyberthreats. Technical measures are important, but farmers and agricultural staff must also learn cybersecurity best practices. Creating a security-conscious culture through training can help all employees understand the importance of data security. Farmers safeguard their data and help stabilize the agricultural sector by investing in these measures.
- *Regulation Compliance*: Farmers can comply with GDPR by using secure transmission methods. These standards help agricultural businesses avoid legal penalties and improve their reputation with consumers and partners. Compliance is essential for operational legitimacy as data protection laws tighten worldwide. Incorrectly handling consumer or supplier personal data can result in large fines and legal action. Security image transmission, which often includes encryption and access controls, protects sensitive data and shows farmers' data privacy commitment. Consumers increasingly prefer ethical data practices, so compliance can give businesses an edge. Farmers can attract conscientious consumers and build brand loyalty by transparently handling data. Compliance with regulations often improves internal processes, boosting operational efficiency for the entire company. In a data-driven market, secure transmission reduces legal risks and benefits agricultural businesses.
- *Efficient Resource Management*: By transmitting only relevant data, secure image transmission helps farmers save resources. Targeted bandwidth reduction and technological tool optimization save money and improve operational efficiency. Farmers can simplify data collection and analysis by transmitting vital data like crop health and moisture levels. In areas with poor internet connectivity, high-resolution image uploads can delay and cost more. Resource efficiency saves money and the environment. Accurate crop health

data can help farmers conserve water, optimize water use, and reduce irrigation. Advanced technologies like precision agriculture tools and IoT devices can be integrated with secure transmission, improving resource efficiency. These technologies require accurate and timely data, making secure transmission essential to modern agriculture. By using secure image transmission to manage resources, farmers can boost productivity and be more environmentally friendly.

- *Advanced Technology Facilitation*: Integrating IoT devices and AI analytics into agriculture requires secure transmission protocols. Precision agriculture is improved by this integration, improving crop and livestock health. Digitalization in agriculture increases the need for interconnected devices and data-driven decision-making. These technologies work seamlessly with secure image transmission. Data accuracy and security are essential for IoT devices that monitor soil moisture, temperature, and crop health. With secure transmission, these devices can share data in real time, allowing farmers to make informed decisions based on current conditions. AI analytics can predict pest outbreaks and optimize fertilizer application using this data. Advanced technology and secure image transmission improve operational efficiency and sustainable agriculture. These technologies help farmers boost productivity and reduce environmental impact, resulting in healthier crops and a more resilient agricultural system.
- *Improved Risk Management*: Pest infestations and weather damage can be monitored with secure image transmission. Farmers can protect their crops and ensure sustainability by using reliable data to develop proactive risk management strategies. The agricultural sector faces risks from pests and diseases to unpredictable weather. Farmers can track these risks and take timely action with secure real-time image transmission. A pest outbreak image can alert farmers to take immediate action and apply targeted pest control. Secure image transmission allows farmers to share important information with agricultural advisors or extension services, promoting risk management collaboration. A cooperative approach can lead to customized strategies to address farm challenges. Secure weather and environmental data transmission is crucial as climate change affects agricultural practices. Farmers can improve their resilience to external threats and sustainability by closely monitoring these variables to make informed planting, irrigation, and crop selection decisions.

Through improved accuracy and dependability of data gathered from multiple sources, including drones, sensors, and satellites, secure image transmission has a substantial impact on agricultural health, which are shown in the figure 2. Farmers can rely on data and images they receive to accurately represent the state of their livestock and crops when strong security measures are in place. In the end, this trust improves yields and sustainability by facilitating prompt decision-making that enables farmers to react swiftly to possible problems like pest infestations or nutrient shortages. By guaranteeing that private information is shielded from unwanted access, secure transmission promotes cooperation between stakeholders, including suppliers and customers. Improved transparency and trust throughout the agricultural supply chain result from farmers being able to confidently share information about their practices. Secure image transfer also makes it possible to integrate cutting-edge technologies, like precision agriculture tools, and manage resources more effectively by preserving data integrity. This improves the resilience and health of agriculture as a whole.

CONCLUSION

In agricultural health monitoring, the significance of secure image transmission cannot be emphasized enough. The security and privacy of this data are vital given the growing dependence on digital tools and technologies for data collection and analysis. Maintaining the integrity of agricultural data is largely dependent on the use of secure transmission techniques like encryption and end-to-end protocols. They improve the accuracy and timeliness of information, enabling farmers to make well-informed decisions. Furthermore, trust-building among agricultural supply chain participants is facilitated by secure transmission, allowing for data sharing and collaboration that can result in better practice and results. Ensuring secure image transmission boosts agricultural operations' overall sustainability and efficiency by safeguarding confidential data from cyber threats, adhering to data regulations, and enabling the integration of cutting-edge technologies. Moreover, it helps farmers to minimize risks and efficiently manage resources, resulting in healthier livestock and crops. There will be an increasing need for more security measures as agricultural practices embrace digital transformation and continue to change. Agricultural data is becoming more digital, and this highlights the need for strong security measures to safeguard this data, which includes environmental monitoring and photos of crop health. It is anticipated that secure image transmission will become more dependableand efficient with the continued development of technologies like blockchain and IoT. A comprehensive security framework will also be essential as data becomes more interconnected across platforms and devices. In order to counter new threats and weaknesses, agricultural stakeholders need to be on the lookout and constantly adjust their security measures. Maintaining the confidentiality and integrity of the data that forms the basis of contemporary farming methods will require the agricultural sector to fully utilize digital technologies, which will require a proactive approach. Looking ahead, securing global food security and sustainable agricultural growth will require significant investments in secure transmission systems.

REFERENCES

Abdullahi, M., Ahmad, A., Pandey, B. K., & Pandey, D. (2024). Digital Currency Adoption: A Comparative Analysis of Global Trends and the Nigerian eNaira Digital Currency. *SN Computer Science*, *5*(5), 1–11. DOI: 10.1007/s42979-024-02882-6

Asghari, P., Rahmani, A. M., & Javadi, H. H. S. (2019). Internet of Things applications: A systematic review. *Computer Networks*, *148*, 241–261. DOI: 10.1016/j.comnet.2018.12.008

Elarmathi, S., Rishabavarthani, P., Sindhuja, M., Elayaraja, P., & Malathi Murugesan, S. (2024). Novel manufacturing systems for cancer diagnosis using ultra-sensitive photonic crystal fiber biosensor with dual-functionalized aptamer-nanocavity. *Microsystem Technologies*, •••, 1–20. DOI: 10.1007/s00542-024-05820-x

George, W. K., Silas, E. I., Pandey, D., & Pandey, B. K. (2024). Utilization of Industry 4.0 Technologies in Nigerian Technical and Vocational Education: A Conundrum for Educators. In *Examining the Rapid Advance of Digital Technology in Africa* (pp. 270–293). IGI Global. DOI: 10.4018/978-1-6684-9962-7.ch014

Islam, S. R., Kwak, D., Kabir, M. H., Hossain, M., & Kwak, K. S. (2015). The internet of things for health care: A comprehensive survey. *IEEE Access : Practical Innovations, Open Solutions*, *3*, 678–708. DOI: 10.1109/ACCESS.2015.2437951

JayaLakshmi. G., Pandey, D., Pandey, B. K., Kaur, P., Mahajan, D. A., & Dari, S. S. (2024). Smart big data collection for intelligent supply chain improvement. In AI and Machine Learning Impacts in Intelligent Supply Chain (pp. 180-195). IGI Global Scientific Publishing.

. Jensen, M. H., & Malter, A. J. (1995). Protected agriculture: a global review.

Kamilaris, A., & Prenafeta-Boldú, F. X. (2018). Deep learning in agriculture: A survey. *Computers and Electronics in Agriculture*, *147*, 70–90. DOI: 10.1016/j.compag.2018.02.016

Kennedy, G. W., Sunday, S. E., Pandey, D., Kabari, A. D., Pandey, B. K., George, A. S., & Dadheech, P. (2024). Building Information Modeling: Harnessing Innovations for Professional Proficiency. In Emerging Engineering Technologies and Industrial Applications (pp. 305-331). IGI Global.

Khadka, M., Sah, M., Chaudhary, R., Sahani, S. K., Sahani, K., Pandey, B. K., & Pandey, D. (2025). Spectroscopic, quantum chemical, and topological calculations of the phenylephrine molecule using density functional theory. *Scientific Reports*, *15*(1), 208. DOI: 10.1038/s41598-024-81633-2 PMID: 39747169

. Konapure, C. G., Pandey, D., Shete, H., Thakar, C. M., Pandey, B. K., & George, A. S. (2025). Artificial Intelligence in Automated Concrete Mix Design Using Computerized Grading Curves. Interdisciplinary Approaches to AI, Internet of Everything, and Machine Learning, 567-586.

. Kumar, B., Pandey, D., Pandey, B. K., & George, A. S. (2024). Higher Education in the Last Four Decades: A Review of Paradigm Shifts in Policy Frameworks. Design and Implementation of Higher Education Learners' Learning Outcomes (HELLO), 333-348.

Kumar, M. S., Prasanna, P. L., Lalitha, M., Joy, M., Jha, S. S., & Pandey, B. K. (2025). Utilizing the Internet of Everything and Artificial Intelligence for Real-Time Workforce Management. In Role of Internet of Everything (IOE), VLSI Architecture, and AI in Real-Time Systems (pp. 153-168). IGI Global Scientific Publishing.

Kumarganesh, S., & Malathi Murugesan, C. (2024). Hybrid plasmonic biosensors with deep learning for colorectal cancer detection. *Plasmonics*, •••, 1–15. DOI: 10.1007/s11468-024-02568-y

Lakshmi, K. V. N., Rajan, R., Pandey, D., & Pandey, B. K. (2024). Circular economy: A catalyst for economic growth-an empirical study. *Circular Economy and Sustainability*, •••, 1–22.

Maheshwari, R., Kumarganesh, S., K v M, S., Gopalakrishnan, A., Selvi, K., Paulchamy, B., Rishabavarthani, P., Sagayam, K. M., Pandey, B. K., & Pandey, D. (2024). Advanced plasmonic resonance-enhanced biosensor for comprehensive real-time detection and analysis of deepfake content. *Plasmonics*, •••, 1–18. DOI: 10.1007/s11468-024-02407-0

Maheshwari, R. U., Paulchamy, B., Pandey, B. K., & Pandey, D. (2024). Enhancing sensing and imaging capabilities through surface plasmon resonance for deepfake image detection. *Plasmonics*, •••, 1–20. DOI: 10.1007/s11468-024-02492-1

Mekala, M. S., & Viswanathan, P. (2017, August). A Survey: Smart agriculture IoT with cloud computing. In 2017 international conference on microelectronic devices, circuits and systems (ICMDCS) (pp. 1-7). IEEE.

Muralidhar, L. B., Lakshmi, K. V. N., Swapna, H. R., Rupani, J., Nethravathi, K., Pandey, B. K., & Pandey, D. (2024). Impact of Organizational Culture on The Level of Corporate Social Responsibility Investments: An Exploratory Study. *Circular Economy and Sustainability*, *4*(3), 1–19. DOI: 10.1007/s43615-024-00371-9

Pandey, B. K., Kanike, U. K., George, A. S., & Pandey, D. (Eds.). (2024d). *AI and machine learning impacts in intelligent supply chain*. IGI Global. DOI: 10.4018/979-8-3693-1347-3

Pandey, B. K., Nassa, V. K., Mukundan, A. P., Mahajan, D. A., Pandey, D., George, A. S., & Dadheech, P. (2024c). An Industry-Focused Traffic System Utilising Internet of Things. In *Emerging Engineering Technologies and Industrial Applications* (pp. 200–213). IGI Global. DOI: 10.4018/979-8-3693-1335-0.ch009

Pandey, B. K., & Pandey, D. (2023). Parametric optimization and prediction of enhanced thermoelectric performance in co-doped CaMnO3 using response surface methodology and neural network. *Journal of Materials Science Materials in Electronics*, *34*(21), 1589. DOI: 10.1007/s10854-023-10954-1

Pandey, B. K., & Pandey, D. (2025). Securing healthcare medical image information using advance morphological component analysis, information hiding systems, and hybrid convolutional neural networks on IoMT. *Computers in Biology and Medicine*, *185*, 109499. DOI: 10.1016/j.compbiomed.2024.109499 PMID: 39642698

Pandey, B. K., Pandey, D., & Lelisho, M. E. (2024a). Face mask identification with enhanced cuckoo optimization and deep learning-based faster regional neural network. *Scientific Reports*, *14*(1), 29719. DOI: 10.1038/s41598-024-78746-z PMID: 39613761

Pandey, B. K., Pandey, D., & Sahani, S. K. (2024b). Autopilot control unmanned aerial vehicle system for sewage defect detection using deep learning. *Engineering Reports*, •••, 12852.

Pandey, B. K., Paramashivan, M. A., Pandey, D., George, A. S., Agarwal, A., Mahajan, D. A., . . . Pramanik, S. (2024e). Future Directions of Digital Twin Architectures for 6G Communication Networks. In Security Issues and Solutions in 6G Communications and Beyond (pp. 197-211). IGI Global.

Pandey, D., Nassa, V. K., Pandey, B. K., Thankachan, B., Dadheech, P., Mahajan, D. A., & George, A. S. (2024a). Artificial Intelligence and Machine Learning and Its Application in the Field of Computational Visual Analysis. In Emerging Engineering Technologies and Industrial Applications (pp. 36-57). IGI Global. DOI: 10.4018/979-8-3693-1335-0.ch003

Pandey, D., & Pandey, B. K. (2022). An efficient deep neural network with adaptive galactic swarm optimization for complex image text extraction. In *Process Mining Techniques for Pattern Recognition* (pp. 121–137). CRC Press. DOI: 10.1201/9781003169550-10

Pandey, D., Pandey, B. K., Nassa, V. K., Mahajan, D. A., George, A. S., & Dadheech, P. (2024c). Optimized Throughput-Based Broadcasting for Next Generation Wireless Networks. In Emerging Engineering Technologies and Industrial Applications (pp. 355-368). IGI Global. DOI: 10.4018/979-8-3693-1335-0.ch018

Pandey, D., Pandey, B. K., Paramashivan, M. A., Mahajan, D. A., Dadheech, P. D., George, A. S., & Hameed, A. S. (2024b). Advanced Digital Data Processing Using Cloud Cryptography: Industrial Applications. In Emerging Engineering Technologies and Industrial Applications (pp. 255-268). IGI Global.

Rai, P. K., Pandey, D., & Pandey, B. K. (2024). The future of enterprise and innovation is compute as a commodity, or CaaC. *Partners Universal International Research Journal*, *3*(2), 89–94.

Ray, P. P. (2018). A survey on Internet of Things architectures. *Journal of King Saud University. Computer and Information Sciences*, *30*(3), 291–319. DOI: 10.1016/j.jksuci.2016.10.003

Saravanakumar, R., TamilSelvi, T., Pandey, D., Pandey, B. K., Mahajan, D. A., & Lelisho, M. E. (2024). Big data processing using hybrid Gaussian mixture model with salp swarm algorithm. *Journal of Big Data*, *11*(1), 167. DOI: 10.1186/s40537-024-01015-3

Satheesh, N., Gopisankar, N., Kumarganesh, S., Anthoniraj, S., Saravanakumar, S., & Martin Sagayam, K. (2025). Advanced AI-driven emergency response systems for enhanced vehicle and human safety. *Iran Journal of Computer Science*, •••, 1–16. DOI: 10.1007/s42044-025-00228-w

Saxena, A., Agarwal, A., Pandey, B. K., & Pandey, D. (2024). Examination of the Criticality of Customer Segmentation Using Unsupervised Learning Methods. *Circular Economy and Sustainability*, *4*(2), 1–14. DOI: 10.1007/s43615-023-00336-4

Shahul, A., Muniandi, B., Paramashivan, M. A., Pandey, D., Pandey, B. K., Dadheech, P., & George, H. (2024). An Analysis of Algorithms and Methods Based on Image Processing for Medical Applications. In *Emerging Engineering Technologies and Industrial Applications* (pp. 173–186). IGI Global. DOI: 10.4018/979-8-3693-1335-0.ch007

Sheela, M. S., Kumarganesh, S., Pandey, B. K., & Lelisho, M. E. (2025). Integration of silver nanostructures in wireless sensor networks for enhanced biochemical sensing. *Discover Nano*, *20*(1), 7. DOI: 10.1186/s11671-024-04159-6 PMID: 39804434

Singh, S., Madaan, G., Swapna, H. R., Singh, A., Pandey, B. K., George, A. S., & Pandey, D. (2025b). Unleashing the Power of AI and Data Analysis: Transforming Insights into Action. In Interdisciplinary Approaches to AI, Internet of Everything, and Machine Learning (pp. 1-24). IGI Global Scientific Publishing.

Singh, S., Madaan, G., Swapna, H. R., Singh, A., Pandey, D., George, A. S., & Pandey, B. K. (2025a). Empowering Connectivity: Exploring the Internet of Things. In Interdisciplinary Approaches to AI, Internet of Everything, and Machine Learning (pp. 89-116). IGI Global Scientific Publishing.

Zarei, M., Mohammadian, A., & Ghasemi, R. (2016). Internet of things in industries: A survey for sustainable development. *International Journal of Innovation and Sustainable Development*, *10*(4), 419–442. DOI: 10.1504/IJISD.2016.079586

Chapter 5
Scientific Progress in Artificial Intelligence for Time-Stamped Interpretation of Camera Images in Medical Safety Systems

Digvijay Pandey
https://orcid.org/0000-0003-0353-174X
Department of Technical Education, Government of Uttar Pradesh, India

Binay Kumar Pandey
https://orcid.org/0000-0002-4041-1213
G.B. Pant University of Agriculture and Technology, India

A. S. Hovan George
Tbilisi State Medical University, Georgia

A. Shaji George
https://orcid.org/0000-0002-8677-3682
Almarai Company, Saudi Arabia

Shyam Sunder
Jaipur Engineering College and Research Centre, India

Ashish Jolly
https://orcid.org/0000-0002-0849-8232
Department of Computer Science, Government PG College Ambala Cantt, India

Shikha Verma
https://orcid.org/0000-0002-2926-6019
Maharishi Markandeshwar University, Mullana, India

ABSTRACT

Security cameras are typical in most systems and come in many varieties. Internet

DOI: 10.4018/979-8-3693-9821-0.ch005

security cameras, or IP cameras, send and receive data. Free smartphone and tablet apps make live video broadcasts easy to access anytime. IP cameras can monitor a facility inside and out. Cameras can also alert guards to suspicious activity so they can investigate. Remote video monitoring using video surveillance is used for safeguarding a property or structure from intruders, theft, and dishonest personnel. CCTV cameras can monitor daily operations, speed them up, and prevent loss. Outdoor CCTV cameras are used to monitor a building. Video surveillance, roving security/protection teams, perimeter fencing, closed gates for cars and pedestrians, and intrusion detection systems can keep this region secure. For safety, CCTV camera pictures are analyzed using machine learning.

INTRODUCTION

Images have developed into an essential element of modern life as a result of the large quantity of information they contain and the important role they play in the distribution of that information to others. In recent years, the fast growth of deep learning technology has led to the introduction of a wide range of different applications related to computer vision. One such application is image-based target categorization and recognition (Pandey, B. K., & Pandey, D., 2025). It is evident that the digital camera on the smartphone used in this study has certain flaws, despite the general improvement in Smartphone photo quality. When a camera capture falls beyond the scope of this investigation, environmental factors are frequently to blame, according to Bikis et al. (2025). It is the responsibility of the computer to restore the scene to its original state. Two of the most common issues that can be discovered in photos that require restoration are noise and a loss of detail (Sheela, M. S. et al., 2025). Pictures are the primary source of data for vision systems; nevertheless, if the images obtained are of low quality and are not accompanied by the proper context, the utility of a computer vision system may be challenged (Satheesh, N. et al., 2025).For this reason, it is crucial to pay close attention to the procedure used to repair seriously damaged images. They are included in a vast array of deep learning models, enabling the choice of which models to use. In order to get a representative estimate, the data from each predictor should be added together. When very disparate network topologies and technologies are combined, the overall effect will be more dependable if the separate models are trustworthy. You might, however, also attempt doing experiments in the other direction. A fresh network model is used at the beginning of each training session, and the final weight is always calculated with a different value. This is a result of the network model's constant updating. It is possible to get around the algorithm's limited capacity for generalization, according to research by Kumar, M. S. et al. (2025), by employing this method iteratively to create a large number of network models and then combining the prediction outcomes from these models.

MACHINE LEARNING

Using data and computational procedures, machine learning (ML), a branch of artificial intelligence (AI) and computer science, attempts to mimic human learning (Konapure, C. G. et al., 2025). Four fundamental approaches may be used in the process of learning new information: reinforcement learning, supervised learning, semi-supervised learning, and unsupervised learning. One important aspect influencing the algorithm that data scientists choose to utilize is the characteristics of the data that they are trying to forecast. The field of machine learning (ML) studies the creation and improvement of automated systems that can "learn," or adapt to new situations, by using previously collected data.

It frequently gets associated with artificial intelligence. Machine learning algorithms may be trained to make judgments and draw conclusions without explicit guidance by providing them with example data (Singh, S. et al., 2025a). The phrase "training data" is frequently used to describe circumstances such as these. When developing traditional algorithms to perform essential tasks in fields like medicine, engineering, virtual reality, agriculture, and CV is either too time-consuming or impracticable, machine learning (ML) algorithms are used in place of conventional algorithms (Singh, S. et al., 2025b).

Computational statistics, which deals with the idea of using computers to generate predictions, has a direct relationship with some subfields of machine learning. Mathematical optimization research has paved the way for new research directions, theoretical frameworks, and application domains in machine learning (Pandey, B. K. et al., 2024a). Analyzing data for exploratory purposes using algorithms based on unsupervised learning is the focus of the computer science discipline known as data mining. Neural networks and data are used in a variety of machine learning techniques that are conceptually similar to how the human brain functions.

When used to address business difficulties, it is known as predictive analytics (Maglietta R., 2022). A kind of machine learning called predictive analytics uses statistical techniques to generate predictions. The most popular and successful model for image categorization is the "Convolutional Neural Network" (commonly abbreviated as "CNN") (Pandey, B. K. et al., 2024b). This technique is based on deep learning. By examining and "training" itself on images of human faces, a computer may learn to recognize faces through a process called deep learning. The system can identify a particular feature of human faces once it has been trained to do so, regardless of whether it appears in any picture. (Maheshwari, R. U. et al.,

2024). The efficacy of the network model will be negatively impacted if the initial data set is not sufficient for training the model. One common practice that is carried out with the goal of improving the model's accuracy is applying processing on the original source image (Maheshwari, R. Uma. et al.,)• The SIFT method for mapping the features is used.

- A random sample of the data is used as the foundation for the RANSAC algorithm, which is used for registering pictures.
- The classification of images via the use of neural networks 1.

The use of convolutional neural networks (CNNs) for the purpose of image classification

IMAGE PROCESSING

Image augmentation, or IA, is a process used to increase a digital image's quality for viewing or studying, according to Saxena et al. (2024). To highlight the shot's primary subject, noise may be removed, edges can be sharpened, and shadows can be brightened (Rai, P. K. et al., 2024). Picture enhancement is the act of enhancing an image's quality in order to accomplish a certain goal, such as making the image more aesthetically pleasing to people (Lakshmi, K. V. N. et al., 2024). The great majority of photo-enhancing techniques are unplanned, and their impact is rarely taken into account. A wide variety of techniques are available for picture enhancement. Among the most popular methods are EE and SF. Any additional efforts to improve the image are made after the generated image has been corrected for geometric and radiometric errors (Kumarganesh, S. et al., 2024). One method that is frequently applied for enhancing images is histogram equalization. Enhancing overall image quality and offering a more realistic representation of a variety of visual material are the goals of this method.

USING MACHINE LEARNING FOR SURVEILLANCE

Image augmentation, or IA, is a process used to increase a digital image's quality for viewing or studying, according to Saxena et al. (2024). To highlight the shot's primary subject, noise may be removed, edges can be sharpened, and shadows can be brightened (Rai, P. K. et al., 2024). Picture enhancement is the act of enhancing an image's quality in order to accomplish a certain goal, such as making the image more aesthetically pleasing to people (Lakshmi, K. V. N. et al., 2024). The great majority of photo-enhancing techniques are unplanned, and their impact is rarely taken into account. (Muralidhar, L. B. et al., 2024). Image augmentation, or IA, is a process used to increase a digital image's quality for viewing or studying, according to Saxena et al. (2024). To highlight the shot's primary subject, noise may be removed, edges can be sharpened, and shadows can be brightened (Rai, P. K. et al., 2024). Picture enhancement is the act of enhancing an image's quality in order to accomplish a certain goal, such as making the image more aesthetically pleasing to people (Lakshmi, K. V. N. et al., 2024). The great majority of photo-enhancing techniques are unplanned, and their impact is rarely taken into account.

Figure 1. Role of surveillance using machine learning

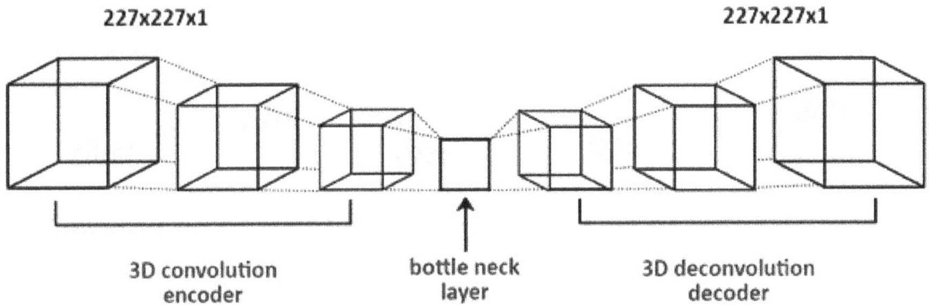

Advances in machine learning (ML) might help safeguard the privacy of people whose images show up in security camera feeds while also increasing the effectiveness of data collection (Pandey, B. K. et al., 2024d). There may be a win-win scenario here. A smart camera that could analyze data internally would be an example of this, doing away with the requirement for data storage and transport. Throughout the process, it can also be smart enough to know what has to be recorded and what it can safely disregard. A smart camera not only increases efficiency but also protects sensitive data from unauthorized or malevolent usage (Elarmathi, S. et al., 2024).

With deep learning software installed, a closed-circuit television system may identify individuals approaching an entrance, decide whether to allow them in, and then delete any relevant footage (Pandey, B. K. et al., 2024e). Once it has achieved its objective, it may "forget" about the information it collects because it is processed locally and does not require transmission or storage. In addition to monitoring a company's parking lot, a camera installed next to a house may be able to see what's happening inside its window (JayaLakshmi, G. et al., 2024). It is possible to set the camera to ignore any input from that area. As a result, the program fixes issues caused by camera placement and stops any accidental or malevolent capture of photos taken elsewhere other than the organization's grounds (George, W. K. et al., 2024).

ROLE OF SURVEILLANCE IN IMAGE PROCESSING FOR SECURITY

One of the many benefits of using artificial intelligence in cybersecurity is that it helps security professionals better analyze, investigate, and comprehend crimes. It improves the tools used to combat fraudsters and safeguard businesses and their clients from fraudulent activities. However, artificial intelligence might occasionally require a lot of resources. Under some conditions, it might not work. Furthermore, hackers may utilize this technology as a new weapon to improve and hone their assaults (Abdullahi, M. et al., 2024). The application of artificial intelligence is also helping the virtual private network sector. Virtual private networks, or VPNs, for all devices might potentially lessen the privacy risk posed by artificial intelligence by utilizing the same technology. Virtual private networks (VPNs) can better defend their clients against potential internet attacks by utilizing machine learning algorithms. Discussions regarding cybersecurity and artificial intelligence are not new. Figure 2 illustrates the importance of surveillance in image processing for safety purposes and may be viewed below.

Figure 2. Role of surveillance in image processing for security

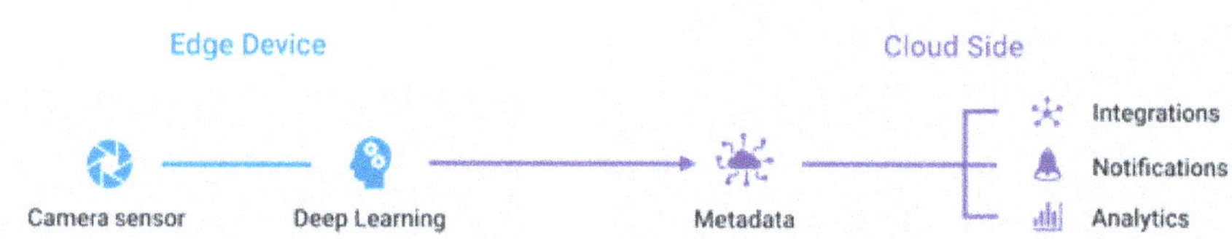

We published research articles that explored how machine learning and artificial intelligence can impact cybersecurity in the future. It is crucial to keep in mind that the foundation of modern cybersecurity solutions is information. It is possible to collect, process, and search video without further jeopardizing privacy security in order to achieve tighter security, better operations, or higher safety. There are several significant privacy and bias issues with the technology currently being utilized to combine cloud-based analytics with cloud-connected security cameras. However, localized, embedded intelligence and analytics are made possible by machine learning software with deep learning capabilities (Kumar, B. et al., 2024). This program helps to strengthen security while preserving the secrecy of personal information since it performs very well while consuming little power. Most of the CCTV video monitoring systems already in use may easily be upgraded to include intelligent video technologies.

ROLE OF MACHINE LEARNING IN IMAGE ENHANCEMENT

A wide range of businesses, including the military, security, healthcare, education, manufacturing, telecommunications, and industrial sectors, are adopting image recognition systems at a rapid pace. The goal of this broad adoption is to increase the processing and analysis speed, accuracy, and efficiency of visual data. But globally, the situation is extremely unstable (Pathania V., 2022). The Retinex algorithm's picture-improving elements work best at extremely small sizes. The Retinex algorithm works effectively even under very hazy conditions. The effect is less obvious as the photo's scale grows, but the colors become more realistic. CNN is incredibly effective in deep learning picture recognition because of its unique mode of operation. Deep neural networks (DNNs) are only one type of machine learning model utilized in state-of-the-art intellectual property approaches nowadays. These methods are used to enhance certain image attributes, add artistic filters, or alter a picture to get optimal quality in order to raise the caliber of computer vision applications. The process of determining what is included in a photograph and its purpose by examining how it is captured is known as "picture recognition" (IR).

LITERATURE REVIEW

The study on IP for human-machine interaction in 3D image processing by A. Sungheetha et al. in 2021 contributed to the field of machine learning. The real world offers a multitude of possible uses for human-robot interaction. The concept of "convergence," where a three-dimensional image is transformed into a two-dimensional projection on a plane, was used to robotic systems using digital visualization to help in item recognition (Pandey, D. et al., 2024a). During the convergence phase, incorrect detection of projections in many planes leads to recognition problems. It is feasible to reduce the rates of identification mistakes by employing an input processing strategy based on a projection methodology.

The conjoining indices may be viewed by projecting the input image in every direction. To increase recognition accuracy and speed up computation, an ML approach was applied. Rather than connecting indices, the intersection was partitioned using a labeled analysis. Finding potential dimension projections where the indices do not correlate is one way to avoid mistakes. Because inputs are labeled and grouped for subsequent use, it is challenging to compare indices and deviations across multiple planes. The suggested model was validated by tests for error, complexity, time, and recognition ratio (Kennedy, G. W. et al., 2024). A used inexpensive cameras to measure and assess the roughness of concrete surfaces (Shahul, A. et al., 2024). In the first implementation, a new index was created to help comprehend the connection between surface area and proportional area. The second approach classifies new pictures based on prior examples using computer vision and machine learning techniques such as data augmentation and transfer learning (Pandey, D. et al., 2024c). Both cases involve 3D laser scanning of blasted concrete, which is based on a proven method. The effectiveness of both methods was confirmed using fresh images of sandblasted surfaces (Pandey, D., & Pandey, B. K., 2022). The results show that both methods predict concrete surface roughness with greater than 93% accuracy.

H. Xiao et al. (2021) reviewed the issue of registering 3D medical images and concentrated on deep learning-based solutions (Pandey, B. K., & Pandey, D., 2023). The goal of this study was to gather the achievements and shortcomings of DL-based 3D picture registration throughout the previous five years. The statistical analysis of the combined research was conducted using registration assessment criteria, image modality, supervision approach, and ROI. The trials were divided into three groups according to whether supervised registration, unsupervised registration, or deep iterative (Ahathiyan, G. S. et al., 2025) registration was utilized.

With an aim of emphasizing the contributions of each particular study, the research is critically analyzed (Pandey, D. et al., 2025). Following a discussion of each methodology's advantages, disadvantages, and new developments, a summary was given. Lastly, they address the problems that affect all communities and provide suggestions for more study.

loss functions with diverse norms to enhance photos captured in poor light. This study offers a novel method for enhancing low-light photos using a DL network with mixed-norm loss functions. A chroma net, illumination-enhancement net, and decomposition net are all combined in this hybrid network. RGB is converted to YCbCr throughout the learning and restoration stages in order to take advantage of the relationship between the RGB channels. The decomposition net and its companion illumination enhancement net help to improve the lighting while also reducing the number of halo artifacts. The reflectance was trained using the illuminance and should subsequently be decoupled from the luminance for a more accurate and less noisy feature map. The chroma-net can also be used independently to adjust color shifts. Each network is trained using a mixed-norm loss function that accounts for chroma quality, illumination, and reflectance in order to increase stability and decrease blurring in the reconstructed image. The experimental results show that the suggested technique outperforms the state-of-the-art DL algorithms.

K. Niu et al. (2021) assessed two-channel deep learning-based night vision picture restoration. Excellent quality and a positive impression are produced by the photos captured with restored night vision. While the values for the FMRB-based DL network-reconstructed enhanced low-light-level night vision image were 3 (MSRCR), the average PSNR and SSIM values for the FMRB-based DL network-reconstructed infrared night vision image were 3.56 dB and 0.0912 higher than those for the image produced by the SRCNN reconstruction algorithm. The purpose of this study was to gather user experiences—both good and bad—with 3D picture registration using DL throughout the last five years. The statistical analysis of the combined experiments made use of registration assessment criteria, imaging modalities, supervision strategies, and ROI.An enhanced DL method for image processing based on SSDs was created. The majority of the items visible in these satellite photos were quite tiny and closely spaced. When CNN is applied to remote sensing pictures, poor recognition results are obtained because the convolution layer lacks sufficient context information (Praveenkumar, T. et al., 2025). This paper proposes an efficient object identification method for ship recognition in remote sensing images based on enhanced SSD to increase detection accuracy while maintaining a steady real-time detection speed. The purpose of this study was to gather user experiences—both good and bad—with 3D picture registration using DL throughout the last five years. The statistical analysis of the studies made use of registration assessment criteria, imaging modalities, supervision strategies, and ROI. Trials were divided into three categories: those where deep iterative registration was utilized, those where supervised registration was used, and those where unsupervised registration was used.

K. Niu et al. Higher-quality picture production has been investigated using generative adversarial networks with improved network performance (Sah, M. et al., 2025). An identical image is first produced in the new space by the enhancement network from the input picture; the generated image is then further improved by the enhancement network; and finally, the discriminator is trained using the generated image as a comparison target by minimizing a loss function that compares the generated image to the original. They used the proposed method on two image datasets and contrasted the outcomes with those of deep learning and more traditional image-enhancing methods. Our experimental results demonstrate that our suggested network successfully enhances pictures in low-light circumstances based on the PNSR and SSIM scores. Two-channel deep learning-based night vision picture restoration. Excellent quality and a positive impression are produced by the photos captured with restored night vision. While the values for the FMRB-based DL network-reconstructed enhanced low-light-level night vision image were 3 (MSRCR), the average PSNR and SSIM values for the FMRB-based DL network-reconstructed infrared night vision image were 3.56 dB and 0.0912 higher than those for the image produced by the SRCNN reconstruction algorithm. The purpose of this study was to gather user experiences—both good and bad—with 3D picture registration using DL throughout the last five years. The statistical analysis of the combined experiments made use of registration assessment criteria, imaging modalities, supervision strategies, and ROI.

In this research, they examined generative adversarial networks, RNNs, and others. A scalable supplementary generation network was presented as part of a model architecture for enhancing rain fog photos with generative countermeasures. The basic issue with picture stacking is examined, and a suggested fix is offered. This method offers strong theoretical assurances for multitasking through adaptive feature learning. In addition to improving computer vision systems' performance, reading this article will improve your visual experience. Low-light photos may have better clarity, texture details, and noise reduction with the use of image enhancing technologies. The first presentation was an analysis of ML and IP techniques for cetacean picture identification. In accordance with the Preferred Reporting Items for Systematic Reviews and Meta-Analyses statement, they conducted a comprehensive examination of statistical and machine learning approaches for cetacean image recognition systems. This article offers a succinct summary of the current explosion in interest in the subject and the diverse range of newly published intelligent systems. Better automated techniques for identifying cetaceans in photos were desperately required, even if several problems still needed to be addressed (Sreedhar, C. et al., 2025).

ReLLIE uses deep RL to improve low-light images in a way that is unique to each viewer. The reward is derived from a carefully constructed set of non-reference loss functions, and the network's weight is kept low to enable it to estimate the lighting curves for a low-light picture input. Unlike one-to-one image translation, ReLLIE learns a strategy to handle a range of low-light measurements and provide highly personalized augmented outputs. Additionally, ReLLIE's plug-and-play denoiser makes it simple to correct real-world photos that contain hybrid corruptions like noise. ReLLIE outperforms state-of-the-art techniques, as shown by extensive testing on a wide range of benchmarks. The present state of DL and medical IP was examined by S. Bhattacharya et al. in 2021 in light of the recent coronavirus (COVID-19) epidemic. A review of the literature on deep learning for COVID-19 medical IPs is presented at the outset, with a focus on the most current and pertinent findings. Secondly, they offer a concise synopsis of the DL sector and its latest medical uses. Next, we provide three distinct case studies from China, Korea, and Canada that demonstrate the application of deep learning for COVID-19 medical IP. Lastly, they highlight a number of difficulties with DL implementations for COVID-19 medical IP, which was supposed to stimulate more research into pandemic management and catastrophe prevention, ultimately resulting in intelligent, healthy societies.. DL that might have a symbolic meaning in IP and signal. In a number of real-world signal and IP challenges, researchers may be able to achieve performance advantages using DNN that were previously unattainable. Despite these developments, deep networks' black-box nature poses challenges to their further advancement and real-world use because of their interpretability issues and requirement for massive amounts of training data.

LIMITATION OF EXISTING RESEARCH

In 2021, A. Sungheetha et al. made a contribution to machine learning by using IP for human-machine interaction in 3D image processing. There are several practical applications for human-robot interaction. "Convergence," which transforms a three-dimensional picture into a two-dimensional projection on a plane, is used in digital visualization in robotic systems to aid in object identification. During convergence, misidentified projections in several planes lead to identification problems. It may be possible to decrease identification errors by implementing projection-based input processing. The conjoining indices are displayed by projecting the input picture in every direction. ML increased recognition accuracy and calculation speed. The intersection was divided by labeled analysis rather than linking indices. Errors may be prevented by identifying dimension projections with mismatched indices. Comparing indices and changes across planes becomes challenging when inputs are labeled and categorized for later use.

used inexpensive cameras to examine the surface roughness of concrete. To better understand surface area and proportional area in the initial implementation, a new index was developed. The second method uses data augmentation and transfer learning to classify new images according to previous examples. In both cases, the tried-and-true technique of 3D laser scanning of blasted concrete was used (Pandey, B. K. et al., 2025). New images of the sandblasted surface were used to test both approaches. Over 93% of concrete surface roughness may be accurately predicted using both approaches.

techniques for 3D medical picture registration based on deep learning. This study looked at the successes and shortcomings of DL-based 3D photo registration during a five-year period. Using registration assessment criteria, image modality, supervision technique, and ROI, the combined investigations were statistically examined. Three groups of trials were created using either supervised, unsupervised, or deep iterative registration. To emphasize the importance of certain findings, the study is critically examined. Each technique's advantages, disadvantages, and emerging trends were examined and compiled. They end with research recommendations and worries for all communities.

To improve low-light images, J. G. Oh et al. (2022) developed a hybrid DL that employs loss functions with mixed norms. In this work, a DL network with mixed-norm loss functions is used to enhance low-light images. Decomposition, illumination enhancement, and chroma nets are all included in this hybrid network. To take use of the RGB channel connection, RGB is transformed to YCbCr during learning and restoration.

With the help of the decomposition-net and its companion illumination-enhancement-net, which improve lighting and lessen halo artifacts, it is feasible to decouple the reflectance from the brightness for a more accurate and noisy feature map. Additionally, the chroma-net has the ability to independently modify color shifts. To improve stability and reduce blurring in the reconstructed picture, each network is trained using a mixed-norm loss function that takes reflectance, illumination, and chroma quality into consideration. The suggested approach works better than existing DL algorithms, according to experimental results.

Two-channel deep learning-based night vision image restoration was tested by K. Niu et al. in 2021. Restored night vision produces stunning, high-quality images. The infrared night vision image had 3.56 dB and 0.0912 higher values than the SRCNN reconstruction algorithm image, while the FMRB-based DL network-reconstructed improved low-light-level night vision image had 3 (MSRCR) PSNR and SSIM values. Over a five-year period, this study gathered both good and negative 3D image registration experiences from DL users. The statistical analysis of the combined investigations used registration assessment criteria, ROI, imaging modalities, and supervision techniques. Depending on whether the trials employed supervised registration, unsupervised registration, or deep iterative registration, three groups were created.

SSD-based DL image processing was improved by L. Jin et al. (2020). The majority of the objects in these satellite images were small and closely spaced. Because the convolution layer lacks context, CNN on remote sensing photos produces subpar identification results. Using an improved SSD, this research offers a great object identification method for ship recognition in remote sensing photos, increasing detection accuracy while preserving real-time detection performance. Over a five-year period, this study gathered both good and negative 3D image registration experiences from DL users. The statistical analysis of the combined investigations used registration assessment criteria, ROI, imaging modalities, and supervision techniques. In the experiments, three registration techniques were used: unsupervised, supervised, and deep iterative.

According to L. Yan et al. (2021), generative adversarial networks that perform better produce photographs of higher quality. The discriminator is trained by minimizing a loss function that compares the created picture to the original image. The enhancement network first produces an identical image in the new space, then refines the generated image. On two picture datasets, they compared the suggested approach to deep learning and conventional image-enhancing techniques. Based on PNSR and SSIM scores, our trials show that our network improves low-light images.

A deep learning-based method for improving photo quality was created by P. Zhang et al. in 2022. This study looked at generative adversarial networks and RNNs. A scalable additional generation network was incorporated into the model method for improving rain fog photos using generative countermeasures. The fundamental problem of picture layering is studied and solved. With robust theoretical guarantees, this multitasking technique makes use of adaptive feature learning. After reading this article, your computer vision system's efficiency and visual experience will both increase. Image enhancement can improve the noise, texture, and clarity of low-light images.

In 2022, ML and IP Techniques for Cetacean Picture Identification were presented by R. Maglietta et al. Following the Preferred Reporting Items for Systematic Reviews and Meta-Analyses statement, they examined the statistical and machine learning techniques used in cetacean picture identification systems. This succinct overview discusses the wide variety of emerging intelligent systems as well as the current surge in coverage of the subject. Automated cetacean detection in photographs needed to be improved, even though certain issues persisted.

According to Zhang et al.'s research from 2021, deep RL aids ReLLIE in making low-light photos better for every viewer. The network's weight is maintained low to predict lighting curves for low-light picture inputs, and the reward is a carefully crafted set of non-reference loss functions. ReLLIE creates a method to manage different low-light measurements and provide highly customized enhanced outputs rather than converting photos one-to-one. ReLLIE can recover real-world photographs with hybrid corruptions like noise because of its plug-and-play denoiser. Experiments on a number of benchmarks demonstrate that ReLLIE performs better than the most advanced methods.

In 2021, S. Bhattacharya et al. looked studied medical IP and DL in the context of COVID-19. Current and noteworthy discoveries are the main topic of the literature study on deep learning for COVID-19 medical IPs. Second, they give a brief overview of the DL industry and its most recent applications in healthcare. Three case studies from China, Korea, and Canada are then presented to demonstrate deep learning for COVID-19 medical IP. Lastly, they point out some challenges with DL implementations for COVID-19 medical IP, which was meant to encourage research into disaster prevention and pandemic management in order to create intelligent, healthy communities.

PROPOSED RESEARCH METHODOLOGY

The methodology describes in great depth the methods and approaches that will be used to complete the assigned task. The development and improvement of the algorithm depend on paying close attention to the subsequent steps. Each of these phrases may be defined as follows in Figure 3:

Figure 3. Research methodology

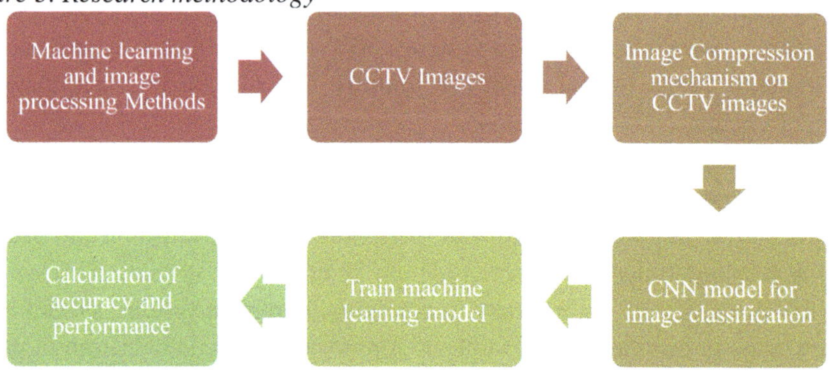

The recommended programming language for putting the suggested image-improvement method into practice is Python. A program called Python may be used to do numerical computations and present the results in a graphical format. A matrix is the most basic form for data storage. Images are handled by Python in the same way as matrices. Python is a software package that comes with an introductory programming language and development environment.

RESULT ANALYSIS OF PROPOSED WORK

Images have been considered at every stage of this research effort to ensure optimal results. Images are preprocessed by scaling them down during the recommended task, and then the CNN model is used to do classification.

Image Compression Before Training

Our goal is to reduce the file size of an image by using LBG Algorithm. There are just a few basic building blocks to the algorithm:

Step 1 First, find the sample mean x1(1) for the entire dataset. The sample mean is proven total mean square distortion for a single prototype.

Step 2 Set $k = 1, l = 1$.

Where l is the index for the iteration and k counts prototypes that have been generated.

Step 3 If $k < M$ split current centroids by adding small offsets. Since if research already has k prototypes, and needs $M - k$ additional prototypes.

If $M - K \geq K$, Split all existing centroids that have been created so far; otherwise research split only $M - K$ of them.

Step 4 For example, to split z1(1) into two centroids

Let $z1(2) = z1(1)$, $z2(2) = z1(1) + \varepsilon$, where ε is a small offset.

Step 5 Use { z1(1), z2(1), ..., zk(1)} as initial prototypes, which include generated centroids and newly split centroids.

Step 6 Check whether prototypes have reached target prototypes.

In other words, if $k < M$, go back to step 3; otherwise, stop.

Simulation of CNN-based Image Training

This kernel's CNNs are based on LeNet5, with a few key enhancements:

- The single 5x5 filter has been replaced with a pair of 3x3 filters. 5x5 nonlinear convolutions are formed.
- The pooling layers are replaced with a convolution with a stride of 2. These evolve into a pooling layer that may be taught.
- In lieu of sigmoid, we use ReLU activation.
- The addition of batch normalization
- Subtraction of Dropout
- An increase in the number of feature maps (channels)
- The ensemble of 15 CNNs uses bagging.

Figure 4 is presenting the CNN model in which different layers are starting as input to the connection layers.

Figure 4. CNN model

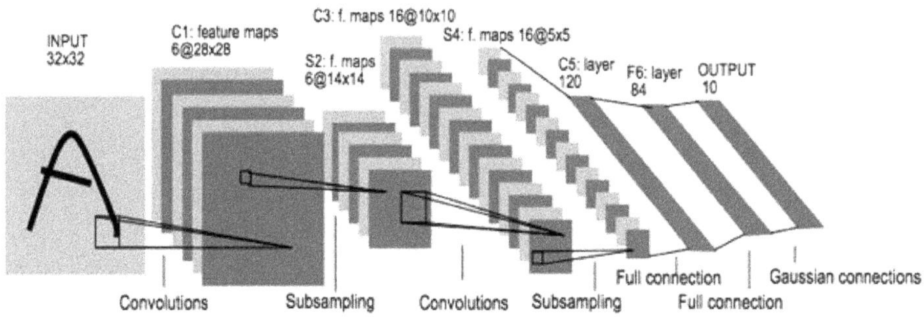

Table 1 presents the simulation of CNN-based image training.

Table 1. Simulation of CNN-based image training

Model Number	Epochs	Train Accuracy	Validation Accuracy
CNN 1	45	0.99621	0.99619
CNN 2	45	0.99616	0.99548
CNN 3	45	0.99592	0.99690
CNN 4	45	0.99624	0.99786
CNN 5	45	0.99573	0.99571
CNN 6	45	0.99626	0.99524
CNN 7	45	0.99640	0.99619
CNN 8	45	0.99608	0.99667
CNN 9	45	0.99637	0.99643
CNN 10	45	0.99621	0.99619
CNN 11	45	0.99610	0.99500
CNN 12	45	0.99648	0.99524
CNN 13	45	0.99605	0.99619
CNN 14	45	0.99663	0.99619
CNN 15	45	0.99658	0.99500

CNN Performance

The highest level of accuracy that could be achieved by a single CNN was 99.81%, with average accuracy being 99.641% & SD being 0.047. An ensemble of fifteen CNNs had an accuracy that reached a high of 99.79%, with an accuracy that averaged 99.745% and a standard deviation of 0.020. Figure 5 presents the CNN performance.

Figure 5. CNN performance

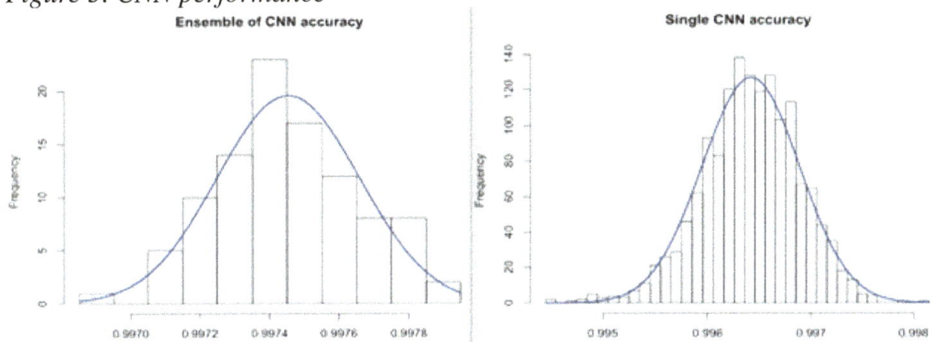

CONCLUSION AND FUTURE SCOPE

A thorough and in-depth explanation of the methods and techniques that will be employed to accomplish the desired outcome is given by methodology. Highlighting the steps that occur after they are completed is one of the most crucial things that must be done in order to enhance and broaden the algorithm. Python is the best programming platform to employ because of its versatility when it comes to implementing the recommended technique for image enhancement. Python is a computer language that is used for both calculating and visually representing numerical quantities. In terms of offering a structure for information storage. A matrix is the most basic and effective choice for offering a structure for information storage. Working with matrices in Python and working with photos both need comparatively comparable procedures. Python is a software product that is sold to clients in packaged form. You can utilize the development environment and programming language included in this package. Both of these components are intuitive enough that even inexperienced programmers may grasp them. Over the course of this study exercise, photographs have been carefully inspected to enhance their quality. Prior to the images being processed by a CNN model for classification, the image is reduced in size during the preprocessing phase of the proposed job. The average accuracy was 99.64 percent, the standard deviation was 0.047 points, and the maximum accuracy for a single CNN was 98 percent. With a standard deviation of 0.020 and an average accuracy of 99.745%, a group of fifteen CNNs demonstrated exceptional performance.

REFERENCES

Abdullahi, M., Ahmad, A., Pandey, B. K., & Pandey, D. (2024). Digital Currency Adoption: A Comparative Analysis of Global Trends and the Nigerian eNaira Digital Currency. *SN Computer Science*, *5*(5), 1–11. DOI: 10.1007/s42979-024-02882-6

Ahathiyan, G. S., Du John, H. V., Moni, D. J., Sagayam, K. M., Pandey, B. K., Pandey, D., & Lelisho, M. E. (2025). Design and simulation of a highly efficient eco-friendly, non-toxic perovskite solar cell. *Discover Nano*, *20*(1), 32. DOI: 10.1186/s11671-025-04190-1 PMID: 39937384

Bhattacharya, S., Reddy Maddikunta, P. K., Pham, Q. V., Gadekallu, T. R., & Krishnan, S. (2020, November). S. R., Chowdhary, C. L., Alazab, M., &JalilPiran, M. (2021). Deep learning and medical image processing for coronavirus (COVID-19) pandemic: A survey. *Sustainable Cities and Society*, *65*, 102589. DOI: 10.1016/j.scs.2020.102589 PMID: 33169099

Bikis, A., Engdaw, M., Pandey, D., & Pandey, B. K. (2025). The impact of urbanization on land use land cover change using geographic information system and remote sensing: A case of Mizan Aman City Southwest Ethiopia. *Scientific Reports*, *15*(1), 12014. DOI: 10.1038/s41598-025-94189-6 PMID: 40199909

Elarmathi, S., Rishabavarthani, P., Sindhuja, M., Elayaraja, P., & Malathi Murugesan, S. (2024). Novel manufacturing systems for cancer diagnosis using ultra-sensitive photonic crystal fiber biosensor with dual-functionalized aptamer-nanocavity. *Microsystem Technologies*, •••, 1–20. DOI: 10.1007/s00542-024-05820-x

George, W. K., Silas, E. I., Pandey, D., & Pandey, B. K. (2024). Utilization of Industry 4.0 Technologies in Nigerian Technical and Vocational Education: A Conundrum for Educators. In *Examining the Rapid Advance of Digital Technology in Africa* (pp. 270–293). IGI Global. DOI: 10.4018/978-1-6684-9962-7.ch014

JayaLakshmi. G., Pandey, D., Pandey, B. K., Kaur, P., Mahajan, D. A., & Dari, S. S. (2024). Smart big data collection for intelligent supply chain improvement. In AI and Machine Learning Impacts in Intelligent Supply Chain (pp. 180-195). IGI Global Scientific Publishing.

Kennedy, G. W., Sunday, S. E., Pandey, D., Kabari, A. D., Pandey, B. K., George, A. S., & Dadheech, P. (2024). Building Information Modeling: Harnessing Innovations for Professional Proficiency. In Emerging Engineering Technologies and Industrial Applications (pp. 305-331). IGI Global.

Konapure, C. G., Pandey, D., Shete, H., Thakar, C. M., Pandey, B. K., & George, A. S. (2025). Artificial Intelligence in Automated Concrete Mix Design Using Computerized Grading Curves. Interdisciplinary Approaches to AI, Internet of Everything, and Machine Learning, 567-586.

Kumar, B., Pandey, D., Pandey, B. K., & George, A. S. (2024). Higher Education in the Last Four Decades: A Review of Paradigm Shifts in Policy Frameworks. Design and Implementation of Higher Education Learners' Learning Outcomes (HELLO), 333-348.

Kumar, M. S., Prasanna, P. L., Lalitha, M., Joy, M., Jha, S. S., & Pandey, B. K. (2025). Utilizing the Internet of Everything and Artificial Intelligence for Real-Time Workforce Management. In Role of Internet of Everything (IOE), VLSI Architecture, and AI in Real-Time Systems (pp. 153-168). IGI Global Scientific Publishing.

Kumarganesh, S., & Malathi Murugesan, C. (2024). Hybrid plasmonic biosensors with deep learning for colorectal cancer detection. *Plasmonics*, •••, 1–15. DOI: 10.1007/s11468-024-02568-y

Lakshmi, K. V. N., Rajan, R., Pandey, D., & Pandey, B. K. (2024). Circular economy: A catalyst for economic growth-an empirical study. *Circular Economy and Sustainability*, •••, 1–22.

Maglietta, R., Carlucci, R., Fanizza, C., & Dimauro, G. (2022). Machine Learning and Image Processing Methods for Cetacean Photo Identification: A Systematic Review. *IEEE Access : Practical Innovations, Open Solutions*, *10*(July), 80195–80207. DOI: 10.1109/ACCESS.2022.3195218

Maheshwari, R., Kumarganesh, S., K v M, S., Gopalakrishnan, A., Selvi, K., Paulchamy, B., Rishabavarthani, P., Sagayam, K. M., Pandey, B. K., & Pandey, D. (2024). Advanced plasmonic resonance-enhanced biosensor for comprehensive real-time detection and analysis of deepfake content. *Plasmonics*, •••, 1–18. DOI: 10.1007/s11468-024-02407-0

Maheshwari, R. U., Paulchamy, B., Pandey, B. K., & Pandey, D. (2024). Enhancing sensing and imaging capabilities through surface plasmon resonance for deepfake image detection. *Plasmonics*, •••, 1–20. DOI: 10.1007/s11468-024-02492-1

Muralidhar, L. B., Lakshmi, K. V. N., Swapna, H. R., Rupani, J., Nethravathi, K., Pandey, B. K., & Pandey, D. (2024). Impact of Organizational Culture on The Level of Corporate Social Responsibility Investments: An Exploratory Study. *Circular Economy and Sustainability*, *4*(3), 1–19. DOI: 10.1007/s43615-024-00371-9

Niu, K., Chen, Y., & Shen, J. (2021). Dual-channel night vision image restoration method based on deep learning. *Computer Applications (Nottingham)*, *41*(6), 10.

Oh, J. G., & Hong, M. C. (2022). Low-Light Image Enhancement Using Hybrid Deep-Learning and Mixed-Norm Loss Functions. *Sensors (Basel)*, *22*(18), 6904. Advance online publication. DOI: 10.3390/s22186904 PMID: 36146252

Pandey, B. K., Kanike, U. K., George, A. S., & Pandey, D. (Eds.). (2024d). *AI and machine learning impacts in intelligent supply chain*. IGI Global. DOI: 10.4018/979-8-3693-1347-3

Pandey, B. K., Nassa, V. K., Mukundan, A. P., Mahajan, D. A., Pandey, D., George, A. S., & Dadheech, P. (2024c). An Industry-Focused Traffic System Utilising Internet of Things. In *Emerging Engineering Technologies and Industrial Applications* (pp. 200–213). IGI Global. DOI: 10.4018/979-8-3693-1335-0.ch009

Pandey, B. K., & Pandey, D. (2023). Parametric optimization and prediction of enhanced thermoelectric performance in co-doped CaMnO3 using response surface methodology and neural network. *Journal of Materials Science Materials in Electronics*, *34*(21), 1589. DOI: 10.1007/s10854-023-10954-1

Pandey, B. K., & Pandey, D. (2025). Securing healthcare medical image information using advance morphological component analysis, information hiding systems, and hybrid convolutional neural networks on IoMT. *Computers in Biology and Medicine*, *185*, 109499. DOI: 10.1016/j.compbiomed.2024.109499 PMID: 39642698

Pandey, B. K., Pandey, D., & Lelisho, M. E. (2024a). Face mask identification with enhanced cuckoo optimization and deep learning-based faster regional neural network. *Scientific Reports*, *14*(1), 29719. DOI: 10.1038/s41598-024-78746-z PMID: 39613761

Pandey, B. K., Pandey, D., & Sahani, S. K. (2024b). Autopilot control unmanned aerial vehicle system for sewage defect detection using deep learning. *Engineering Reports*, •••, 12852.

Pandey, B. K., Pandey, D., & Sahani, S. K. (2025). Autopilot control unmanned aerial vehicle system for sewage defect detection using deep learning. *Engineering Reports*, *7*(1), e12852. DOI: 10.1002/eng2.12852

Pandey, B. K., Paramashivan, M. A., Pandey, D., George, A. S., Agarwal, A., Mahajan, D. A., . . . Pramanik, S. (2024e). Future Directions of Digital Twin Architectures for 6G Communication Networks. In Security Issues and Solutions in 6G Communications and Beyond (pp. 197-211). IGI Global.

Pandey, D., Nassa, V. K., Pandey, B. K., Thankachan, B., Dadheech, P., Mahajan, D. A., & George, A. S. (2024a). Artificial Intelligence and Machine Learning and Its Application in the Field of Computational Visual Analysis. In Emerging Engineering Technologies and Industrial Applications (pp. 36-57). IGI Global. DOI: 10.4018/979-8-3693-1335-0.ch003

Pandey, D., & Pandey, B. K. (2022). An efficient deep neural network with adaptive galactic swarm optimization for complex image text extraction. In *Process Mining Techniques for Pattern Recognition* (pp. 121–137). CRC Press. DOI: 10.1201/9781003169550-10

Pandey, D., Pandey, B. K., Nassa, V. K., Mahajan, D. A., George, A. S., & Dadheech, P. (2024c). Optimized Throughput-Based Broadcasting for Next Generation Wireless Networks. In Emerging Engineering Technologies and Industrial Applications (pp. 355-368). IGI Global. DOI: 10.4018/979-8-3693-1335-0.ch018

Pandey, D., Pandey, B. K., Paramashivan, M. A., Mahajan, D. A., Dadheech, P. D., George, A. S., & Hameed, A. S. (2024b). Advanced Digital Data Processing Using Cloud Cryptography: Industrial Applications. In Emerging Engineering Technologies and Industrial Applications (pp. 255-268). IGI Global.

Pandey, D., Sharma, M., Talwar, R., & Pandey, B. K. (2025). A compact quintuple band miniaturized elliptical planar monopole antenna for 5G/6G wireless systems. *Analog Integrated Circuits and Signal Processing*, *122*(3), 1–16. DOI: 10.1007/s10470-025-02310-6

Praveenkumar, T., Anthoniraj, S., Kumarganesh, S., Somaskandan, M., Martin Sagayam, K., Pandey, B. K., Pandey, D., & Sahani, S. K. (2025). Enhanced Circuit Board Analysis: Infrared Image Segmentation Utilizing Markov Random Field (MRF) and Level Set Techniques. *Engineering Reports*, *7*(3), e70029. DOI: 10.1002/eng2.70029

Rai, P. K., Pandey, D., & Pandey, B. K. (2024). The future of enterprise and innovation is compute as a commodity, or CaaC. *Partners Universal International Research Journal*, *3*(2), 89–94.

Sah, M., Chaudhary, R., Sahani, S. K., Sahani, K., Pandey, B. K., Pandey, D., & Lelisho, M. E. (2025). Quantum physical analysis of caffeine and nicotine in CCL4 and DMSO solvent using density functional theory. *Scientific Reports*, *15*(1), 10372. DOI: 10.1038/s41598-025-91211-9 PMID: 40140665

Saravanakumar, R., TamilSelvi, T., Pandey, D., Pandey, B. K., Mahajan, D. A., & Lelisho, M. E. (2024). Big data processing using hybrid Gaussian mixture model with salp swarm algorithm. *Journal of Big Data*, *11*(1), 167. DOI: 10.1186/s40537-024-01015-3

Satheesh, N., Gopisankar, N., Kumarganesh, S., Anthoniraj, S., Saravanakumar, S., & Martin Sagayam, K. (2025). Advanced AI-driven emergency response systems for enhanced vehicle and human safety. *Iran Journal of Computer Science*, •••, 1–16. DOI: 10.1007/s42044-025-00228-w

Saxena, A., Agarwal, A., Pandey, B. K., & Pandey, D. (2024). Examination of the Criticality of Customer Segmentation Using Unsupervised Learning Methods. *Circular Economy and Sustainability*, *4*(2), 1–14. DOI: 10.1007/s43615-023-00336-4

Shahul, A., Muniandi, B., Paramashivan, M. A., Pandey, D., Pandey, B. K., Dadheech, P., & George, H. (2024). An Analysis of Algorithms and Methods Based on Image Processing for Medical Applications. In *Emerging Engineering Technologies and Industrial Applications* (pp. 173–186). IGI Global. DOI: 10.4018/979-8-3693-1335-0.ch007

Sheela, M. S., Kumarganesh, S., Pandey, B. K., & Lelisho, M. E. (2025). Integration of silver nanostructures in wireless sensor networks for enhanced biochemical sensing. *Discover Nano*, *20*(1), 7. DOI: 10.1186/s11671-024-04159-6 PMID: 39804434

Singh, S., Madaan, G., Swapna, H. R., Singh, A., Pandey, B. K., George, A. S., & Pandey, D. (2025b). Unleashing the Power of AI and Data Analysis: Transforming Insights into Action. In Interdisciplinary Approaches to AI, Internet of Everything, and Machine Learning (pp. 1-24). IGI Global Scientific Publishing.

Singh, S., Madaan, G., Swapna, H. R., Singh, A., Pandey, D., George, A. S., & Pandey, B. K. (2025a). Empowering Connectivity: Exploring the Internet of Things. In Interdisciplinary Approaches to AI, Internet of Everything, and Machine Learning (pp. 89-116). IGI Global Scientific Publishing.

Sreedhar, C., Kallam, S., Ghantasala, G. P., Anthoniraj, S., Kumarganesh, S., Sagayam, K. M., & Pandey, D. (2025). Enhancing healthcare data security using RFE and CRHSM for big data. *Computers in Biology and Medicine*, *190*, 110063. DOI: 10.1016/j.compbiomed.2025.110063 PMID: 40154199

Yan, L., Fu, J., Wang, C., Ye, Z., Chen, H., & Ling, H. (2021). Enhanced network optimized generative adversarial network for image enhancement. *Multimedia Tools and Applications*, *80*(9), 14363–14381. DOI: 10.1007/s11042-020-10310-z

Zhang, P. (2022). Image Enhancement Method Based on Deep Learning. *Mathematical Problems in Engineering*, *2022*, 1–9. Advance online publication. DOI: 10.1155/2022/6797367 PMID: 35781947

Zhang, R., Guo, L., Huang, S., & Wen, B. (2021). ReLLIE: Deep reinforcement learning for customized low-light image enhancement.In *Proceedings of the 29th ACM international conference on multimedia*, pp. 2429-2437. DOI: 10.1145/3474085.3475410

Chapter 6

Integrating Machine Learning With Secure Telemedicine Image Transmission

Sneha Suhasrao Palimkar
https://orcid.org/0000-0001-8014-0342
College of Engineering, Pune Technological University, Pune, India

Sulakshana Sagar Malwade
Dr. Vishwanath Karad MIT World Peace University, Pune, India

Farhadeeba Ilyas Shaikh
Dr. Vishwanath Karad MIT World Peace University, Pune, India

B. Nagalakshmi
Department of Information Technology, Lords Institute of Engineering and Technology, Telangana, India

L. K. Joshila Grace
https://orcid.org/0000-0003-2220-9035
Computer Science and Engineering, Sathyabama Institute of Science and Technology, Chennai, India

Kawerinder Singh Sidhu
https://orcid.org/0000-0002-8910-6279
Uttaranchal Institute of Management, Uttaranchal University, Dehradun, India

ABSTRACT

The rapid development of telemedicine has resulted in the emergence of significant challenges concerning the transmission of medical images in a secure manner. Given the growing reliance of the healthcare industry on digital platforms for diagnosis and treatment, it is of the utmost importance to protect the confidentiality and integrity of sensitive patient data. The application of machine learning (ML) in the context of improving the safety and effectiveness of telemedicine image transmission. By

DOI: 10.4018/979-8-3693-9821-0.ch006

utilizing advanced machine learning techniques, such as dynamic encryption algorithms, real-time anomaly detection, and adaptive security protocols, healthcare providers are able to better protect themselves against cybersecurity threats while simultaneously ensuring that they have timely access to high-quality medical images.

INTRODUCTION

Telemedicine is a crucial component of healthcare since it allows patients to share their medical records with medical professionals, facilitating remote diagnosis, consultations, and treatment. Transmission of diagnostic images, including MRIs, CT scans, and X-rays, is a crucial aspect of telemedicine (Pandey, B. K., & Pandey, D., 2025). The accuracy of diagnosis depends on these images, but in order to protect patient privacy and data integrity, secure and effective transmission methods are needed. Resolving the issues of privacy, efficiency, and transmission speed through the integration of machine learning (ML) with secure telemedicine image transmission is becoming increasingly apparent. Health-related photos are a prime target for cyberattacks because they hold extremely sensitive data. Traditionally, these transmissions have been secured via encryption techniques like RSA or the Advanced Encryption Standard (AES). Yet, these traditional encryption methods can be computationally costly and susceptible to sophisticated attacks, particularly when handling massive amounts of data in real-time. Machine learning can be useful in this situation. ML can improve encryption techniques by allowing more resilient and adaptable protection against data breaches by dynamically modifying security protocols based on real-time threat analysis. Machine learning also increases image transmission efficiency in addition to security. Reducing the bandwidth needed for transmission by compressing medical images without sacrificing quality is possible with machine learning algorithms, especially in the field of image processing. doctors can work with clearer images by optimizing image quality using deep learning techniques like convolutional neural networks (CNNs), which reduce noise and enhance critical features. The speed and dependability of telemedicine services are increased by these ML-driven procedures, which also enhance the diagnostic value of images by cutting down on transmission times. To further identify and stop cybersecurity risks during picture transmission, machine learning can be incorporated into telemedicine platform. Anomaly detection algorithms allow for real-time threat detection and response by scanning data streams for anomalous patterns that might point to a cyberattack. The dynamic adaptation of security measures, such as encryption and data protection, can be ensured by using reinforcement learning models in response to emerging threats. In order to protect private medical data from potential hackers, this provides an additional layer of security to the telemedicine ecosystem.

Limitations in Telemedicine Image Transmission Security

- *Vulnerability to Cyberattacks*: Medical images conveyed through telemedicine platforms are prime targets for cyberattacks, including hacking, data breaches, and ransomware. These platforms manage sensitive patient information, such as medical history and diagnostic images, rendering them appealing targets for cybercriminals aiming to exploit the value of healthcare data. Man-in-the-middle attacks, in which adversaries intercept and potentially modify medical data during transmission, present considerable risks. An altered image may result in erroneous diagnoses or postponed treatments, adversely affecting patient care. The increase in ransomware attacks within the healthcare sector underscores the susceptibility of telemedicine platforms. Perpetrators encrypt medical images and demand ransom payments for access restoration. These incidents not only disrupt healthcare services but also subject healthcare organizations to financial losses, legal repercussions, and reputational harm. Numerous telemedicine platforms lack robust defenses against these intricate attacks, rendering them susceptible to data exfiltration and operational disruptions.
- *Inadequate Encryption Standards*: Numerous telemedicine platforms continue to employ obsolete or inadequate encryption protocols that fail to ensure the necessary security for safeguarding sensitive medical information. Despite the availability of more advanced encryption methods such as TLS (Transport Layer Security), encryption techniques like SSL (Secure Sockets Layer), which possess known vulnerabilities, continue to be utilized. Inadequate encryption enables attackers to exploit vulnerabilities and obtain unauthorized access to sensitive information, jeopardizing patient confidentiality. Encryption techniques that are presently considered secure may become susceptible as computational capabilities advance. The emergence of quantum computing (Khadka, M. et al., 2025) poses a significant risk to conventional encryption techniques, such as RSA, which depends on the complexity of factoring large integers. Telemedicine platforms face the risk of compromise from future technological advancements if they do not adopt quantum-resistant encryption techniques (Pryor, L. et al., 2021).
- *Latency and Computational Costs*: Encryption algorithms intended to safeguard medical images frequently entail heightened computational expenses. Advanced encryption techniques, although exceptionally secure, necessitate considerable processing power to encrypt and decrypt extensive medical images in real-time (Sheela, M. S. et al., 2025). This leads to heightened latency, particularly for high-resolution images such as MRIs and CT scans, resulting in transmission delays and potentially hindering patient care. Many

telemedicine platforms encounter the dilemma of balancing security and performance. Besides latency, these computational demands can impose a significant burden on system resources (Satheesh, N. et al., 2025), especially for smaller healthcare facilities or telemedicine platforms with constrained infrastructure. This complicates the scalability of these platforms without substantial investment in high-performance computing resources (Kumar, M. S. et al., 2025), thereby increasing operational costs. Consequently, certain platforms may utilize inferior encryption techniques to prevent performance decline, thereby jeopardizing data security (Konapure, C. G. et al., 2025).

- *Data Integrity Risks*: Maintaining data integrity during transmission poses a significant challenge for telemedicine platforms. Medical images may be compromised, modified, or entirely lost during transmission due to network complications, file compression inaccuracies, or malicious interference (Singh, S. et al., 2025a). Corrupted images can result in misinterpretation by healthcare providers, leading to misdiagnosis or unsuitable treatments. For instance, absent or modified data in an X-ray may lead a physician to neglect a fracture or tumor. Threats to data integrity (Singh, S. et al., 2025b) are not always readily apparent, and healthcare providers may inadvertently base decisions on erroneous data. Platforms devoid of robust integrity-checking mechanisms, such as hash functions or digital signatures, are especially susceptible. In the absence of these safeguards, medical images may be altered during transit, whether inadvertently or with intent, resulting in diminished diagnostic quality and jeopardizing patient safety (Siddiqui, N. et al., 2021).
- *Interoperability Problems*: Telemedicine platforms frequently employ various communication protocols, encryption techniques, and security standards. The absence of standardization results in interoperability challenges when medical images must be exchanged among various healthcare systems or platforms (Pandey, B. K. et al., 2024a). For example, if one platform employs an outdated encryption standard while another utilizes more sophisticated protocols, the secure transmission of data between these platforms becomes challenging, thereby heightening the risk of vulnerabilities (Pandey, B. K. et al., 2024b). Interoperability challenges impede the transfer of medical data, as systems may necessitate supplementary processing to convert files or re-encrypt data to adhere to varying security standards. This not only jeopardizes security but also postpones essential diagnoses and treatments, especially in emergencies where rapid decision-making is imperative (Maheshwari, R. U. et al., 2024). A cohesive strategy for encryption and data transmission standards in telemedicine would alleviate these risks

Figure 1. Telemedicine image transmission security limitations

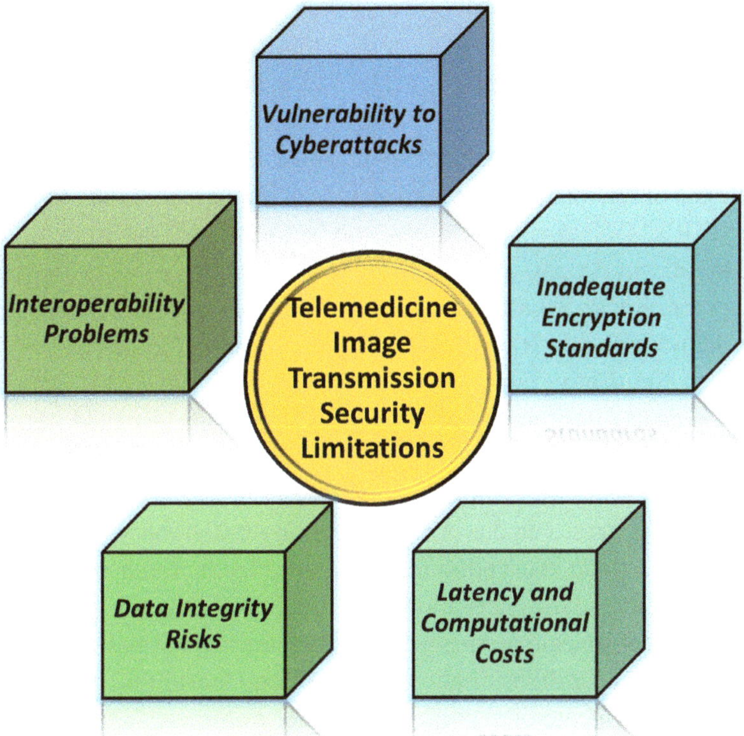

There are a number of limitations that are associated with the security of telemedicine image transmission. These limitations, which are illustrated in Figure 1, pose risks to patient data and privacy. One of the most significant problems is the susceptibility to cyberattacks, which can result in data breaches and the disclosure of sensitive information if these attacks are carried out without authorization. Interoperability issues are caused by the fact that different systems use different standards and protocols, which makes it more difficult to exchange data (Maheshwari, R. Uma. et al., 2024) in a secure manner. Inadequate encryption standards can make it possible for information to be intercepted while images are being transmitted (Saxena, A. et al., 2024). In addition, there is a possibility that data integrity will be compromised if images are changed while they are being transmitted, which could result in incorrect diagnoses. The latency and computational costs that are associated with security measures may impede the transmission of images in real time, which will have an effect on the overall efficiency of telemedicine services.

Transforming Security and Efficiency in Transmission

Machine learning (ML) (Rai, P. K. et al., 2024) is quickly becoming a game-changer in the field of telemedicine, helping to address many of the challenges that traditional methods are unable to effectively manage (Lakshmi, K. V. N. et al., 2024). This includes both the efficiency of transmission and the security of the data. Through the use of telemedicine, sensitive medical information, such as diagnostic images like MRIs, CT scans, and X-rays, can be transmitted securely. In order to protect the privacy of patients and maintain the integrity of their data, these images are necessary for remote diagnosis; however, these images require stringent security measures (Saravanakumar, R. et al., 2024). Additionally, the large size of these medical images frequently results in slow transmission speeds, which can make it difficult to implement real-time consultations and emergency medical interventions. In order to improve the safety and effectiveness of image transmission, machine learning provides potentially useful solutions. Traditional methods of encryption are less adaptable and less resilient than machine learning-based encryption algorithms. When compared to static encryption methods, machine learning models have the ability to dynamically adjust encryption protocols in response to evolving threats.

This provides real-time protection against cyberattacks such as data breaches and ransomware. Other capabilities of anomaly detection algorithms that are powered by machine learning include the ability to monitor transmission activity, identify irregular patterns, and flag potential threats before they compromise sensitive data. ML-driven image compression techniques have the potential to significantly reduce the size of medical images (Kumarganesh, S. et al., 2024) without compromising their quality, which is a significant performance improvement. The utilization of bandwidth is optimized as a result of this, which guarantees faster transmission times. This is especially important in time-sensitive situations such as emergency care. There are also other deep learning techniques, such as convolutional neural networks (CNNs) that are used to improve image quality. These techniques include reducing noise and sharpening critical features, as well as improving diagnostic accuracy while maintaining fast and secure data transmission throughout the process (Shreyas, K. K. et al., 2017).

TECHNOLOGICAL LANDSCAPE OF TELEMEDICINE

Development of Telemedicine Platforms

The development of telemedicine platforms has revolutionized the delivery of healthcare by making it possible to conduct diagnostics and consultations remotely. In the beginning, telemedicine was a crude form of communication that relied on basic technologies such as telephone calls and fax machines to transmit medical information (Muralidhar, L. B. et al., 2024). The functionality of these early systems was restricted, and they offered only a minimal level of integration with clinical workflows. As a result, patient care was frequently fragmented. Telemedicine platforms have evolved to incorporate video conferencing tools and secure messaging systems as technology has advanced. This has made it possible for patients and healthcare providers to interact in real time with one another (Pandey, B. K. et al., 2024c). This change was a significant improvement because it made it possible to conduct consultations that were more comprehensive. Because of the proliferation of internet-based platforms (Pandey, B. K. et al., 2024d), healthcare providers now have access to a wider variety of tools to manage patient care. These tools include electronic health records (EHRs) and patient management systems. The integration of these technologies was frequently restricted, which resulted in problems with interoperability and inefficiencies in the exchange of patient data. Cloud-based architectures made it possible to create solutions that were both scalable and flexible, which in turn enabled healthcare organizations to safely store and access vast amounts of data (Elarmathi, S. et al., 2024). Mobile applications further expanded access by enabling patients to participate in virtual visits using their mobile devices, such as smartphones or tablets. Because of these developments, there was a significant increase in the utilization of telehealth, particularly during the COVID-19 pandemic, when remote consultations became indispensable for the continuation of healthcare delivery. Artificial intelligence (AI), machine learning (ML), and data analytics are some of the advanced features that are now being incorporated into modern telemedicine platforms in order to improve patient care (Shelton, J. et al., 2018). These platforms make use of algorithms that are driven by artificial intelligence to perform tasks such as triaging patients, automating appointment scheduling, and analyzing medical images in order to make diagnoses more quickly (Pandey, B. K. et al., 2024e). Additionally, the utilization of interoperable standards and protocols, such as HL7 and DICOM, has resulted in an improvement in the seamless exchange of medical data across various systems, which has led to an increase in the level of collaboration among healthcare providers.

Medical Images Transmitted in Telemedicine

When it comes to facilitating remote diagnosis, treatment, and patient monitoring, telemedicine is dependent on the transmission of a wide variety of medical images (JayaLakshmi, G. et al., 2024). When it comes to patient care, each type of image serves a distinct purpose, and it is essential for medical professionals to have access to all of these images in order to make educated decisions. Figure 2 shows the primary categories of medical images that are typically transmitted through telemedicine. Telemedicine encompasses a wide range of medical images, each of which plays an important part in the treatment of patients. As a result of the efficient transmission of these images, medical professionals will be able to make precise diagnoses and administer treatment in a timely manner, which will ultimately lead to improved patient outcomes.

1. *X-rays*: In the field of telemedicine, X-rays are among the most frequently employed imaging techniques. They are primarily employed for the purpose of diagnosing bone fractures, infections, and other conditions that affect the skeletal system. Because they can be obtained in a reasonable amount of time and can be transmitted in an effective manner, they are suitable for use in remote consultations. Because digital X-ray technology enables immediate image acquisition and sharing, it is an indispensable tool in emergency situations where prompt diagnosis is of the utmost importance (George, W. K. et al., 2024). Furthermore, developments in image enhancement technologies have made it possible for medical professionals to obtain images that are clearer, which has led to an increase in the diagnostic accuracy of remote evaluations.
2. *Computerized Tomography (CT) scans*: By providing detailed cross-sectional images of the body, computed tomography (CT) scans make it possible to visualize internal organs, tissues, and structures. On the other hand, they are especially helpful in the diagnosis of conditions such as tumors, internal injuries, and infections. Because CT images are larger in size than X-rays, it is necessary to use transmission methods that are both secure and efficient in order to preserve their quality. High-resolution images (Abdullahi, M. et al., 2024) obtained from computed tomography (CT) scans can assist radiologists in recognizing subtle variations in tissue density, which is essential for making accurate diagnoses. In addition, recent developments in cloud computing and telehealth platforms have made it possible for healthcare providers to quickly share CT images with one another. This has made it easier for healthcare providers to work together and make decisions in a timely manner (Istiaque Ahmed, K. et al., 2021).

3. *Magnetic resonance imaging* (MRI): In order to generate detailed images of organs and soft tissues, magnetic resonance imaging (MRI) makes use of powerful magnetic fields and radio waves. When it comes to diagnosing neurological disorders, injuries to the musculoskeletal system, and other internal conditions, it is of great value. As a result of their large file sizes, the high-resolution images that are produced by magnetic resonance imaging (MRI) machines are essential for accurate diagnosis; however, they can present difficulties when it comes to transmission. In order to overcome these challenges, sophisticated compression algorithms are frequently utilized to reduce the size of the file without compromising the quality of the image. Furthermore, remote access to MRI images enables specialists located in different locations to work together on complex cases, which improves the quality of patient care and the planning of treatment.
4. *Ultrasound Images*: The use of sound waves to create images of soft tissues and organs is what makes ultrasound imaging a diagnostic tool that is both non-invasive and versatile. In addition to its use in cardiology, urology, and other fields, it is frequently employed in the field of obstetrics for the purpose of monitoring the development of the fetus. As a result of their small size and the speed with which they can be transmitted, ultrasound images are ideally suited for use in telemedicine applications. It is possible for medical professionals to conduct point-of-care ultrasounds, which enables them to evaluate patients in real time during virtual consultations. Developments in mobile ultrasound technology have made it possible for medical professionals to capture and transmit high-quality images directly from the location of the patient, which has resulted in an increase in access to care.
5. *Pathology Slides*: The process of digital pathology involves transforming conventional glass slides into digital images that can be analyzed remotely by pathologists. Due to the fact that they enable a more in-depth examination of tissue samples, these images are extremely important for the diagnosis of diseases such as cancer. In order to maintain diagnostic accuracy, the transmission of pathology images must ensure a high resolution. This is because even minute details in the architecture of the tissue can have a significant impact on the diagnosis. By facilitating collaborative reviews, digital pathology platforms make it possible for pathologists located in different locations to consult on difficult cases and share their insights. Additionally, the incorporation of machine learning algorithms into digital pathology can be of assistance in recognizing patterns and irregularities in tissue samples, thereby enhancing the diagnostic efficiency and accuracy (Lütkepohl, H., 2010).

6. *Electrocardiograms*, (ECGs): The fact that they are not conventional images, electrocardiograms (ECGs) offer vital information regarding the electrical activity of the heart. These signals can be transmitted as graphical representations, which enables medical professionals to evaluate the health of the heart from a remote location. Continuous electrocardiogram monitoring can be an essential component for patients who are experiencing cardiovascular issues, as it enables timely interventions. The transmission of electrocardiogram (ECG) data in real time is made possible by telemedicine platforms. This data can then be analyzed by cardiologists in order to identify irregularities such as arrhythmias or signs of ischemia. The capability of remotely monitoring the heart health of patients reduces the need for in-person visits and makes it possible to take preventative measures to manage cardiovascular conditions.
7. *Dermatological Images*: It is possible to transmit high-resolution images of skin lesions, rashes, or other dermatological conditions in order to conduct distance consultations with dermatologists. The diagnosis of skin conditions, the determination of whether or not additional treatment is required, and the monitoring of the efficacy of treatments are all aided by these images. Patients are able to submit images in a secure manner through tele dermatology platforms, which enables dermatologists to review and provide feedback without the need for an in-person visit. This method is especially helpful for patients who live in remote areas and have limited access to specialized medical care. Through the analysis of images and the provision of preliminary evaluations based on predetermined criteria, the application of AI algorithms in dermatology can also be of assistance in the diagnosis of conditions.
8. *Retinal Images*: Fundus photography is a technique that takes pictures of the retina and other parts of the eye's interior surface. When it comes to diagnosing conditions such as diabetic retinopathy and macular degeneration, these images are absolutely necessary. Through the use of telemedicine, retinal images can be evaluated remotely, which makes timely interventions possible and reduces the likelihood of vision loss. Innovative imaging technologies, such as optical coherence tomography (OCT), offer even more granularity, which enables medical professionals to evaluate the layers of the retina and identify the earliest indications of disease. Patients are able to receive comprehensive eye care without having to travel long distances thanks to the incorporation of teleophthalmology into telemedicine platforms. This helps to significantly improve access to specialized services.

Figure 2. Telemedicine medical image types

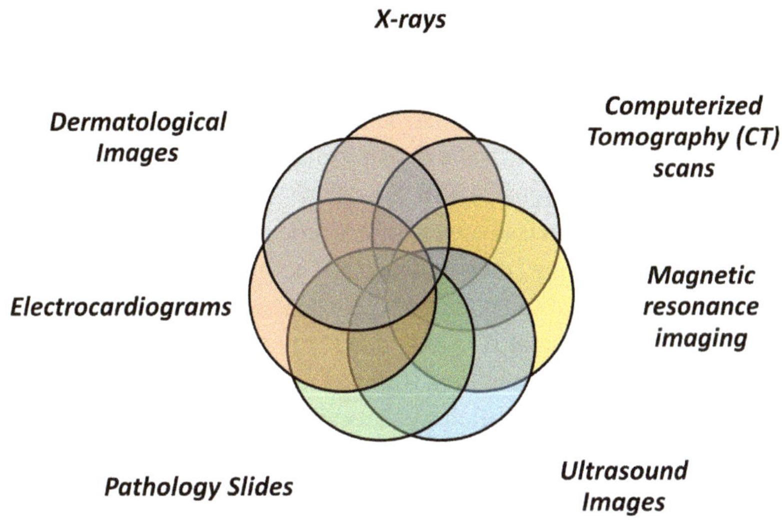

Digital Communication Protocols in Telemedicine

Digital communication protocols (Kumar, B. et al., 2024) are essential for medical image and data exchange in telemedicine's fast-changing landscape. These protocols allow healthcare providers to communicate, collaborate, and access vital information remotely. DICOM and PACS are dominant standards in this field. Modern telemedicine infrastructure relies on these frameworks to improve healthcare delivery. Medical image storage, transmission, and retrieval are governed by DICOM. To promote medical imaging device and software interoperability, NEMA created DICOM. Before DICOM, medical imaging was unstandardized, making it difficult to share and access images across systems, which slowed diagnosis and cooperative care. The DICOM standard allows X-ray, CT, MRI, and ultrasound images to be shared (Pandey, D. et al., 2024a). Multiple manufacturers' devices can work together because the standard specifies file formats and network protocols. Each DICOM file contains the image, patient data, acquisition parameters, and image orientation. This comprehensive data packaging lets healthcare providers access image details for clinical decision-making. Multiple imaging and treatment modalities are one of DICOM's advantages. It is compatible with digital radiography, computed tomography, magnetic resonance imaging, and nuclear medicine. This flexibility lets healthcare institutions add new imaging modalities without major system changes.

DICOM supports the transfer of non-image data like radiology reports and patient demographics, improving healthcare system communication. DIC allows efficient integration with other healthcare information systems like EHRs and LIS by standardizing data format and communication protocols.

Complex PACS stores, transmits, and manages medical images and data. Healthcare providers can access images from various imaging modalities in it. Telemedicine relies on PACS to remotely access and share images as well as collaborate with specialists in different locations. A PACS system's core is its DICOM-compliant imaging device interface. Images are captured, processed, and stored in PACS using DICOM standards during imaging studies. The integration organizes images, making patient data retrieval and review easy for healthcare providers. Clinical staff can search for images by patient ID, study date, or modality type in PACS systems' user-friendly interfaces.By eliminating film and manual image handling, PACS is a major benefit. In traditional radiology, developing, storing, and retrieving film images was laborious. Automating these processes with PACS speeds up diagnosis and image access. Rapid image access can improve patient outcomes in emergencies, making efficiency crucial.

Advanced PACS features include image manipulation and analysis. Radiologists can use these tools to set contrast, zoom in, and apply filters to improve image clarity. More accurate interpretations improve remote diagnostic services. By letting healthcare professionals' access and share images from anywhere with an internet connection (Pandey, D. et al., 2024b), PACS systems enable multi-disciplinary collaboration. Telemedicine allows specialists to review cases remotely, making this capability useful. Images can be shared securely and quickly between radiologists, primary care physicians, and other specialists to improve patient evaluations and treatment plans.

Integrating DICOM and PACS has changed telemedicine by allowing medical images to be shared across healthcare settings. In telemedicine, DICOM secures and standardizes image transmission, while PACS stores and retrieves them. DICOM and PACS streamline workflows, allowing healthcare providers to quickly locate patient data. A primary care doctor can refer a patient to a specialist. Through PACS, the primary care provider can share the patient's imaging studies with the specialist before the consultation. After this pre-evaluation, the telemedicine visit can focus on specific questions and examination. The integration of AI and machine learning with DICOM and PACS is also improving telemedicine. AI algorithms (Kennedy, G. W. et al., 2024) can help radiologists spot anomalies in medical images. Automation improves diagnostic accuracy and frees up doctors to treat more complex cases. Although DICOM and PACS have many benefits in telemedicine, they also have drawbacks. Internet transmission of sensitive patient data raises data security and privacy concerns (Shahul, A. et al., 2024). Patient data must be protected during transmission and storage by encryption and secure access protocols in healthcare organizations. When hospitals use multiple PACS vendors, system interoperability can be difficult. Continuous stakeholder collaboration is needed to achieve widespread interoperability, but standardization efforts are underway to improve compatibility and system communication.

MACHINE LEARNING IN MEDICAL IMAGE OPTIMIZATION

ML for Image Denoising, Compression, and Storage

Image processing has undergone a revolution thanks to ML for image denoising, compression, and storage optimization machine learning (ML), which provides cutting-edge methods for compression, storage optimization, and image denoising. These applications are especially important for telemedicine, where precise diagnosis and effective data management depend on high-quality images. When it comes to medical imaging, where clarity is crucial, denoising tries to eliminate noise from images without sacrificing any significant details. Image integrity is frequently compromised by traditional denoising techniques, particularly when signal-to-noise ratios are low. Nevertheless, machine learning (ML) algorithms in particular, deep learning models like convolutional neural networks (CNNs) have demonstrated impressive success in this field. Large datasets of both clean and noisy images are used to train these models so they can distinguish between noise and actual image features (Pandey, D. et al., 2024c). They can therefore efficiently restore high-quality images, improving telemedicine's diagnostic precision. Machine learning has a big impact on image compression, which is necessary for the effective transmission and storage of medical images. Especially in high-resolution images, conventional compression methods like JPEG and PNG can lose significant information. Conversely, machine learning (ML)-based techniques for compression, like autoencoders and generative adversarial networks (GANs), maximize compression by discovering the inherent structures in the data (Pandey, D., & Pandey, B. K., 2022). These methods can reduce bandwidth usage and storage requirements in telemedicine applications by achieving higher compression ratios without sacrificing image quality. Healthcare organizations can better manage their resources by using machine learning (ML) algorithms to forecast future storage requirements and analyze usage patterns in the field of storage optimization. Organizations can optimize storage costs and improve overall system performance by implementing intelligent data management systems that prioritize the storage of frequently accessed images while archiving less critical data.

Image Clarity and Reducing Noise with ML

Artificial neural network (Pandey, B. K., & Pandey, D., 2023) has emerged as a transformative influence in medical imaging, especially in enhancing image clarity and minimizing noise, which are essential for attaining superior diagnostic results. Noise in medical images can obscure critical details, hindering healthcare professionals' ability to accurately interpret results. Utilizing advanced machine learning algorithms, medical professionals can augment image quality, thereby enhancing diagnostic precision and patient care. A principal method utilized in machine learning for image denoising is the application of convolutional neural networks (CNNs). These networks are engineered to discern hierarchical patterns in data and can proficiently distinguish between noise and significant image features. Throughout the training process, CNNs are presented with pairs of noisy and pristine images, allowing them to acquire the ability to restore the original clarity of the images. Upon completion of training, these models can eliminate noise from new images while maintaining essential details, a capability that is especially beneficial in radiology, pathology, and other domains where accuracy is crucial. Machine learning algorithms can adjust to the distinct attributes of various imaging modalities, including MRI, CT, and ultrasound. Every modality possesses distinct noise profiles and artifacts, which can complicate the denoising procedure. By customizing machine learning models to the distinct needs of each imaging modality, healthcare providers can realize substantial enhancements in image quality. Improved image clarity enables more precise diagnoses, allowing physicians to easily detect abnormalities, evaluate disease progression, and track treatment efficacy. Enhancing image quality via machine learning not only improves diagnostic results but also optimizes the overall workflow in clinical environments. Enhanced imaging allows radiologists and other specialists to minimize the duration required for result interpretation, resulting in expedited turnaround times for patient diagnoses and treatment strategies. This efficiency is particularly vital in emergency situations where prompt decisions can greatly influence patient outcomes.

Integrating ML with Edge Computing

Medical imaging and telemedicine have advanced by combining machine learning (ML) with edge computing for on-device image processing. Data is processed closer to the source with edge computing rather than cloud servers. In healthcare, real-time image processing is crucial, so this method has many benefits. Latency reduction is a major benefit of edge computing. In time-sensitive medical applications like remote diagnostics and tele-surgery, even minor delays can be disastrous. Healthcare providers can get immediate feedback by processing images on smartphones, tablets, or portable imaging equipment. Clinicians can act quickly based on image insights with this capability. Edge computing with ML improves real-time image analysis. Edge devices can perform image classification, segmentation, and denoising without internet connectivity using advanced algorithms. A portable ultrasound machine can analyze images on its own, identifying abnormalities and pathologies and providing immediate results to the clinician. This is especially useful in rural or underserved areas with unreliable internet access. On-device processing also improves patient data security and privacy. Process sensitive medical images locally to reduce data breaches during transmission to centralized servers. In healthcare, HIPAA compliance is essential. Minimizing data transfer and processing locally helps healthcare organizations control patient data. Integrating ML with edge computing allows it to operate in resource-constrained environments. Not all healthcare facilities, especially in developing countries, have powerful cloud infrastructure. These conditions allow healthcare providers to use advanced imaging technologies without IT support or infrastructure using edge devices with ML algorithms. Evolutionary machine learning models can be optimized for edge computing environments to remain lightweight and efficient. Model pruning, quantization, and knowledge distillation allow edge devices to run robust ML models without sacrificing performance. This adaptability lets devices with limited computational power use advanced ML image processing algorithms.

ML-DRIVEN ENCRYPTION AND IMAGE SECURITY

Dynamic encryption algorithms in medical image transmission can now be improved with the help of deep learning techniques. It's possible that static algorithms used in traditional encryption techniques won't change to meet new cybersecurity threats. Deep learning, on the other hand, can make encryption systems more resilient and adaptable. With the ability to examine enormous volumes of data and spot trends and abnormalities, deep learning models can dynamically modify encryption settings in response to threats as they arise. To detect changes in data patterns that might point to a security breach, for example, convolutional neural networks (CNNs) can be trained. This allows the system to adjust its encryption keys or algorithms appropriately. Patient data is shielded from unwanted access thanks to this dynamic approach, which improves the security of private medical images during transmission. Since any unauthorized access or data tampering can have serious consequences, real-time anomaly detection is essential for spotting suspicious activities in medical image transmission. By continuously observing data transmission patterns, machine learning algorithms can be trained to create a baseline of typical activity. Models can be trained from labeled datasets with both normal and anomalous behavior using techniques like supervised learning. After they are put into use, these models can identify when patterns change, highlighting anomalous behavior like illegal access attempts, corrupted data, or anomalous data transfer volumes. Healthcare companies can reduce the risk of data breaches and guarantee the integrity of transmitted medical images by promptly responding to possible threats by implementing real-time anomaly detection. By enabling systems to learn from their interactions with the environment, reinforcement learning (RL) provides a novel way to improve adaptive security in telemedicine protocols. Using RL, security protocols in telemedicine can be optimized based on continuous threat and vulnerability assessments. For instance, an RL agent can monitor security conditions continuously and modify data-sharing permissions, encryption levels, and access controls in response to real-time risk identification.

Telemedicine systems can react proactively to new threats thanks to this adaptive security approach, which guarantees the security of patient data. Furthermore, reinforcement learning can lessen the impact of upcoming cybersecurity threats in telemedicine by learning from previous incidents and modifying strategies accordingly. Medical image data can be used to predict and prevent emerging cybersecurity threats with the help of artificial intelligence (AI) models. AI algorithms are able to predict potential security risks and vulnerabilities by analyzing historical data and identifying trends. Incoming data streams can be examined for indications of possible threats using techniques like anomaly detection, predictive analytics, and machine learning classification. For example, a model may identify an anomalous pattern in the medical image data access logs and raise the alarm for a possible security breach, thereby triggering an instant investigation. By automating reactions to threats detected, such as temporarily blocking access to sensitive data or notifying security personnel, AI can improve preventive measures. Healthcare companies can reinforce their defenses against new and emerging threats by incorporating AI models into their cybersecurity plans. This will guarantee that medical image data is kept safe and only available to authorized personnel.

ML IN TRANSMISSION SPEED AND DATA REDUCTION

Enhancing bandwidth utilization is a paramount issue in medical imaging, where substantial file sizes can impede effective data transmission. Compression techniques powered by machine learning provide novel solutions to this challenge. Conventional compression techniques frequently encounter difficulties in achieving a balance between minimizing file size and maintaining image quality. Nonetheless, machine learning algorithms, especially deep learning methodologies, can evaluate image attributes and acquire optimal compression techniques. Autoencoders and generative adversarial networks (GANs) can be employed to compress medical images by discerning and preserving critical features while discarding superfluous data. This adaptive compression method not only diminishes file sizes but also preserves essential diagnostic information. By optimizing bandwidth utilization, healthcare providers can facilitate expedited image transmission, thereby enhancing collaboration and improving patient care. Real-time image encoding and decoding are crucial for facilitating rapid and efficient transmission of medical images. Convolutional neural networks (CNNs) are being utilized to substantially improve this process. Conventional encoding methods frequently utilize intricate algorithms that may cause delays in image transmission. However, deep learning models can streamline the encoding and decoding processes by learning to process and compress images more efficiently. For instance, CNNs can be trained to directly encode images into lower-dimensional representations while maintaining essential features, facilitating faster transmission times. These models can swiftly reconstruct high-quality images from compressed data, reducing delays and enhancing the overall efficiency of telemedicine applications. Healthcare organizations can leverage deep learning for real-time encoding and decoding to guarantee prompt access to essential medical images, facilitating expedited clinical decisions.

Generative models are essential for error correction in the transmission of medical images, tackling issues of data corruption and loss. Errors may arise during image transmission over networks due to bandwidth fluctuations or interference, potentially compromising the integrity of the received images. Generative models, specifically Generative Adversarial Networks (GANs) and Variational Autoencoders (VAEs), can be utilized to address these challenges. These models can acquire the ability to produce credible images from training data, enabling them to reconstruct or rectify corrupted images during transmission. For example, if an image is afflicted with artifacts or is partially compromised, a generative model can evaluate the intact sections and generate the absent or damaged areas based on acquired patterns. This feature guarantees that healthcare providers obtain superior images for diagnosis, even in difficult transmission conditions. Achieving a balance between image quality and transmission speed is essential in medical imaging, particularly in situations necessitating rapid access to high-resolution images. Machine learning methodologies provide novel solutions to attain this equilibrium.

Through the utilization of adaptive algorithms, machine learning can dynamically modify image compression levels in accordance with network conditions and the significance of the transmitted images. In high-demand scenarios, such as emergency care, the system can enhance speed by applying greater compression to non-essential images, while maintaining superior quality for critical diagnostic images. This capability to concurrently optimize image quality and transmission speed guarantees that clinicians receive timely information, thereby enhancing patient outcomes and improving the efficiency of telemedicine services.

CONCLUSION

Image transmission security and efficiency have been greatly improved by machine learning, which has become a revolutionary force in the field of telemedicine. Machine learning (ML) tackles the inherent challenges that are associated with medical image data, such as ensuring that data integrity is maintained, optimizing bandwidth usage, and maintaining high image quality. This is accomplished through the utilization of complex algorithms and analytical methods. The integration of ML into telemedicine platforms strengthens security measures and protects sensitive patient data through real-time anomaly detection systems that identify suspicious activities and dynamic encryption techniques that adjust to threats in real-time. Real-time encoding and decoding skills and compression techniques enabled by machine learning (ML) enhance image transmission efficiency, guaranteeing healthcare providers timely access to vital diagnostic data. With machine learning and artificial intelligence developing at a rapid pace, telemedicine and secure healthcare platforms will likely change in the future. Improved capabilities in anomaly detection, predictive analytics, and adaptive security measures are to be expected as these technologies advance. Strong and safe telemedicine solutions will also be required due to the rising demand for remote healthcare services, which has been exacerbated by recent global health incidents. Healthcare companies can protect their systems from new cybersecurity threats and continue to offer patients high-quality care by utilizing machine learning. Future healthcare delivery will probably look different as a result of the continued integration of ML in telemedicine, which is expected to streamline clinical workflows, improve patient outcomes, and create a more secure environment.

REFERENCES

Abdullahi, M., Ahmad, A., Pandey, B. K., & Pandey, D. (2024). Digital Currency Adoption: A Comparative Analysis of Global Trends and the Nigerian eNaira Digital Currency. *SN Computer Science*, *5*(5), 1–11. DOI: 10.1007/s42979-024-02882-6

Elarmathi, S., Rishabavarthani, P., Sindhuja, M., Elayaraja, P., & Malathi Murugesan, S. (2024). Novel manufacturing systems for cancer diagnosis using ultra-sensitive photonic crystal fiber biosensor with dual-functionalized aptamer-nanocavity. *Microsystem Technologies*, •••, 1–20. DOI: 10.1007/s00542-024-05820-x

George, W. K., Silas, E. I., Pandey, D., & Pandey, B. K. (2024). Utilization of Industry 4.0 Technologies in Nigerian Technical and Vocational Education: A Conundrum for Educators. In *Examining the Rapid Advance of Digital Technology in Africa* (pp. 270–293). IGI Global. DOI: 10.4018/978-1-6684-9962-7.ch014

Istiaque Ahmed, K., Tahir, M., Hadi Habaebi, M., Lun Lau, S., & Ahad, A. (2021). Machine learning for authentication and authorization in iot: Taxonomy, challenges and future research direction. *Sensors (Basel)*, *21*(15), 5122. DOI: 10.3390/s21155122 PMID: 34372360

JayaLakshmi. G., Pandey, D., Pandey, B. K., Kaur, P., Mahajan, D. A., & Dari, S. S. (2024). Smart big data collection for intelligent supply chain improvement. In AI and Machine Learning Impacts in Intelligent Supply Chain (pp. 180-195). IGI Global Scientific Publishing.

Kennedy, G. W., Sunday, S. E., Pandey, D., Kabari, A. D., Pandey, B. K., George, A. S., & Dadheech, P. (2024). Building Information Modeling: Harnessing Innovations for Professional Proficiency. In Emerging Engineering Technologies and Industrial Applications (pp. 305-331). IGI Global.

Khadka, M., Sah, M., Chaudhary, R., Sahani, S. K., Sahani, K., Pandey, B. K., & Pandey, D. (2025). Spectroscopic, quantum chemical, and topological calculations of the phenylephrine molecule using density functional theory. *Scientific Reports*, *15*(1), 208. DOI: 10.1038/s41598-024-81633-2 PMID: 39747169

. Konapure, C. G., Pandey, D., Shete, H., Thakar, C. M., Pandey, B. K., & George, A. S. (2025). Artificial Intelligence in Automated Concrete Mix Design Using Computerized Grading Curves. Interdisciplinary Approaches to AI, Internet of Everything, and Machine Learning, 567-586.

. Kumar, B., Pandey, D., Pandey, B. K., & George, A. S. (2024). Higher Education in the Last Four Decades: A Review of Paradigm Shifts in Policy Frameworks. Design and Implementation of Higher Education Learners' Learning Outcomes (HELLO), 333-348.

Kumar, M. S., Prasanna, P. L., Lalitha, M., Joy, M., Jha, S. S., & Pandey, B. K. (2025). Utilizing the Internet of Everything and Artificial Intelligence for Real-Time Workforce Management. In Role of Internet of Everything (IOE), VLSI Architecture, and AI in Real-Time Systems (pp. 153-168). IGI Global Scientific Publishing.

Kumarganesh, S., & Malathi Murugesan, C. (2024). Hybrid plasmonic biosensors with deep learning for colorectal cancer detection. *Plasmonics*, •••, 1–15. DOI: 10.1007/s11468-024-02568-y

Lakshmi, K. V. N., Rajan, R., Pandey, D., & Pandey, B. K. (2024). Circular economy: A catalyst for economic growth-an empirical study. *Circular Economy and Sustainability*, •••, 1–22.

Lütkepohl, H. (2010). *Impulse response function*. DOI: 10.1057/9780230280830_16

Maheshwari, R., Kumarganesh, S., K v M, S., Gopalakrishnan, A., Selvi, K., Paulchamy, B., Rishabavarthani, P., Sagayam, K. M., Pandey, B. K., & Pandey, D. (2024). Advanced plasmonic resonance-enhanced biosensor for comprehensive real-time detection and analysis of deepfake content. *Plasmonics*, •••, 1–18. DOI: 10.1007/s11468-024-02407-0

Maheshwari, R. U., Paulchamy, B., Pandey, B. K., & Pandey, D. (2024). Enhancing sensing and imaging capabilities through surface plasmon resonance for deepfake image detection. *Plasmonics*, •••, 1–20. DOI: 10.1007/s11468-024-02492-1

Muralidhar, L. B., Lakshmi, K. V. N., Swapna, H. R., Rupani, J., Nethravathi, K., Pandey, B. K., & Pandey, D. (2024). Impact of Organizational Culture on The Level of Corporate Social Responsibility Investments: An Exploratory Study. *Circular Economy and Sustainability*, *4*(3), 1–19. DOI: 10.1007/s43615-024-00371-9

Pandey, B. K., Kanike, U. K., George, A. S., & Pandey, D. (Eds.). (2024d). *AI and machine learning impacts in intelligent supply chain*. IGI Global. DOI: 10.4018/979-8-3693-1347-3

Pandey, B. K., Nassa, V. K., Mukundan, A. P., Mahajan, D. A., Pandey, D., George, A. S., & Dadheech, P. (2024c). An Industry-Focused Traffic System Utilising Internet of Things. In *Emerging Engineering Technologies and Industrial Applications* (pp. 200–213). IGI Global. DOI: 10.4018/979-8-3693-1335-0.ch009

Pandey, B. K., & Pandey, D. (2023). Parametric optimization and prediction of enhanced thermoelectric performance in co-doped CaMnO3 using response surface methodology and neural network. *Journal of Materials Science Materials in Electronics, 34*(21), 1589. DOI: 10.1007/s10854-023-10954-1

Pandey, B. K., & Pandey, D. (2025). Securing healthcare medical image information using advance morphological component analysis, information hiding systems, and hybrid convolutional neural networks on IoMT. *Computers in Biology and Medicine, 185*, 109499. DOI: 10.1016/j.compbiomed.2024.109499 PMID: 39642698

Pandey, B. K., Pandey, D., & Lelisho, M. E. (2024a). Face mask identification with enhanced cuckoo optimization and deep learning-based faster regional neural network. *Scientific Reports, 14*(1), 29719. DOI: 10.1038/s41598-024-78746-z PMID: 39613761

Pandey, B. K., Pandey, D., & Sahani, S. K. (2024b). Autopilot control unmanned aerial vehicle system for sewage defect detection using deep learning. *Engineering Reports*, •••, 12852.

Pandey, B. K., Paramashivan, M. A., Pandey, D., George, A. S., Agarwal, A., Mahajan, D. A., . . . Pramanik, S. (2024e). Future Directions of Digital Twin Architectures for 6G Communication Networks. In Security Issues and Solutions in 6G Communications and Beyond (pp. 197-211). IGI Global.

Pandey, D., Nassa, V. K., Pandey, B. K., Thankachan, B., Dadheech, P., Mahajan, D. A., & George, A. S. (2024a). Artificial Intelligence and Machine Learning and Its Application in the Field of Computational Visual Analysis. In Emerging Engineering Technologies and Industrial Applications (pp. 36-57). IGI Global. DOI: 10.4018/979-8-3693-1335-0.ch003

Pandey, D., & Pandey, B. K. (2022). An efficient deep neural network with adaptive galactic swarm optimization for complex image text extraction. In *Process Mining Techniques for Pattern Recognition* (pp. 121–137). CRC Press. DOI: 10.1201/9781003169550-10

Pandey, D., Pandey, B. K., Nassa, V. K., Mahajan, D. A., George, A. S., & Dadheech, P. (2024c). Optimized Throughput-Based Broadcasting for Next Generation Wireless Networks. In Emerging Engineering Technologies and Industrial Applications (pp. 355-368). IGI Global. DOI: 10.4018/979-8-3693-1335-0.ch018

Pandey, D., Pandey, B. K., Paramashivan, M. A., Mahajan, D. A., Dadheech, P. D., George, A. S., & Hameed, A. S. (2024b). Advanced Digital Data Processing Using Cloud Cryptography: Industrial Applications. In Emerging Engineering Technologies and Industrial Applications (pp. 255-268). IGI Global.

Pryor, L., Dave, R., Seliya, J., & Boone, E. S. (2021, December). Machine learning algorithms in user authentication schemes. In *2021 International Conference on Electrical, Computer and Energy Technologies (ICECET)* (pp. 1-6). IEEE. DOI: 10.1109/ICECET52533.2021.9698440

Rai, P. K., Pandey, D., & Pandey, B. K. (2024). The future of enterprise and innovation is compute as a commodity, or CaaC. *Partners Universal International Research Journal, 3*(2), 89–94.

Saravanakumar, R., TamilSelvi, T., Pandey, D., Pandey, B. K., Mahajan, D. A., & Lelisho, M. E. (2024). Big data processing using hybrid Gaussian mixture model with salp swarm algorithm. *Journal of Big Data, 11*(1), 167. DOI: 10.1186/s40537-024-01015-3

Satheesh, N., Gopisankar, N., Kumarganesh, S., Anthoniraj, S., Saravanakumar, S., & Martin Sagayam, K. (2025). Advanced AI-driven emergency response systems for enhanced vehicle and human safety. *Iran Journal of Computer Science*, •••, 1–16. DOI: 10.1007/s42044-025-00228-w

Saxena, A., Agarwal, A., Pandey, B. K., & Pandey, D. (2024). Examination of the Criticality of Customer Segmentation Using Unsupervised Learning Methods. *Circular Economy and Sustainability, 4*(2), 1–14. DOI: 10.1007/s43615-023-00336-4

Shahul, A., Muniandi, B., Paramashivan, M. A., Pandey, D., Pandey, B. K., Dadheech, P., & George, H. (2024). An Analysis of Algorithms and Methods Based on Image Processing for Medical Applications. In *Emerging Engineering Technologies and Industrial Applications* (pp. 173–186). IGI Global. DOI: 10.4018/979-8-3693-1335-0.ch007

Sheela, M. S., Kumarganesh, S., Pandey, B. K., & Lelisho, M. E. (2025). Integration of silver nanostructures in wireless sensor networks for enhanced biochemical sensing. *Discover Nano, 20*(1), 7. DOI: 10.1186/s11671-024-04159-6 PMID: 39804434

Shelton, J., Rice, C., Singh, J., Jenkins, J., Dave, R., Roy, K., & Chakraborty, S. (2018, August). Palm print authentication on a cloud platform. In 2018 International Conference on Advances in Big Data, Computing and Data Communication Systems (icABCD) (pp. 1-6). IEEE. DOI: 10.1109/ICABCD.2018.8465479

Shreyas, K. K., Rajeev, S., Panetta, K., & Agaian, S. S. (2017, April). Fingerprint authentication using geometric features. In *2017 IEEE International Symposium on Technologies for Homeland Security (HST)* (pp. 1-7). IEEE.

Siddiqui, N., Pryor, L., & Dave, R. (2021). User authentication schemes using machine learning methods—a review. In Proceedings of International Conference on Communication and Computational Technologies: ICCCT 2021 (pp. 703-723). Springer Singapore. DOI: 10.1007/978-981-16-3246-4_54

Singh, S., Madaan, G., Swapna, H. R., Singh, A., Pandey, D., George, A. S., & Pandey, B. K. (2025a). Empowering Connectivity: Exploring the Internet of Things. In Interdisciplinary Approaches to AI, Internet of Everything, and Machine Learning (pp. 89-116). IGI Global Scientific Publishing.

Singh, S., Madaan, G., Swapna, H. R., Singh, A., Pandey, B. K., George, A. S., & Pandey, D. (2025b). Unleashing the Power of AI and Data Analysis: Transforming Insights into Action. In Interdisciplinary Approaches to AI, Internet of Everything, and Machine Learning (pp. 1-24). IGI Global Scientific Publishing.

Chapter 7
Enhancing Machine Learning Efficiency Through Secure Medical Image Sharing

M. Rajkumar
Vellore Institute of Technology, India

Niladri Maiti
https://orcid.org/0000-0001-8014-0342
School of Dentistry, Central Asian University, Tashkent, Uzbekistan

Riddhi Chawla
School of Dentistry, Central Asian University, Tashkent, Uzbekistan

Ripal Ranpara
https://orcid.org/0000-0002-5823-5406
Faculty of Computer Application, Marwadi University, India

R. Yogitha
https://orcid.org/0000-0001-9880-8750
Sathyabama Institute of Science and Technology, India

Pallavi Sagar Deshpande
https://orcid.org/0000-0002-2203-5867
Bharati Vidyapeeth, India

Aakifa Shahul
SRM Medical College, India

ABSTRACT

The development of machine learning applications in the healthcare industry depends on safe medical image sharing. Protecting patient privacy is more difficult but necessary as medical imaging data grows. This paper investigates how to integrate encryption techniques and secure data-sharing methods, like blockchain, to facilitate cross-organizational collaboration while maintaining data privacy. Sensitive patient data is kept in local systems thanks to collaborative models like federated learning,

DOI: 10.4018/979-8-3693-9821-0.ch007

which enable institutions to train machine learning algorithms on decentralized datasets. This strategy makes use of the variety of data available across healthcare facilities while protecting the privacy of medical records. The creation of machine learning models for diagnosis and treatment planning that are more reliable and accurate is made possible by the safe interchange of medical images.

INTRODUCTION

Machine learning models are being used more and more in medical image analysis to diagnose diseases and plan treatments. However, access to sizable, varied datasets is necessary for these models to function well and be accurate (Pandey, B. K., & Pandey, D., 2025). Strict privacy laws pertaining to medical data, like HIPAA and GDPR, which restrict the sharing of patient information, including medical images, present a significant obstacle to the creation of such datasets. Beyond these constraints, secure medical image sharing is critical to improving machine learning effectiveness. Encryption techniques, which safeguard patient privacy and guarantee that only authorized parties can access medical images, are among the main solutions for safe sharing. Federated learning is a newer method that allows collaboration without direct data sharing by training machine learning models locally at different healthcare facilities. This decentralized setup (Khadka, M. et al., 2025) preserves privacy while still allowing institutions to benefit from larger datasets because only model updates rather than the actual data are shared between them. Artificial neural network (Pandey, B. K., & Pandey, D., 2023) based blockchain technology also provides a means of guaranteeing traceable, transparent, and safe image sharing amongst healthcare systems. Data integrity is maintained by recording any modifications or access to medical images on blockchain's immutable ledger. Another method that enables multiple institutions to work together on machine learning model training while maintaining the privacy of their data is secure multi-party computation (MPC) (Sheela, M. S. et al., 2025). Secure medical image sharing improves the performance of machine learning models by providing access to larger datasets. This is essential for developing more generalized models that are capable of identifying illnesses in a range of demographics. A greater variety of data sources improves convergence and model accuracy, increasing the overall effectiveness of machine learning (Satheesh, N. et al., 2025) in medical diagnostics. In the end, safe medical image sharing will spur advancements in artificial intelligence in healthcare, guaranteeing improved patient outcomes and more precise diagnostic instruments

Machine Learning in Improving Diagnostic Accuracy

The application of artificial intelligence (Kumar, M. S. et al., 2025) is causing a revolution in the field of diagnostics by making it possible to conduct analyses of medical data that are both more accurate and more quickly. The capability of this technology to recognize intricate patterns in a variety of medical images, including X-rays, MRIs, and CT scans, makes it possible to detect diseases earlier and with greater precision. In areas such as cancer detection, where early diagnosis plays a pivotal role in improving patient outcomes, this takes on an especially important role. In some cases, the performance of expert radiologists can be surpassed by the capabilities of advanced algorithms that have been trained on extensive datasets. These algorithms (Konapure, C. G. et al., 2025) are able to identify subtle signs of tumors or abnormalities that human specialists potentially overlook. One of the most important advantages of these systems is their capacity to acquire new knowledge and become more advanced over time. It is possible for them to maintain a level of alignment with the ever-evolving body of medical knowledge (Ali, A., et al., 2021) because their accuracy and diagnostic capabilities continue to improve as they are exposed to new data. The dynamic integration of various types of information, such as patient records, laboratory results, and genetic data, is what makes these systems different from static tools. As a result, they are able to provide more individualized and accurate diagnoses for each individual patient. A significant reduction in the amount of time required to arrive at conclusions is one of the many benefits that these cutting-edge diagnostic tools offer (Singh, S. et al., 2025a). With these systems, information can be processed quickly, allowing medical professionals to make decisions more quickly. Traditional methods, on the other hand, frequently require manual examinations that are labour-intensive. When time-sensitive decisions are essential, such as in emergency care, this is especially helpful because it allows for a more expedient response (Liu, J. et al., 2018).

Accessing Medical Data Due to Privacy

Privacy concerns make it difficult to access medical data for clinical and research purposes. One of the main problems is the strict laws governing patient data, like the General Data Protection Regulation (GDPR) in Europe and the Health Insurance Portability and Accountability Act (HIPAA) in the United States. The purpose of these laws is to safeguard patient privacy and guarantee the secure handling of personal health data. On the other hand, they may make it more difficult for academics and medical professionals to exchange and use data efficiently (Singh, S. et al., 2025b). Sensitive patient information may be compromised by data breaches, which presents another difficulty. Even in cases where data sharing could result in major medical advancements, institutions are reluctant to share information because of the fear of unauthorized access to personal health records. This worry is especially strong when it comes to delicate conditions, like infectious diseases or mental health issues, because the stigma associated with these conditions may prevent people from agreeing to the use of their data (Pandey, B. K. et al., 2024a). Accessibility problems can also arise from data standardization. Hospitals, clinics, and laboratories are just a few of the places where medical data is frequently obtained, and each uses a different format and system for information storage. Research efforts may be further hampered by the inability to aggregate and analyze data thoroughly due to this lack of standardization. Getting patients informed consent to share their data can be a difficult procedure. Patients may refuse to participate in studies or give their data because they are hesitant about how their information will be used (Hameed, K. et al., 2016).

OBSTACLES IN MEDICAL IMAGE

Data Privacy and Security Concerns

In the healthcare industry, concerns regarding data privacy and security are of the utmost importance, particularly when it comes to the management of sensitive patient information. The vast amount of medical data that is generated from a variety of sources, such as electronic health records, imaging, and wearable devices, presents a unique set of challenges when it comes to protecting the confidentiality of patients. A significant cause for concern is the possibility of data breaches, which can result in the disclosure of sensitive personal health information to individuals who are not authorized to receive it. Theft of identity, financial fraud (Pandey, B. K. et al., 2024b), and significant damage to a patient's reputation are all potential outcomes of incidents of this nature. In order to protect themselves from cyberattacks and guarantee that patient information is kept confidential, healthcare organizations need to put in place stringent security measures. The Health Insurance Portability and Accountability Act (HIPAA) in the United States and the General Data Protection Regulation (GDPR) in Europe are two examples of regulatory frameworks that impose stringent guidelines on the manner in which patient data should be handled. These regulations have the intention of protecting the privacy of individuals; however, they may also create obstacles that prevent the sharing of data and collaboration in clinical practices and research. Keeping up with these regulations frequently necessitates a significant amount of administrative work, which can slow down the process of utilizing data (Maheshwari, R. U. et al., 2024) for the development of innovative healthcare solutions. The requirement that patients give their informed consent before their data can be used for research or shared with third parties is another obstacle that must be overcome. A great number of people are reluctant to take part in research projects or to grant access to their data because they are concerned about the ways in which their information will be utilized (Maheshwari, R. Uma. et al., 2024). Because of this reluctance, the availability of valuable datasets that are necessary for advancing medical research and improving patient outcomes may be restricted. Additional security concerns are brought up as a result of the growing prevalence of cloud-based storage solutions and digital health technologies. When it comes to storing and managing data, relying on third-party providers can result in vulnerabilities if these entities do not adhere to stringent security protocols (Kim, H. et al., 2019).

Interoperability, Data Standardization

Technical impediments to efficient data sharing and collaboration in the healthcare industry include interoperability and data standardization. These difficulties may make it more difficult to integrate different systems and may restrict the use of data for innovative research and practical clinical uses. The ability of various health information systems, tools, and applications to interface, exchange, and correctly interpret shared data is known as interoperability (Saxena, A. et al., 2024). The electronic health record (EHR) systems used by many healthcare providers are dissimilar and not built to function well together. Healthcare practitioners may find it challenging to obtain the comprehensive data required for well-informed decision-making as a result of this incompatibility, which may lead to fragmentate patient information (Rai, P. K. et al., 2024). Care coordination is hampered and error risk rises when systems are unable to communicate effectively. An additional major challenge is data standardization. Many formats, structures, and terminologies can be used to record medical data, which can result in discrepancies that make data sharing and analysis more challenging. For example, coding systems that differ from ICD-10 for diagnoses and LOINC for lab tests may be present in clinical data. Analyses that are meaningful can be limited by the complexity and time required to aggregate data from various sources when there are no standard formats in place. Differences in the patient population and data gathering techniques may make standardization initiatives even more challenging (Lakshmi, K. V. N. et al., 2024). Contradictions that may impact the quality of data can arise, for instance, from disparities in how various institutions record patient histories, vital signs, and treatment regimens. Development and implementation of sophisticated analytical tools and artificial intelligence applications can also be impeded by the lack of interoperability standards and standardized data formats. Model effectiveness and generalizability are limited when training on heterogeneous datasets due to the lack of a cohesive methodology.

Healthcare providers, tech companies, and government agencies must work together to overcome these technological obstacles (Saravanakumar, R. et al., 2024). A better way to encourage interoperability and make the integration of disparate systems easier is to develop and implement common standards for data exchange, like Fast Healthcare Interoperability Resources (FHIR). The healthcare industry can facilitate better data exchange, improve patient care, and support more extensive research projects by resolving these obstacles (Jiang, S. et al., 2019).

Lack of Unified Protocols for Secure Sharing

Sensitive patient data protection is severely hampered by the absence of standard protocols for safe data sharing in the healthcare industry. Standardized guidelines and procedures that guarantee the safe transfer of data across multiple platforms and organizations are referred to as unified protocols. On the other hand, various systems, each with its own security measures, are employed by various healthcare organizations to make up the current landscape. It is challenging to create a trustworthy framework for secure communication because of this variance, which results in inconsistent data sharing. Vulnerability to data breaches and unauthorized access is increased in the absence of a common framework. Healthcare companies run the risk of unintentionally disclosing private patient information to unauthorized parties in the absence of standard security procedures, which also increases the likelihood of data theft. Furthermore, patient data is further put at risk by the disparate security protocols used by various organizations, which leave holes that can be exploited. In this disjointed environment, following regulations also becomes difficult. The General Data Protection Regulation (GDPR) in Europe and the Health Insurance Portability and Accountability Act (HIPAA) in the United States are two examples of the various regions' and nations' unique data protection laws. Due to the intricate web of legal requirements that organizations must manage, the implementation of secure data-sharing practices is made more difficult by these disparate regulations. The potential for cooperation and innovation in healthcare research and practice is also restricted by this inconsistency, which also has an impact on data security (Chen, X. et al., 2018). Building trust in data-sharing initiatives requires addressing the absence of standardized protocols. The ability of healthcare organizations to securely and efficiently share data while maintaining patient privacy can be improved by establishing uniform security guidelines. The healthcare industry can support research, stimulate innovation, and enhance patient outcomes while maintaining the security of sensitive data by establishing a unified framework for safe data exchange.

SECURE MEDICAL IMAGE SHARING

Blockchain in Facilitating Secure and Transparent Data Exchange

Through the provision of a decentralized and unchangeable system, which is illustrated in figure 1, blockchain technology plays a significant part in ensuring the secure and transparent sharing of data. Because patient information is stored across multiple nodes in the healthcare industry, for example, it is extremely difficult to change or otherwise manipulate records (Kumarganesh, S. et al., 2024). All authorized participants are able to access the same data thanks to the transparency of blockchain technology, which helps to foster trust while maintaining one's privacy. Further automation of data access controls is provided by smart contracts, which ensures that only authorized parties are able to view sensitive information. Through the implementation of this strategy, security is improved, the likelihood of data breaches is decreased, and the sharing of data across industries is made more collaborative and effective (Muralidhar, L. B. et al., 2024).

- *Tamper-Proof Record*: Data recorded in the blockchain is encrypted and interconnected with preceding entries, forming an unalterable chain. This feature is vital in healthcare, where preserving precise patient records is crucial for effective treatment. Modifications to patient data, including alterations in medical history or treatment plans, are documented in a manner that preserves previous versions, ensuring they remain intact and accessible. Once data is documented, it cannot be modified or erased, thereby preserving the integrity of sensitive information, including patient health records. This immutability is also beneficial in legal contexts, where precise and unaltered records are essential for litigation or compliance. Blockchain improves accountability in healthcare organizations by offering a transparent and irrefutable record of data modifications (Pandey, B. K. et al., 2024c).
- *Transparency*: All participants in the blockchain network possess access to identical data and transaction histories. This transparency is especially advantageous in clinical trials, allowing researchers to oversee study progress and guarantee accurate data reporting. It aids in detecting potential biases or inconsistencies in data reporting (Pandey, B. K. et al., 2024d), thereby enhancing the reliability of research outcomes. This transparency cultivates trust among stakeholders, enabling the verification of information accuracy and legitimacy. Patients can be confident that their data is neither manipulated nor misrepresented, thereby increasing their propensity to disclose sensitive information for research purposes. This trust is essential for fostering

a collaborative environment in which stakeholders cooperate to achieve improved patient outcomes.

- *Patient Control*: Patients possess the authority to regulate their data by permitting or rescinding access to their medical records. This control is crucial regarding data privacy issues, as patients increasingly seek greater autonomy over their health information (Elarmathi, S. et al., 2024). Through the implementation of blockchain technology, patients can designate individuals who may access their data and the intended purposes, in accordance with their preferences and comfort levels. This obviates the necessity for intermediaries, granting patients greater autonomy over their health information. This transition to patient-centered data management can enhance engagement and involvement in their healthcare journeys. Patients who perceive greater control are more inclined to engage actively in their treatment regimens and communicate candidly with healthcare professionals.
- *Smart Contracts*: Self-executing contracts automate procedures such as data access requests and consent administration. These contracts may encompass established regulations that govern the access and timing of data retrieval, thereby ensuring adherence to consent agreements. A smart contract could autonomously limit access to a patient's data until explicit consent is obtained, thereby safeguarding privacy. Smart contracts guarantee that only authorized individuals can access particular information, thereby improving adherence to data protection regulations. Automating these processes enables healthcare organizations to alleviate administrative burdens and diminish the likelihood of human error in data access management. This efficient method also enables quicker response times for data requests (Pandey, B. K. et al., 2024e), advantageous for both providers and patients.
- *Decentralization*: Data is distributed across numerous nodes within the network, thereby diminishing the likelihood of centralized data breaches. In a conventional centralized system, a singular point of failure may result in disastrous data breaches. Conversely, the decentralized architecture of blockchain ensures that if a single node is compromised, the integrity of the remaining network is preserved, significantly complicating the efforts of attackers to obtain comprehensive datasets (JayaLakshmi, G. et al., 2024). Should a single node be compromised, the overall integrity of the system remains unblemished, thereby enhancing its resilience to attacks. This resilience is especially critical in the healthcare sector, where data breaches can significantly impact patient privacy and safety. Blockchain enhances security by distributing data across multiple nodes, a feature absents in conventional systems.
- *Augmented Security*: The encryption and decentralized characteristics of blockchain markedly diminish the likelihood of unauthorized access to con-

fidential information. Every transaction is safeguarded by cryptographic algorithms, rendering it exceedingly challenging for hackers to alter or access information without appropriate authorization (George, W. K. et al., 2024). This degree of security is essential for safeguarding patient information against progressively advanced cyber threats. Ongoing surveillance of the network can identify and address security threats instantaneously. Automated alerts can be established to inform stakeholders of anomalous activity, facilitating prompt intervention prior to any substantial harm transpiring. This proactive security strategy improves patient data safety and strengthens trust in the healthcare system.

- *Facilitating Collaboration*: Secure and transparent data sharing facilitates enhanced collaboration among healthcare providers, researchers, and patients. Access to a unified, immutable data source enables healthcare professionals to coordinate care more efficiently (Abdullahi, M. et al., 2024), resulting in enhanced patient outcomes. This collaboration is crucial in multidisciplinary treatment environments, where diverse specialists must exchange insights regarding a patient's care. This may result in enhanced patient care and progress in medical research via shared insights. Researchers can access a more extensive dataset for analysis, enabling the identification of novel treatments and insights into disease patterns. The collaborative framework promoted by blockchain can stimulate innovation and expedite the creation of novel healthcare solutions.

Figure 1. Blockchain's role in secure data sharing

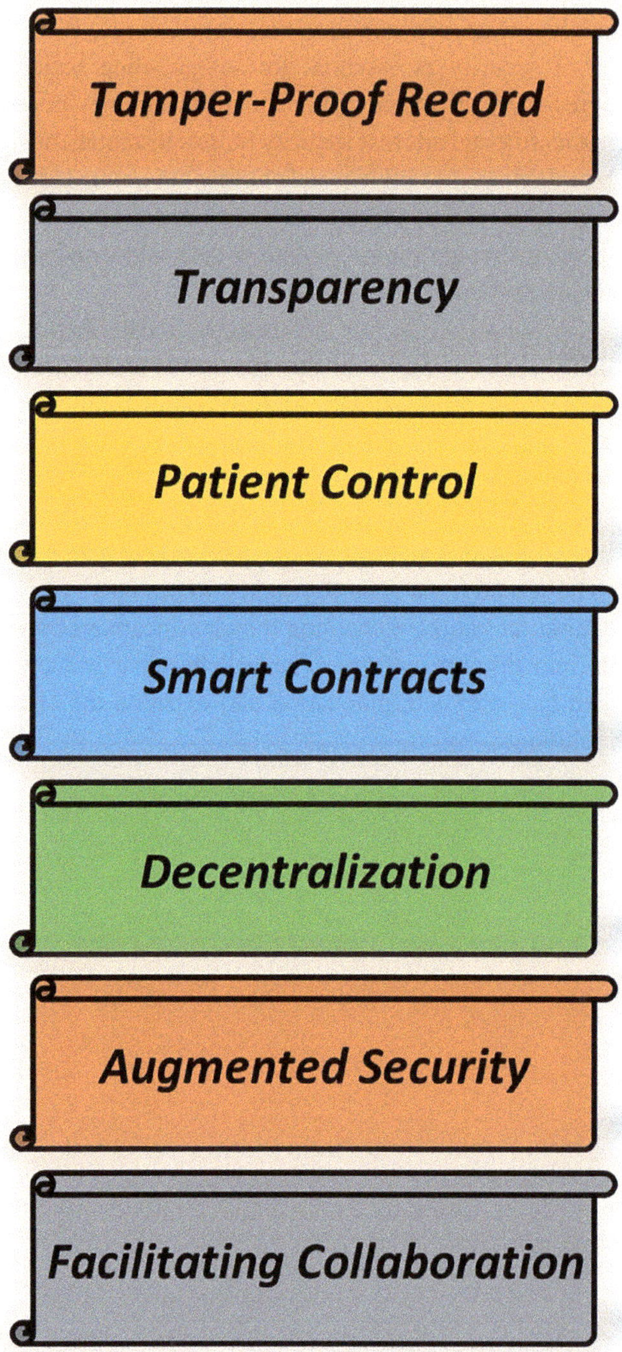

Secure Multi-Party Computation (MPC)

Data sharing is crucial in many industries, especially healthcare, in the digital age. When handling sensitive patient data (Kumar, B. et al., 2024), secure and transparent information sharing is crucial. Blockchain technology can solve data sharing issues. Its decentralization and strong security make it a promising solution for data protection and stakeholder collaboration. Healthcare organizations generate massive amounts of patient, treatment, and medical image data daily. Research and high-quality care require this information (Pandey, D. et al., 2024a). This data is sensitive and requires strict security to prevent unauthorized access and breaches. Patient privacy and data integrity are often compromised by traditional data sharing methods. Several factors emphasize secure data sharing. Medical professionals must safeguard patient data by law and ethics. Identity theft, financial fraud, and patient reputation damage can result from breaches. Second, diagnosis and treatment require accurate and reliable data. Unauthorized changes can endanger patients. Third, organizations must follow data handling regulations like HIPAA in the US. Finally, healthcare providers need secure data sharing to collaborate. Centralized systems that are vulnerable (Pandey, D. et al., 2024b) to security threats make traditional data-sharing methods difficult. Single points of failure in centralized databases allow hackers to compromise large amounts of sensitive data. Intermediaries may not have strong security, adding to data transfer risks. Healthcare data fragmentation is another issue. Different healthcare providers may use incompatible systems, making data sharing difficult (Kennedy, G. W. et al., 2024). Lack of interoperability can cause incomplete patient records and treatment delays. Variations in data formats and coding can complicate sharing and cause errors that can harm patient care. Blockchain technology could solve these issues. By creating a decentralized, tamper-proof ledger, it secures data while allowing authorized users access. Each transaction on a blockchain is nearly impossible to change or delete, preserving data integrity. Healthcare relies on accurate, unaltered records for treatment and legal compliance. Blockchain is notable for its data transparency. Patients, healthcare providers, and researchers trust the network because all participants can see transaction histories. Transparency allows users to verify information, encouraging patient care collaboration and innovation. Patients gain data control and transparency with blockchain. Individuals can grant or revoke access to their medical records, allowing them to control sensitive information. This patient-centered approach improves privacy and health management engagement. When patients feel in control of their data, they are more likely to participate in their treatment plans and communicate with their doctors. Smart contracts improve data sharing security and efficiency in blockchain technology. Smart contracts execute automatically based on coded terms. Data access requests and consent management can be automated by these contracts to restrict access to specific information (Shahul, A. et al., 2024).

Healthcare organizations can reduce administrative burdens and human error by automating these workflows. The decentralized nature of blockchain reduces centralized data breaches. Since data is stored across multiple network nodes, the system remains intact if one node fails. In a time of widespread data breaches, this data distribution improves security and resilience against cyberattacks. Healthcare data sharing using blockchain technology addresses regulatory compliance issues. Blockchain is transparent and auditable, helping organizations meet legal requirements. Keeping track of data access and changes helps healthcare providers comply with regulations, simplifying audits and reducing penalties. Demand for secure, efficient, and transparent data sharing will rise as healthcare evolves. Blockchain technology can meet these growing needs. Blockchain helps stakeholders collaborate, improve patient care, and innovate healthcare research by protecting sensitive patient data. Blockchain implementation in healthcare data sharing can streamline clinical trials and research. Privacy and regulatory issues make data access (Pandey, D. et al., 2024c) difficult for researchers. Blockchain gives researchers a larger dataset while protecting patient privacy. This can boost research results and speed up treatment development. Global healthcare benefits from blockchain's characteristics. Data sharing must be standardized as healthcare systems become more interconnected across borders. Blockchain allows secure data sharing across jurisdictions, protecting patient privacy. This capability is crucial in a globalized world where patients seek care in multiple countries. Technological infrastructure for blockchain implementation is another issue. Some healthcare organizations lack the resources or technical expertise to integrate blockchain solutions into their systems. Thus, healthcare blockchain deployment requires technology and training investments. Also important is interoperability. Blockchain can enable data sharing between organizations, but it must be compatible with EHRs. Blockchain technology can improve patient care, healthcare stakeholder collaboration, and medical research as demand for secure and efficient data sharing grows. By removing adoption barriers and unifying data sharing, the healthcare industry can maximize blockchain's potential to improve patient and provider outcomes.

TECHNOLOGICAL SOLUTIONS FOR SECURE SHARING

Frameworks and Tools for Data Encryption

For the purpose of protecting sensitive data across a wide range of applications and industries, encryption frameworks and tools are, as shown in figure 2, absolutely necessary. Notable frameworks include the Advanced Encryption Standard (AES), which provides robust security by means of symmetric encryption, and homomorphic encryption, which enables computations to be performed on encrypted data without exposing the confidentiality of the data. The encryption of communication channels between clients and servers is accomplished by tools such as Secure Socket Layer (SSL), which safeguards data while it is being transmitted. Users of Windows can benefit from full-disk encryption with BitLocker, while users of macOS can reap the same benefits with FileVault. The utilization of these tools and frameworks not only improves data privacy but also assists organizations in meeting regulatory requirements. This helps to guarantee that sensitive information is protected from unauthorized access and breaches (Pandey, D., & Pandey, B. K., 2022).

Figure 2. Encryption frameworks and tools

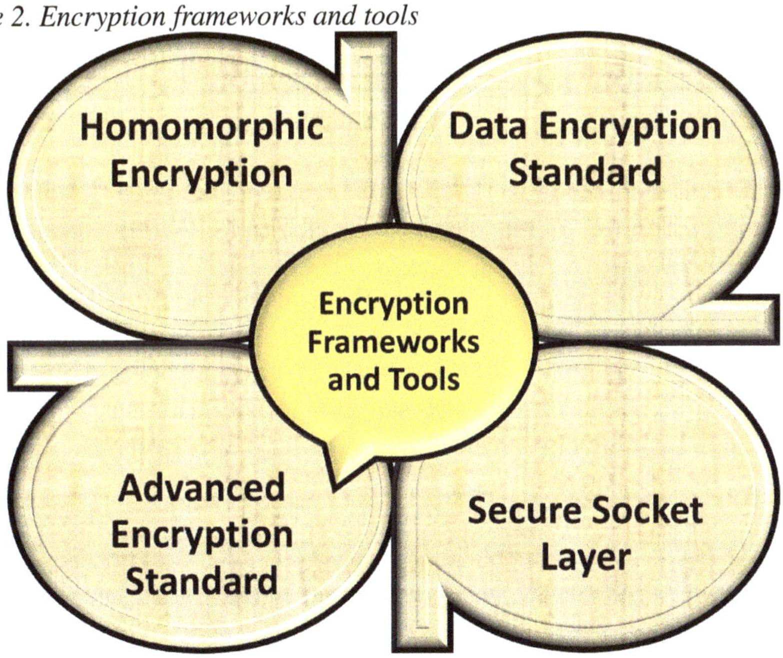

- *Homomorphic Encryption*: Homomorphic encryption is a sophisticated cryptographic technique that enables computations on encrypted data without prior decryption. This functionality is especially advantageous in cloud computing settings, where sensitive information is frequently handled externally. Homomorphic encryption enables organizations to utilize cloud-based analytics while preserving the confidentiality and security of their data. Healthcare providers can examine patient data while safeguarding individual records, thereby ensuring adherence to privacy regulations like HIPAA. Nonetheless, homomorphic encryption is computationally demanding and may present performance challenges, necessitating careful consideration for particular applications where data privacy is critical.
- *Data Encryption Standard (DES)*: The Data Encryption Standard (DES) is a symmetric-key algorithm that was extensively utilized for data encryption in the late 20th century. DES encrypts data in 64-bit blocks utilizing a 56-bit key, rendering it appropriate for safeguarding diverse forms of sensitive information. Although DES was instrumental in data security, advancements in computational power ultimately made it susceptible to brute-force attacks. As a result, it has predominantly been supplanted by more secure algorithms such as the Advanced Encryption Standard (AES). Although its usage is waning, comprehending DES is crucial for historical context and for acknowledging the progression of encryption technologies throughout history.
- *Advanced Encryption Standard (AES)*: The Advanced Encryption Standard (AES) is a symmetric encryption algorithm instituted by the U.S. National Institute of Standards and Technology (NIST) in 2001. It has emerged as the benchmark for encrypting sensitive data owing to its robust security attributes and efficiency. AES accommodates key lengths of 128, 192, and 256 bits, enabling organizations to select the security level that aligns with their requirements. The algorithm functions on fixed-size blocks of 128 bits and is extensively utilized in diverse applications, ranging from securing communications to safeguarding data at rest. AES is recognized for its rapidity and efficacy in both hardware and software applications, rendering it a favored option for information security across various sectors.
- *Secure Socket Layer (SSL)*: Secure Socket Layer (SSL) is a protocol that guarantees secure communication across a computer network. SSL encrypts data transmitted between web browsers and servers, ensuring confidentiality and integrity for sensitive information, including passwords, credit card numbers, and personal data. SSL safeguards data from eavesdroppers and man-in-the-middle attacks during transmission by creating an encrypted connection. Despite being largely supplanted by Transport Layer Security (TLS), SSL established the foundation for secure web communications. Numerous

websites continue to employ SSL certificates to signify secure connections, usually denoted by "https://" in the URL, thereby assuring users of the safety of their online transactions.

Implementation of Blockchain Platforms

Many industries are adopting blockchain platforms like Ethereum and Hyperledger to improve data security and transparency. Decentralised applications (dApps) and smart contracts can transform how organisations manage and exchange information using these platforms. Smart contract capabilities make Ethereum a popular blockchain platform. Instead of intermediaries, developers can create dApps that automate processes and enforce agreements. This feature helps in trust- and efficiency-driven industries like finance, supply chain management, and healthcare. In healthcare, Ethereum can secure patient records and manage consent transparently through smart contracts. By giving patients control over their sensitive data, this reduces data breaches and improves patient privacy. The Hyperledger consortium develops enterprise-specific blockchain frameworks and tools. Hyperledger uses privileges to access blockchains, unlike Ethereum, which uses public blockchains. Businesses that want more data and participant control benefit from this approach. Top framework Hyperledger Fabric lets companies build private networks to meet their needs. Data privacy, consensus mechanisms, and enterprise system integration are possible with this flexibility. To implement blockchain platforms, governance, scalability, and interoperability must be considered. For decision-making and regulatory compliance, organizations need clear governance structures. Public blockchains like Ethereum face scalability issues due to network congestion, which slows transaction speeds and costs.

CONCLUSION

Secure sharing of medical images is crucial for improving healthcare delivery and increasing the efficacy of data-driven methodologies in medical practice. By protecting sensitive patient information while permitting access to essential data, healthcare providers can ensure regulatory compliance and uphold patient trust. The significance of secure sharing is amplified as the quantity of medical imaging data increases, requiring strong data protection mechanisms. The incorporation of secure sharing techniques with collaborative machine learning markedly enhances the efficacy of model training and deployment. When organizations can exchange images and associated data without jeopardizing privacy, they can create more precise and resilient algorithms. This partnership enhances diagnostic capabilities and customizes treatment plans, thereby improving patient care. The significance of secure medical image sharing on healthcare innovation is paramount. The ongoing evolution of technology will enable secure sharing and analysis of medical images, thereby promoting innovative research and the creation of new therapeutic strategies. This will consequently result in improved patient outcomes and a more efficient healthcare system overall. By emphasizing security in data sharing, the healthcare sector can fully leverage advanced analytics and machine learning, facilitating a healthier future.

REFERENCES

Abdullahi, M., Ahmad, A., Pandey, B. K., & Pandey, D. (2024). Digital Currency Adoption: A Comparative Analysis of Global Trends and the Nigerian eNaira Digital Currency. *SN Computer Science*, *5*(5), 1–11. DOI: 10.1007/s42979-024-02882-6

Ali, A., Rahim, H. A., Pasha, M. F., Dowsley, R., Masud, M., Ali, J., & Baz, M. (2021). Security, privacy, and reliability in digital healthcare systems using blockchain. *Electronics (Basel)*, *10*(16), 2034. DOI: 10.3390/electronics10162034

. Chen, X., Ji, J., Luo, C., Liao, W., & Li, P. (2018, December). When machine learning meets blockchain: A decentralized, privacy-preserving and secure design. In 2018 IEEE international conference on big data (big data) (pp. 1178-1187). IEEE.

Elarmathi, S., Rishabavarthani, P., Sindhuja, M., Elayaraja, P., & Malathi Murugesan, S. (2024). Novel manufacturing systems for cancer diagnosis using ultra-sensitive photonic crystal fiber biosensor with dual-functionalized aptamer-nanocavity. *Microsystem Technologies*, •••, 1–20. DOI: 10.1007/s00542-024-05820-x

George, W. K., Silas, E. I., Pandey, D., & Pandey, B. K. (2024). Utilization of Industry 4.0 Technologies in Nigerian Technical and Vocational Education: A Conundrum for Educators. In *Examining the Rapid Advance of Digital Technology in Africa* (pp. 270–293). IGI Global. DOI: 10.4018/978-1-6684-9962-7.ch014

Hameed, K., Ali, A., Naqvi, M. H., Jabbar, M., Junaid, M., & Haider, A. (2016, August). Resource management in operating systems-a survey of scheduling algorithms. In *Proceedings of the International Conference on Innovative Computing (ICIC)*, Lanzhou, China (pp. 2-5).

JayaLakshmi. G., Pandey, D., Pandey, B. K., Kaur, P., Mahajan, D. A., & Dari, S. S. (2024). Smart big data collection for intelligent supply chain improvement. In AI and Machine Learning Impacts in Intelligent Supply Chain (pp. 180-195). IGI Global Scientific Publishing.

. Jiang, S., Cao, J., McCann, J. A., Yang, Y., Liu, Y., Wang, X., & Deng, Y. (2019, July). Privacy-preserving and efficient multi-keyword search over encrypted data on blockchain. In 2019 IEEE international conference on Blockchain (Blockchain) (pp. 405-410). IEEE.

Kennedy, G. W., Sunday, S. E., Pandey, D., Kabari, A. D., Pandey, B. K., George, A. S., & Dadheech, P. (2024). Building Information Modeling: Harnessing Innovations for Professional Proficiency. In Emerging Engineering Technologies and Industrial Applications (pp. 305-331). IGI Global.

Khadka, M., Sah, M., Chaudhary, R., Sahani, S. K., Sahani, K., Pandey, B. K., & Pandey, D. (2025). Spectroscopic, quantum chemical, and topological calculations of the phenylephrine molecule using density functional theory. *Scientific Reports*, *15*(1), 208. DOI: 10.1038/s41598-024-81633-2 PMID: 39747169

Kim, H., Kim, S. H., Hwang, J. Y., & Seo, C. (2019). Efficient privacy-preserving machine learning for blockchain network. *IEEE Access : Practical Innovations, Open Solutions*, *7*, 136481–136495. DOI: 10.1109/ACCESS.2019.2940052

Konapure, C. G., Pandey, D., Shete, H., Thakar, C. M., Pandey, B. K., & George, A. S. (2025). Artificial Intelligence in Automated Concrete Mix Design Using Computerized Grading Curves. Interdisciplinary Approaches to AI, Internet of Everything, and Machine Learning, 567-586.

Kumar, B., Pandey, D., Pandey, B. K., & George, A. S. (2024). Higher Education in the Last Four Decades: A Review of Paradigm Shifts in Policy Frameworks. Design and Implementation of Higher Education Learners' Learning Outcomes (HELLO), 333-348.

Kumar, M. S., Prasanna, P. L., Lalitha, M., Joy, M., Jha, S. S., & Pandey, B. K. (2025). Utilizing the Internet of Everything and Artificial Intelligence for Real-Time Workforce Management. In Role of Internet of Everything (IOE), VLSI Architecture, and AI in Real-Time Systems (pp. 153-168). IGI Global Scientific Publishing.

Kumarganesh, S., & Malathi Murugesan, C. (2024). Hybrid plasmonic biosensors with deep learning for colorectal cancer detection. *Plasmonics*, •••, 1–15. DOI: 10.1007/s11468-024-02568-y

Lakshmi, K. V. N., Rajan, R., Pandey, D., & Pandey, B. K. (2024). Circular economy: A catalyst for economic growth-an empirical study. *Circular Economy and Sustainability*, •••, 1–22.

Liu, J., Li, X., Ye, L., Zhang, H., Du, X., & Guizani, M. (2018, December). BPDS: A blockchain based privacy-preserving data sharing for electronic medical records. In *2018 IEEE Global Communications Conference (GLOBECOM)* (pp. 1-6). IEEE. DOI: 10.1109/GLOCOM.2018.8647713

Maheshwari, R., Kumarganesh, S., K v M, S., Gopalakrishnan, A., Selvi, K., Paulchamy, B., Rishabavarthani, P., Sagayam, K. M., Pandey, B. K., & Pandey, D. (2024). Advanced plasmonic resonance-enhanced biosensor for comprehensive real-time detection and analysis of deepfake content. *Plasmonics*, •••, 1–18. DOI: 10.1007/s11468-024-02407-0

Maheshwari, R. U., Paulchamy, B., Pandey, B. K., & Pandey, D. (2024). Enhancing sensing and imaging capabilities through surface plasmon resonance for deepfake image detection. *Plasmonics*, •••, 1–20. DOI: 10.1007/s11468-024-02492-1

Muralidhar, L. B., Lakshmi, K. V. N., Swapna, H. R., Rupani, J., Nethravathi, K., Pandey, B. K., & Pandey, D. (2024). Impact of Organizational Culture on The Level of Corporate Social Responsibility Investments: An Exploratory Study. *Circular Economy and Sustainability*, *4*(3), 1–19. DOI: 10.1007/s43615-024-00371-9

Pandey, B. K., Kanike, U. K., George, A. S., & Pandey, D. (Eds.). (2024d). *AI and machine learning impacts in intelligent supply chain*. IGI Global. DOI: 10.4018/979-8-3693-1347-3

Pandey, B. K., Nassa, V. K., Mukundan, A. P., Mahajan, D. A., Pandey, D., George, A. S., & Dadheech, P. (2024c). An Industry-Focused Traffic System Utilising Internet of Things. In *Emerging Engineering Technologies and Industrial Applications* (pp. 200–213). IGI Global. DOI: 10.4018/979-8-3693-1335-0.ch009

Pandey, B. K., & Pandey, D. (2023). Parametric optimization and prediction of enhanced thermoelectric performance in co-doped CaMnO3 using response surface methodology and neural network. *Journal of Materials Science Materials in Electronics*, *34*(21), 1589. DOI: 10.1007/s10854-023-10954-1

Pandey, B. K., & Pandey, D. (2025). Securing healthcare medical image information using advance morphological component analysis, information hiding systems, and hybrid convolutional neural networks on IoMT. *Computers in Biology and Medicine*, *185*, 109499. DOI: 10.1016/j.compbiomed.2024.109499 PMID: 39642698

Pandey, B. K., Pandey, D., & Lelisho, M. E. (2024a). Face mask identification with enhanced cuckoo optimization and deep learning-based faster regional neural network. *Scientific Reports*, *14*(1), 29719. DOI: 10.1038/s41598-024-78746-z PMID: 39613761

Pandey, B. K., Pandey, D., & Sahani, S. K. (2024b). Autopilot control unmanned aerial vehicle system for sewage defect detection using deep learning. *Engineering Reports*, •••, 12852.

Pandey, B. K., Paramashivan, M. A., Pandey, D., George, A. S., Agarwal, A., Mahajan, D. A., . . . Pramanik, S. (2024e). Future Directions of Digital Twin Architectures for 6G Communication Networks. In Security Issues and Solutions in 6G Communications and Beyond (pp. 197-211). IGI Global.

Pandey, D., Nassa, V. K., Pandey, B. K., Thankachan, B., Dadheech, P., Mahajan, D. A., & George, A. S. (2024a). Artificial Intelligence and Machine Learning and Its Application in the Field of Computational Visual Analysis. In Emerging Engineering Technologies and Industrial Applications (pp. 36-57). IGI Global. DOI: 10.4018/979-8-3693-1335-0.ch003

Pandey, D., & Pandey, B. K. (2022). An efficient deep neural network with adaptive galactic swarm optimization for complex image text extraction. In *Process Mining Techniques for Pattern Recognition* (pp. 121–137). CRC Press. DOI: 10.1201/9781003169550-10

Pandey, D., Pandey, B. K., Nassa, V. K., Mahajan, D. A., George, A. S., & Dadheech, P. (2024c). Optimized Throughput-Based Broadcasting for Next Generation Wireless Networks. In Emerging Engineering Technologies and Industrial Applications (pp. 355-368). IGI Global. DOI: 10.4018/979-8-3693-1335-0.ch018

Pandey, D., Pandey, B. K., Paramashivan, M. A., Mahajan, D. A., Dadheech, P. D., George, A. S., & Hameed, A. S. (2024b). Advanced Digital Data Processing Using Cloud Cryptography: Industrial Applications. In Emerging Engineering Technologies and Industrial Applications (pp. 255-268). IGI Global.

Rai, P. K., Pandey, D., & Pandey, B. K. (2024). The future of enterprise and innovation is compute as a commodity, or CaaC. *Partners Universal International Research Journal*, *3*(2), 89–94.

Saravanakumar, R., TamilSelvi, T., Pandey, D., Pandey, B. K., Mahajan, D. A., & Lelisho, M. E. (2024). Big data processing using hybrid Gaussian mixture model with salp swarm algorithm. *Journal of Big Data*, *11*(1), 167. DOI: 10.1186/s40537-024-01015-3

Satheesh, N., Gopisankar, N., Kumarganesh, S., Anthoniraj, S., Saravanakumar, S., & Martin Sagayam, K. (2025). Advanced AI-driven emergency response systems for enhanced vehicle and human safety. *Iran Journal of Computer Science*, •••, 1–16. DOI: 10.1007/s42044-025-00228-w

Saxena, A., Agarwal, A., Pandey, B. K., & Pandey, D. (2024). Examination of the Criticality of Customer Segmentation Using Unsupervised Learning Methods. *Circular Economy and Sustainability*, *4*(2), 1–14. DOI: 10.1007/s43615-023-00336-4

Shahul, A., Muniandi, B., Paramashivan, M. A., Pandey, D., Pandey, B. K., Dadheech, P., & George, H. (2024). An Analysis of Algorithms and Methods Based on Image Processing for Medical Applications. In *Emerging Engineering Technologies and Industrial Applications* (pp. 173–186). IGI Global. DOI: 10.4018/979-8-3693-1335-0.ch007

Sheela, M. S., Kumarganesh, S., Pandey, B. K., & Lelisho, M. E. (2025). Integration of silver nanostructures in wireless sensor networks for enhanced biochemical sensing. *Discover Nano*, *20*(1), 7. DOI: 10.1186/s11671-024-04159-6 PMID: 39804434

Singh, S., Madaan, G., Swapna, H. R., Singh, A., Pandey, D., George, A. S., & Pandey, B. K. (2025a). Empowering Connectivity: Exploring the Internet of Things. In Interdisciplinary Approaches to AI, Internet of Everything, and Machine Learning (pp. 89-116). IGI Global Scientific Publishing.

Singh, S., Madaan, G., Swapna, H. R., Singh, A., Pandey, B. K., George, A. S., & Pandey, D. (2025b). Unleashing the Power of AI and Data Analysis: Transforming Insights into Action. In Interdisciplinary Approaches to AI, Internet of Everything, and Machine Learning (pp. 1-24). IGI Global Scientific Publishing.

Chapter 8

Machine Learning and Secure Image Transmission for Disease Forecasting

Angotu Saida
https://orcid.org/0009-0000-6030-7424
Department of Electronics and Communication Engineering, KG Reddy College of Engineering and Technology, India

Mallareddy Adudhodla
Department of IT, CVR College of Engineering, Telangana, India

Niladri Maiti
Central Asian University, Tashkent, Uzbekistan

Krishna Murthy Inumula
https://orcid.org/0000-0002-4556-549X
Symbiosis International University, Pune, India

G. Kalaiarasi
https://orcid.org/0009-0003-9792-3214
Department of Computer Science and Engineering, Sathyabama Institute of Science and Technology, Chennai, India

Lakshmi Chandrakanth Kasireddy
https://orcid.org/0009-0002-0392-739X
ThoughtSpot Inc., USA

ABSTRACT

The transformative potential of machine learning (ML) in disease forecasting is emphasizes how crucial secure transmission techniques are to maintaining the integrity of patient data. With the growing reliance of healthcare on sophisticated data analytics, machine learning (ML) models have become indispensable instruments for forecasting disease outbreaks and enhancing patient results. ML algorithms are able to detect patterns and trends that help with early detection and intervention in a variety of health conditions by examining large datasets that include clinical data, medical images, and environmental factors. But considering the increasing

DOI: 10.4018/979-8-3693-9821-0.ch008

frequency of cyberattacks and data breaches in the healthcare industry, it is critical that this sensitive data be transmitted securely.

□INTRODUCTION

The rising incidence of infectious and non-communicable diseases has made global health issues more urgent. Diseases that spread quickly across borders, overwhelming healthcare systems and causing widespread social and economic disruption, are infectious diseases like COVID-19 and other viral outbreaks. Non-communicable diseases (NCDs), such as diabetes, cancer, and heart disease, continue to be significant causes of death worldwide. These conditions are made worse by aging populations and changes in lifestyle. When taken as a whole, these health risks place a heavy burden on healthcare systems around the globe, necessitating the urgent need for creative solutions that can recognize and treat these illnesses early. Lack of funding, a lack of qualified personnel, and inadequate infrastructure frequently make it difficult for healthcare systems, particularly in low- and middle-income nations, to deliver quality treatment. The burden on these systems is compounded by the fact that delayed disease diagnosis raises treatment costs and degrades patient outcomes. Reducing morbidity and mortality for many infectious and chronic diseases requires prompt diagnosis and treatment. People in many nations, however, are left vulnerable to both sudden outbreaks and slowly progressing illnesses due to a lack of resources for early screening and real-time disease surveillance. Improving patient outcomes requires early disease detection. Early diagnosis frequently results in more efficient treatments, better control over the course of the disease, and cheaper medical expenses. For example, early detection greatly improves the chances of survival in cancer cases because patients can receive less intrusive treatments. On the other hand, late-stage diagnosis frequently necessitates more aggressive interventions with lower recovery rates. Preventing the rapid spread of epidemics is another benefit of early detection of infectious diseases. This is because health authorities (Pandey, B. K., & Pandey, D., 2025) can take targeted actions like vaccination campaigns, quarantines, and public health advisories before outbreaks get out of control. Early detection systems that can predict future outbreaks are critical to stopping the spread of disease. Quick detection of disease indicators in populations allows for prompt public health interventions, preventing the spread of infectious illnesses. Technology (Khadka, M. et al., 2025).) is essential in this situation. Medical data can be analysed in great quantities using data-driven methods like machine learning, which can identify patterns that point to the beginning of a disease. Similarly, early indicators of diseases like diabetic retinopathy or lung cancer are being identified by medical imaging technologies in conjunction with artificial intelligence, enabling earlier and more precise diagnosis. Healthcare systems can effectively address the challenges presented by both established and emerging diseases by prioritizing early detection, which could ultimately result in lifesaving measures and enhance global health outcomes.

Machine Learning in Disease Forecasting

Machine learning (ML) (Satheesh, N. et al., 2025) is a key part of health data analysis because it helps healthcare professionals find useful information in huge amounts of data. ML can find patterns, predict outcomes, and help doctors diagnose diseases by using algorithms that learn from past patient records, clinical data, and imaging studies. This technology makes it easier to make choices, which leads to more personalized treatment plans and better care for patients. ML models can also look at real-time data from wearable tech (Kumar, M. S. et al., 2025), which lets doctors keep an eye on patients' health all the time. As more healthcare systems use machine learning, the chances of better disease management, early detection, and better use of resources keep growing. The application of machine learning (ML) (Konapure, C. G. et al., 2025) to the analysis of large datasets to find patterns and trends greatly improves the prediction of disease. ML's Role in Disease Prediction are shown in Figure 1.

Figure 1. ML's role in disease prediction

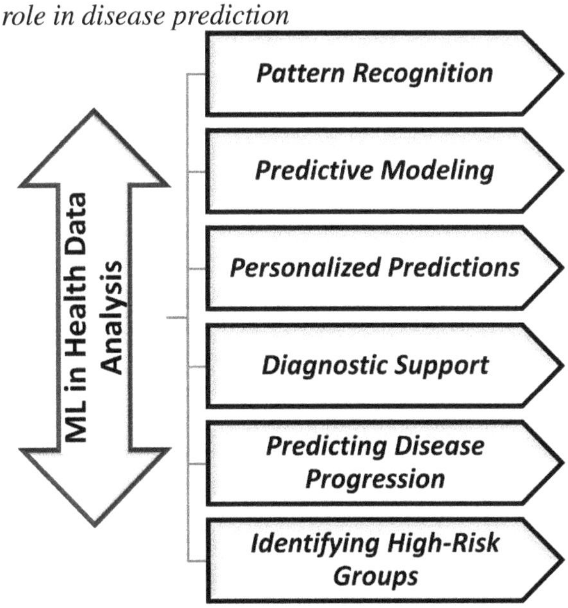

- *Pattern Recognition*: Machine learning (ML) is an effective method for detecting diseases at an early stage because it is particularly adept at recognizing intricate patterns within large datasets (Singh, S. et al., 2025a). Algorithms that use machine learning can uncover subtle correlations that may be missed by human analysis by analysing patient data, which includes medical histories, genetic information, and lifestyle factors. In the case of diseases such as diabetes or cancer, for example, machine learning has the ability to identify patterns in biomarkers or imaging data (Singh, S. et al., 2025b), thereby detecting early signs of these diseases long before symptoms become apparent. It is possible to take a more proactive approach to healthcare by recognizing patterns, which can lead to improved outcomes through earlier interventions.
- *Predictive Modeling*: Machine learning makes it possible to develop predictive models that can forecast disease outbreaks or evaluate the risks of infectious diseases for individuals. In order to generate accurate forecasts, these models are able to examine historical health data, information gathered from real-time monitoring (Pandey, B. K. et al., 2024a), environmental factors, and similar data. An example of this would be the utilization of predictive models for the purpose of predicting the spread of infectious diseases such as influenza or COVID-19. These models analyses patterns in population movement, climate, and infection rates. The likelihood of developing diseases such as cardiovascular conditions can be predicted by these models on an individual level based on the specific health profile of a patient, which can then be used to guide preventative care strategies (Provenzano, S. et al., 2019).
- *Personalized Predictions*: Machine learning's capacity to provide personalized disease predictions is one of the most revolutionary aspects of its application in the healthcare industry. This is accomplished through the analysis of individual data (Pandey, B. K. et al., 2024b), which may include genetic markers, lifestyle choices, and previous health conditions. Machine learning provides personalized predictions for each individual patient. By way of illustration, machine learning algorithms have the capability to forecast how an individual might react to a particular treatment based on their genetic composition. This paves the way for therapies that are both more personalized and more effective. Because treatments can be tailored to meet the specific requirements of the individual, this individualized approach is beneficial in the management of chronic diseases and in lowering the risk of complications.
- *Diagnostic Support*: For the purpose of assisting medical professionals with diagnostics, machine learning systems are becoming increasingly important, particularly in the field of medical imaging. An example of this would be the ability of machine learning algorithms to analyze MRI, CT, or X-ray images in order to detect abnormalities such as tumors, fractures, or lesions with a

high degree of precision (Maheshwari, R. U. et al., 2024). These systems provide radiologists with a second opinion, which helps to improve diagnostic precision and reduce the likelihood of errors caused by human intervention. When it comes to oncology, cardiology, and neurology, diagnostic tools that are powered by machine learning have the ability to analyze lab results and patient symptoms in order to provide support for clinical decision-making. This helps to improve the speed and accuracy of diagnoses in these areas (Maheshwari, R. Uma. et al., 2024).

- *Predicting Disease Progression*: In order to monitor and adjust treatment plans as required, clinicians are able to use machine learning to model and predict the progression of diseases over time. As an illustration, machine learning algorithms (Saxena, A. et al., 2024) have the capability to forecast the progression of neurodegenerative diseases such as Alzheimer's disease or predict how a cancer might develop based on a patient's response to its treatment. Physicians are able to improve patient outcomes by staying ahead of the progression of the disease thanks to these predictions (Rai, P. K. et al., 2024), which allow them to optimize care by adjusting treatments in real time. In addition, continuous monitoring through wearables and electronic health records provides data that is fed back into these machine learning systems, which helps to refine the predictive accuracy of these systems (Lakshmi, K. V. N. et al., 2024).
- *Identifying High-Risk Groups*: The use of machine learning allows for the efficient analysis of vast amounts of population health data, which can then be used to identify groups that are at a higher risk of developing particular diseases (Saravanakumar, R. et al., 2024). The field of public health, for example, makes use of machine learning to identify populations that are more likely to be affected by conditions such as diabetes, hypertension, or infectious diseases. This is accomplished by taking into account factors such as geographic location, socioeconomic status, and genetic predisposition. The most vulnerable individuals can be targeted with targeted public health interventions, such as vaccination campaigns or early screening programs, which ultimately leads to more effective disease prevention and control. These insights help direct these interventions (Kumarganesh, S. et al., 2024).

MACHINE LEARNING MODEL TYPES FOR FORECASTING DISEASES

Figure 2. Types of machine learning models for disease forecasting

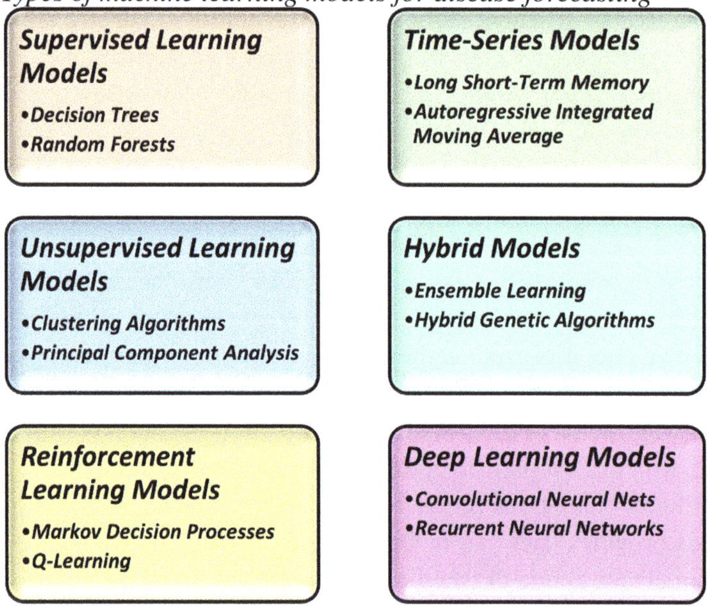

Figure 2 shows several machine learning models used for disease forecasting, each with its own strengths. Supervised learning models, like logistic regression and support vector machines, predict specific disease outcomes based on labelled datasets (Muralidhar, L. B. et al., 2024). Unsupervised learning models, like clustering algorithms, group similar patient data without labels, revealing hidden patterns (Pandey, B. K. et al., 2024c).

1. *Supervised Learning Models*: Because supervised learning makes predictions about new, unseen data based on historical data, it is the most popular kind of machine learning for disease prediction. Using a labeled dataset as its learning source, the model can forecast future cases based on patterns that are similar to the output (such as the occurrence or non-occurrence of a disease) (Pandey, B. K. et al., 2024d).
   a. *Decision Trees*: Decision trees divide a dataset into smaller subsets by classifying the data through a series of yes/no questions. Utilizing patient symptoms, lifestyle, and genetic data, they are helpful in identifying disease risk factors in disease forecasting (Elarmathi, S. et al., 2024).). Based on variables like age, family history, and BMI, decision trees, for instance, can

categorize patients into risk groups for diabetes or cardiovascular disease. In the healthcare industry, where comprehension of the reasoning behind predictions is critical, decision trees are especially useful due to their simplicity and interpretability.

   b. *Random Forests*: To increase generalization and prediction accuracy, random forests synthesize results from several decision trees. Complex medical datasets are a good fit for this ensemble approach because it improves robustness and minimizes overfitting. Through the process of aggregating decisions from multiple trees, each taking into account distinct patient features, random forests can be used in disease forecasting to predict a patient's chance of developing chronic illnesses. For instance, random forests can create a thorough prediction for heart disease by analyzing a variety of variables, including blood pressure, cholesterol, and exercise routines.

2. *Unsupervised Learning Models*: If the data has no labels or obvious results, unsupervised learning is applied. These algorithms are meant to search through the data for buried trends, groupings, or patterns. Finding new disease subtypes or unidentified disease patterns is especially helpful in the healthcare industry.
   a. *Clustering Algorithms*: Similarity-based clustering algorithms divide data into groups. These algorithms can be applied to disease forecasting in order to identify novel disease patterns or divide patients into various risk groups. Cluster analysis, for example, can be used to find patient groups with shared symptoms or genetic profiles. This information can be used to track the spread of diseases across different geographic areas or to identify new disease subtypes. Patient demographics such as age, lifestyle, and biomarkers are frequently used to create groups using K-Means, one of the most widely used clustering techniques (JayaLakshmi, G. et al., 2024).
   b. *Principal Component Analysis*: The dimensionality reduction technique known as Principal Component Analysis (PCA) reduces the number of variables in complex datasets while maintaining the most crucial information. With PCA, genetic or biomarker data can be made less complex for use in disease forecasting, which facilitates the identification of important variables that influence disease risk. To focus on the most important genes that are correlated with the advancement of the disease, researchers can use PCA to reduce the dimensionality of genetic data in cancer research, for instance.
3. *Reinforcement Learning Models*: Through the use of rewards and penalties based on the model's performance, reinforcement learning (RL) teaches a model to make a series of decisions. When making decisions sequentially, as in disease management or treatment planning, reinforcement learning is especially helpful.

a. *Markov Decision Processes (MDPs)*: In reinforcement learning, Markov Decision Processes (MDPs) are utilized to simulate decision-making scenarios in which the decision-maker has some control over the outcome and some randomness. MDPs have applications in the healthcare industry that help optimize treatment regimens for long-term conditions like cancer and diabetes. Making adjustments to future decisions to optimize long-term health outcomes, the model takes into account past decisions' outcomes (e.g., a patient's reaction to a treatment).
b. *Q-Learning*: One type of reinforcement learning that aids in making decisions in real time is called Q-Learning. As a patient's health changes, it is frequently utilized in personalized medicine to forecast the best course of action. Q-Learning is a useful tool in disease forecasting because it can forecast the course of a disease and recommend treatments that will optimize patient outcomes, like the best time to schedule surgery or prescribe a medication.

4. *Deep Learning Models*: Many-layered artificial neural networks are used by deep learning models, a subset of machine learning, to process large and complicated datasets. With unstructured data, such as text, images, and time-series data, these models are very good at generating predictions.
   a. *Convolutional Neural Nets (CNNs)*: As CNNs are trained to analyze image data, they are perfect for deciphering medical images from CT, MRI, and X-ray scans, among other tests. CNNs (George, W. K. et al., 2024) have a broad application in radiology for early disease detection, including cancer forecasting. By spotting tumors that human radiologists might overlook, CNNs can, for instance, evaluate mammograms to find early indicators of breast cancer and thereby greatly increase diagnosis accuracy. Skin lesions can be identified and classified as benign or malignant in dermatology using CNNs.
   b. *Recurrent Neural Networks (RNNs)*: RNNs are made for sequential data, which makes them appropriate for time-series analysis, like tracking the course of a disease over time. By tracking blood sugar levels in diabetic patients, for example, RNNs are used in disease forecasting to forecast how a patient's condition will change over time based on past health data (Abdullahi, M. et al., 2024). In order to model long-term dependencies in time-series data and make more precise predictions about future health events like heart attacks or strokes, RNNs with long short-term memory (LSTM) are especially helpful.
5. *Hybrid Models*: A single model type's limitations are addressed and forecasting accuracy is increased with hybrid models, which integrate several machine learning techniques. Hybrid methods can produce predictions that are more accurate

and dependable by combining the advantages of several models (Kumar, B. et al., 2024).

a. *Ensemble Learning*: To increase prediction accuracy, ensemble learning techniques like bagging and boosting combine the results of several different models. The predictions of different models (e.g., decision trees, neural networks, and logistic regression) are often combined in ensemble methods to produce more reliable forecasts in the field of disease forecasting (Pandey, D. et al., 2024a). As an illustration, an ensemble model may use spatial clustering and time-series analysis to forecast the location and timing of outbreaks of infectious diseases like the flu.
b. *Hybrid Genetic Algorithms*: Genetic algorithms (GAs) can be combined with machine learning models to optimize the search for the best model parameters. In disease forecasting, hybrid models with GAs are used to fine-tune prediction models by simulating the process of natural selection, ensuring that only the best-performing models or features are used (Pandey, D. et al., 2024b). This approach is useful for complex medical problems, like predicting multi-factorial diseases, where optimal combinations of variables need to be discovered.

6. *Time-Series Models*: When it comes to predicting data trends that change over time, time-series models are especially helpful (Kennedy, G. W. et al., 2024). By tracking and projecting the future trajectory of diseases using past data, these models are extensively employed in disease forecasting.
   a. *Long Short-Term Memory*: The Long Short-Term Memory (LSTM) RNN type is intended to manage time-series data with long-term dependencies. LSTM networks are used in disease forecasting to make long-term predictions about the course of a disease by evaluating past patient data. Examples of this include forecasting the likelihood of an asthma attack based on environmental data or hypothesizing blood sugar trends in patients with diabetes.
   b. *Autoregressive Integrated Moving Average*: The statistical model known as Autoregressive Integrated Moving Average (ARIMA) is utilized in epidemiology, particularly for forecasting short-term diseases. For example, ARIMA models can be used to forecast the number of new flu cases in a given region by analyzing historical data to predict future trends (Shahul, A. et al., 2024). Health officials can better plan interventions like vaccination drives or quarantines by using ARIMA, which is widely used in public health to predict disease outbreaks.

IMAGE-BASED DATA IN PREDICTION

Utilization of Diagnostic Imaging

Diagnostic imaging is essential in contemporary medicine, offering non-invasive methods to visualize the body's internal structures and functions. Early disease detection, diagnosis, and treatment planning are crucial across various medical disciplines, including oncology, cardiology, and neurology. Advanced imaging technologies enable healthcare providers to precisely evaluate medical conditions, direct surgical interventions, and track disease progression, thereby reducing the necessity for invasive procedures. X-ray imaging is a prevalent and essential diagnostic technique utilized for identifying bone fractures, infections, and pulmonary conditions such as pneumonia or tuberculosis. X-rays offer rapid and distinct images of dense structures such as bones, establishing them as a primary instrument in both emergency and routine medical care. Computed tomography (CT) scans, an advanced variant of X-ray technology, provide intricate cross-sectional images of the body. CT scans are especially effective for diagnosing internal injuries, identifying cancers, and evaluating the severity of heart disease by providing detailed visualization of organs, blood vessels, and tissues. Magnetic resonance imaging (MRI) is a potent diagnostic instrument that yields highly detailed images of soft tissues without employing radiation. MRIs are particularly effective in identifying neurological disorders, including brain tumors, strokes, and spinal cord irregularities, as well as orthopedic issues such as ligament tears or joint degeneration. The capacity to accurately distinguish among various tissue types renders MRI the gold standard for numerous intricate diagnoses. Ultrasound imaging is a prevalent, non-invasive method that employs sound waves to generate images (Pandey, D. et al., 2024c) of the body's internal organs and structures.

It is commonly utilized in obstetrics to assess fetal development during gestation, while also serving a crucial function in diagnosing conditions associated with the heart, blood vessels, and abdominal organs. In contrast to X-rays or CT scans, ultrasound employs non-ionizing radiation, rendering it a safer alternative for repeated applications, especially in vulnerable groups such as pregnant women and infants. Positron emission tomography (PET) scans, frequently integrated with CT or MRI, are employed to identify metabolic and biochemical alterations in tissues. PET scans are crucial in oncology for detecting malignant cells, assessing the degree of cancer dissemination, and evaluating treatment efficacy. PET imaging can identify diseases at their initial stages by emphasizing regions of heightened metabolic activity, even prior to the manifestation of structural alterations. The amalgamation of diagnostic imaging with artificial neural network (Pandey, B. K., & Pandey, D., 2023) is revolutionizing the domain (Pandey, D., & Pandey, B. K., 2022). AI-driven systems can evaluate medical images with exceptional accuracy, facilitating expedited and precise diagnoses. AI algorithms are employed to identify tumors in mammograms and lung abnormalities in chest X-rays with superior sensitivity compared to conventional methods. This enhances diagnostic precision while alleviating the burden on radiologists, facilitating more prompt patient care (Guidance, W. H. O., 2021).

Feature Extraction for Early Detection

Feature extraction from medical images is essential for improving early disease detection by identifying critical characteristics or patterns that may be undetectable to the human eye. This procedure entails isolating and quantifying distinct attributes, including shape, texture, intensity, and contrast, from imaging data such as X-rays, MRIs, or CT scans. The extracted features are subsequently analyzed to identify abnormalities that may signify the early presence of a disease. Feature extraction facilitates earlier and more accurate diagnoses by offering a detailed and precise evaluation of medical images, which is essential for effective treatment and enhanced patient outcomes. A notable advantage of feature extraction is its capacity to identify subtle anomalies that may be overlooked during visual examination. In mammography, minute calcifications or anomalies in breast tissue may serve as early indicators of breast cancer. Automated feature extraction can elucidate these patterns, facilitating earlier detection and intervention. Likewise, chest X-rays can more accurately identify small nodules or asymmetries that may indicate early-stage lung cancer.

The ability to detect subtle details can greatly influence patient survival rates by enabling treatment at a stage when the disease is more controllable. Feature extraction facilitates quantitative analysis of medical images, offering a uniform and objective methodology for diagnosis. Transforming visual data into numerical values enables the measurement, tracking, and comparison of attributes such as size, shape, and texture over time. This quantitative analysis diminishes the subjectivity of human interpretation and guarantees more dependable diagnoses. In cancer diagnosis, the assessment of tumor size and texture over time via extracted features enables physicians to identify changes promptly, facilitating timely treatment modifications (Palaniappan, S., V, R., & David, B., 2022). The efficacy of feature extraction is significantly enhanced when integrated with machine learning algorithms. Machine learning models can be trained on extracted features to identify patterns indicative of particular diseases. Machine learning-analyzed MRI scans can distinguish between benign and malignant tumors by evaluating extracted features such as texture and irregularity. These algorithms exhibit heightened sensitivity to early disease indicators, facilitating swifter and more precise detection compared to conventional diagnostic techniques. Feature extraction is particularly adept at identifying micro-level alterations that may indicate the emergence of diseases such as Alzheimer's, cancer, or cardiovascular disorders. Subtle alterations in brain tissue identified via texture analysis in MRIs can indicate early signs of neurodegeneration prior to substantial structural damage. In ophthalmology, extracting features from retinal images can reveal subtle alterations in blood vessel patterns, potentially signaling the onset of diabetic retinopathy prior to the manifestation of symptoms. This early identification facilitates prompt intervention, enhancing the likelihood of effective treatment and averting additional disease advancement. The incorporation of multimodal imaging, utilizing feature extraction across various imaging modalities such as CT, MRI, and PET, offers a holistic perspective on a patient's health. Integrating anatomical characteristics from CT scans with metabolic data from PET scans can facilitate the earlier identification of cancers by revealing both structural anomalies and metabolic activity. This holistic method is essential for early diagnosis, especially in intricate diseases such as cancer, where prompt intervention can be lifesaving (Roy, S. et al., 2021).

SECURITY THREATS IN TRANSMISSION

Risks of Cyberattacks on Healthcare Data Systems

Ransomware and data theft pose serious threats to patient safety, data privacy, and the operational stability of healthcare institutions. Concerns regarding cyberattacks on healthcare data systems have become increasingly prevalent in recent years. Cybercriminals who are looking to make a financial gain or gain unauthorized access to critical data are increasingly targeting healthcare systems because of their increasing reliance on digital infrastructure to store and manage sensitive patient information. These kinds of attacks can have devastating effects, including the compromise of patient care, the loss of financial resources, and the impairment of an organization's reputation over the long term. The number of ransomware attacks, in particular, has increased significantly over the past few years, affecting healthcare facilities all over the world.

The goal of these attacks is to make critical data inaccessible by encrypting it after cybercriminals have gained access to the network (Sheela, M. S. et al., 2025) of a healthcare system. Finally, in order to decrypt the files, they demand a ransom, which is typically paid in cryptocurrency. There is the potential for ransomware to have a devastating effect. Surgical procedures, diagnostic tests, and access to electronic health records (EHRs) could be among the routine operations that hospitals are compelled to halt. The care of patients may be delayed or disrupted as a result of this, which may result in potentially life-threatening circumstances. The fear of losing patient data or experiencing prolonged downtime, which only encourages further attacks, is a common reason why healthcare institutions feel pressured to pay the ransom. Data theft is another significant risk that exists in addition to ransomware. Big amounts of sensitive information, such as personal identification details, medical histories, insurance information, and payment data, are stored in the databases of healthcare information systems. Cybercriminals who engage in identity theft, fraud, or even the sale of stolen data on the black market tend to target healthcare organizations because of the wealth of information that they possess. Individuals may experience long-term repercussions as a result of the theft of patient data, including the exposure of private medical conditions, the theft of their identities, and financial fraud. In addition, healthcare providers who fail to adequately protect patient information have the potential to face regulatory consequences as well as financial penalties under laws such as the Health Insurance Portability and Accountability Act (HIPAA). There is also a significant worry regarding the possibility of medical devices and systems that are connected being compromised. Critical systems, such as insulin pumps, pacemakers, or diagnostic tools, are susceptible to cyberattacks as the integration of healthcare technology continues to increase. These attacks can have direct repercussions for the health and safety of potential patients. It is possible for attackers to manipulate or disable these devices, putting people's lives in danger (Ghannam, R. B., & Techtmann, S. M., 2021).

Legal and Ethical Concerns

Legal and ethical issues arise when medical images are accessed without permission due to the sensitivity of healthcare data. X-rays, MRIs, and CT scans are subject to strict privacy and ethical standards because they often contain patient data. When unauthorized parties access these images, patient confidentiality, personal data misuse, and trust between patients and healthcare providers can be violated. Unauthorized access has legal and ethical consequences for patient care. Accessing medical images without permission violates patient privacy laws. In many countries, healthcare providers must follow strict data collection, storage, and transmission regulations. In the US, HIPAA sets strict guidelines for protecting personal health information (PHI), including medical images. Accessing, sharing, or using these images without permission can result in steep fines and legal action against the healthcare provider or organization that breached. According to the European General Data Protection Regulation (GDPR), healthcare organizations must protect personal data from unauthorized access. Medical image breaches can lead to fines, lawsuits, and reputational damage to institutions, emphasizing the importance of legal compliance. Unauthorised access to medical images violates patient autonomy, confidentiality, and trust. Patients trust doctors to protect their medical data, including images (Atkinson, A. et al., 2023). When unauthorized access violates trust, healthcare system confidence can suffer. Inappropriate sharing or misuse of sensitive medical conditions in these images may make patients feel vulnerable and exposed. The confidentiality of medical images is essential to medical ethics because unauthorized disclosure can lead to stigma or discrimination. Unauthorized access to medical images of stigmatized illnesses may lead to social or workplace discrimination, making patients more vulnerable. Uninformed consent before sharing or using medical images is another ethical issue. Medical images are usually used for diagnosis or treatment with patient consent. The unauthorised use of these images for research, commercial gain, or cybercrime violates their autonomy. Patients' data use and access are protected by informed consent, a cornerstone of healthcare ethics. Unauthorized access breaches this principle, leaving patients powerless over their personal data and its misuse. Healthcare providers must responsibly secure patient data, including medical images. Security breaches or unauthorized access to these systems are ethical violations. Providers must store, transmit, and restrict access to medical images. Over and above technical safeguards, healthcare organizations must train staff on data security and ethical data handling to promote accountability and vigilance (Roth, J. A. et al., 2018).

INNOVATIVE SECURE TRANSMISSION TECHNIQUES

Advanced secure transmission methods are essential for safeguarding sensitive medical images and maintaining patient confidentiality in the swiftly advancing realm of healthcare technology. With the rise of cyber threats, the necessity for stringent security protocols in medical data transmission has become critical. Among these techniques, advanced encryption standards (AES) and homomorphic encryption have become vital instruments for protecting medical images during transmission. Advanced Encryption Standards (AES) is a widely utilized encryption protocol that offers a robust level of security for data both at rest and in transit. AES employs symmetric key encryption, signifying that the identical key is utilized for both encryption and decryption. This method is both efficient and effective, rendering it optimal for securing medical images during network transmission. Encrypting images prior to transmission enables healthcare providers to safeguard data from unauthorized access, even in the event of interception. Homomorphic encryption enables computations to be executed on encrypted data without prior decryption. This feature is especially advantageous in healthcare, facilitating collaborative analysis of medical images while safeguarding patient privacy. Researchers can utilize encrypted images to create disease forecasting models while ensuring the security of patient data, thereby enabling data sharing between institutions without compromising confidentiality. Another innovative method for secure transmission is Secure Multi-Party Computation (SMPC), which allows multiple parties to jointly compute functions based on their inputs while maintaining the confidentiality of those inputs. Within the framework of collaborative disease forecasting, SMPC enables healthcare professionals to examine and exchange insights derived from medical images while safeguarding sensitive patient information from disclosure. This method promotes institutional collaboration, improving the capacity to discern patterns and trends in disease progression while safeguarding individual patient privacy. Utilizing SMPC enables organizations to provide significant data for collective analyses while ensuring compliance with privacy regulations, thereby enhancing disease management strategies (Stewart, L. A. et al., 2015). Quantum cryptography offers a promising prospect for safeguarding medical communications in the future. In contrast to conventional cryptographic techniques, quantum cryptography utilizes the principles of quantum mechanics to establish secure communication channels. Quantum Key Distribution (QKD) is a highly promising application that enables two parties to generate a shared, secret key utilizing quantum bits (qubits). The distinctive characteristics of qubits guarantee that any effort to intercept the communication would disrupt the quantum state, notifying the parties of a security violation. The healthcare sector's growing dependence on digital communication necessitates the integration of quantum cryptography, which could offer an unparalleled level of security for the transmission of sensitive medical images, rendering unauthorized access nearly impossible.

REMOTE HEALTHCARE AND ML

Telemedicine and Secure Image Transmission

Healthcare professionals can now provide prompt and efficient care through digital technologies and remote consultations thanks to telemedicine, which has become a revolutionary force in disease forecasting. The secure transmission of diagnostic images is at the heart of this evolution and is essential for improving overall health monitoring, treatment planning, and patient assessment. Protecting private medical information while it is being transmitted is becoming more and more important as telemedicine becomes the norm. Allowing for instant access to expert consultations is a major benefit of telemedicine in the context of disease forecasting. Many times, in order to diagnose conditions like tumors or fractures, patients may need to be evaluated immediately using diagnostic imaging methods like CT or MRI scans. These images can be safely sent via telemedicine to medical professionals who can administer assessments in real time, suggest additional testing, or start treatment plans right away. For prompt interventions, especially when a prompt diagnosis has a direct impact on patient outcomes, having instant access to expert opinions can be vital. By enabling continued patient monitoring for patients with chronic conditions, telemedicine also facilitates continuity of care. To monitor the course of their diseases, patients with conditions like diabetes or heart disease frequently need routine imaging. Early problem identification is made easier by telemedicine, which enables medical professionals to gather and analyze diagnostic images continuously over time. The uninterrupted availability of vital information for decision-making is ensured by the secure transmission of these images, enabling medical teams to make proactive modifications to treatment plans and lower the chance of patient worsening. The possibility of patient participation in their healthcare journey is also increased by telemedicine. In order to give their healthcare providers the most up-to-date information, patients can actively manage their health by uploading diagnostic images through secure platforms. Due to their increased involvement in treatment choices, patients are encouraged to feel more accountable and own their health. Furthermore, by safely exchanging their photos with several medical professionals, patients can obtain specialized care or second opinions, improving the general standard of their health care. Public health programs can benefit from the use of telemedicine in disease forecasting. Healthcare companies are able to recognize new disease trends and outbreaks by examining patterns in diagnostic images that are transmitted from different areas. The safe gathering of imaging data, for example, from several medical facilities can provide information about the frequency of specific ailments, like infectious outbreaks or respiratory ailments. Public health professionals are able to better allocate resources, carry out preventive measures, and enhance community health outcomes overall thanks to this data-driven approach. The efficiency and accuracy of disease forecasting are further improved by the integration of telemedicine with electronic health record (EHR) systems. By ensuring that diagnostic images are securely transmitted, an entire view of a patient's medical history can be viewed and seamlessly integrated into their electronic health record (EHR). Healthcare professionals can make more accurate diagnoses and treatment plans thanks to this integrated approach, which gives them access to a comprehensive dataset on which to base their decisions. The ability to access past imaging data also supports proactive disease management strategies by enabling the tracking of changes in a patient's condition over time.

Real-Time Forecasting with Secure Data

Enhancing remote patient monitoring systems with real-time forecasting and secure data channels improves healthcare delivery, especially for chronically ill patients. Reliable monitoring and timely interventions require real-time data analysis and secure communication as healthcare becomes more patient-centered. Remote patient monitoring systems' real-time forecasting lets doctors rapidly assess a patient's health. Chronic diseases like diabetes, hypertension, and heart disease require this ability because vital signs can indicate complications. They use advanced analytics and machine learning algorithms to spot trends or anomalies in patient data, alerting healthcare providers to potential health issues before they worsen. Continuous glucose monitoring systems can alert patients and providers if blood sugar levels reach dangerous levels, allowing them to take immediate action to avoid problems. In remote monitoring systems, secure data channels are necessary to protect patient data. Due to the sensitivity of health data, strong security measures are needed to prevent abuse. Sending vital signs and medical histories to healthcare providers is secure with advanced encryption protocols. By restricting access to sensitive data to authorized personnel, authentication mechanisms improve patient privacy and monitoring system trust. Active forecasting and secure data transmission improve patient engagement in healthcare management. Patients with monitoring devices can make informed care decisions based on immediate health feedback. Heart failure patients may use remote weight, blood pressure, and heart rate monitoring. A concerning trend, such as rapid weight gain due to fluid retention, can prompt the patient to adjust their medication or contact their doctor. Proactive care empowers patients to manage their health and collaborate with their doctors. Better remote patient monitoring systems can also help healthcare providers coordinate care. When patient data is securely transmitted in real time, multiple healthcare professionals can access it. More informed decision-making and collaborative treatment planning are possible in complex cases that require multiple specialists. The primary care physician, surgeon, and physical therapist may monitor a post-surgery patient. These providers can better coordinate care by sharing real-time data, ensuring the patient receives overall support during recovery.

CROSS-BORDER DISEASE SURVEILLANCE

Cross-border disease surveillance is increasingly vital in a globalized world, where diseases can swiftly disseminate across nations. As global partnerships for disease outbreak forecasting expand, the utilization of secure transmission techniques and machine learning (ML) models is essential. This facilitates prompt forecasting and safeguards sensitive data exchanged between nations. Nonetheless, challenges such as data standardization and the assurance of secure transmission across diverse jurisdictions must be resolved for effective global health initiatives. International collaborations are essential for detecting and forecasting disease outbreaks, especially in response to global health threats such as pandemics. The exchange of diagnostic images, genomic data, and epidemiological information internationally enables health authorities to identify patterns and make informed decisions. Nonetheless, this data-sharing procedure must be secure to avert breaches that could jeopardize patient privacy or result in data misuse. Encryption and blockchain technologies are being employed to safeguard sensitive information in these collaborations through secure transmission protocols. Countries involved in a global disease surveillance network may exchange real-time diagnostic images for collaborative analysis; however, ensuring secure transmission is essential to prevent unauthorized access and uphold compliance with international privacy regulations such as GDPR and HIPAA. Machine learning models are progressively utilized in global forecasting networks to anticipate disease outbreaks, monitor infection dissemination, and identify vulnerable populations. These machine learning models examine extensive datasets from various regions, encompassing diagnostic images, patient information, and environmental variables. Ensuring the safeguarding of this sensitive information while utilizing these models internationally is a primary concern. Homomorphic encryption facilitates computations on encrypted data, permitting healthcare organizations and governments to collaborate on disease forecasting without revealing raw data to potential breaches. Secure multi-party computation (SMPC) enables nations to collaborate on analyses while preserving the confidentiality of their respective datasets. A major challenge in cross-border disease surveillance is the absence of standardization in the secure transmission of medical images and health data across various healthcare systems. Countries frequently possess disparate regulations, security protocols, and technical infrastructures, which can obstruct seamless data sharing. Standardizing these processes internationally is essential for establishing a unified global response to disease outbreaks. For instance, while some nations may employ specific encryption standards for transmitting medical images, others may utilize disparate protocols or antiquated systems, resulting in vulnerabilities in the shared data. Implementing international standards for secure image transmission potentially spearheaded by entities like the World Health Organization (WHO) may address these challenges and enhance global disease surveillance initiatives. Discrepancies in privacy legislation among nations introduce an additional layer of complexity to the standardization of secure transmission. Conflicting data protection requirements across various regions complicate the establishment of a standardized system for sharing medical images. Establishing a framework that adheres to local privacy regulations while guaranteeing data security is crucial for successful collaboration. This may entail the establishment of universal encryption standards and secure cloud-based systems that enable countries to exchange encrypted data in real time without the risk of breaches.

CONCLUSION

The field of disease forecasting has witnessed a significant transformation due to the application of machine learning (ML), which has introduced novel approaches for early diagnosis, prediction, and treatment of medical conditions. Machine learning models have improved disease outbreak predictions by speeding up and increasing accuracy by sifting through massive datasets and finding patterns that would be hard for humans to notice. This has improved patient care both locally and globally. It is impossible to overstate the significance of secure data transmission, though. Privacy laws must be followed and patient trust must be preserved by protecting patient data when medical images and other health-related information are exchanged. Robust security measures, such as encryption, secure multi-party computation, or homomorphic encryption, are required to protect sensitive health information from cyber threats and unauthorized access. There is a lot of potential for future advancements in health forecasting systems when AI is combined with secure transmission techniques. Global health crises can be avoided by healthcare systems with increased ability to anticipate disease outbreaks, remotely manage patient care, and work together internationally as these technologies advance. In the end, more proactive and effective healthcare solutions will result from the continued development of AI-powered health systems and stronger data security measures.

REFERENCES

Abdullahi, M., Ahmad, A., Pandey, B. K., & Pandey, D. (2024). Digital Currency Adoption: A Comparative Analysis of Global Trends and the Nigerian eNaira Digital Currency. *SN Computer Science*, *5*(5), 1–11. DOI: 10.1007/s42979-024-02882-6

Atkinson, A., Ellenberger, B., Piezzi, V., Kaspar, T., Salazar-Vizcaya, L., Endrich, O., Leichtle, A. B., & Marschall, J. (2023). Extending outbreak investigation with machine learning and graph theory: Benefits of new tools with application to a nosocomial outbreak of a multidrug-resistant organism. *Infection Control and Hospital Epidemiology*, *44*(2), 246–252. DOI: 10.1017/ice.2022.66 PMID: 36111457

Elarmathi, S., Rishabavarthani, P., Sindhuja, M., Elayaraja, P., & Malathi Murugesan, S. (2024). Novel manufacturing systems for cancer diagnosis using ultra-sensitive photonic crystal fiber biosensor with dual-functionalized aptamer-nanocavity. *Microsystem Technologies*, •••, 1–20. DOI: 10.1007/s00542-024-05820-x

George, W. K., Silas, E. I., Pandey, D., & Pandey, B. K. (2024). Utilization of Industry 4.0 Technologies in Nigerian Technical and Vocational Education: A Conundrum for Educators. In *Examining the Rapid Advance of Digital Technology in Africa* (pp. 270–293). IGI Global. DOI: 10.4018/978-1-6684-9962-7.ch014

Ghannam, R. B., & Techtmann, S. M. (2021). Machine learning applications in microbial ecology, human microbiome studies, and environmental monitoring. *Computational and Structural Biotechnology Journal*, *19*, 1092–1107. DOI: 10.1016/j.csbj.2021.01.028 PMID: 33680353

Guidance, W. H. O. (2021). *Ethics and governance of artificial intelligence for health*. World Health Organization.

JayaLakshmi. G., Pandey, D., Pandey, B. K., Kaur, P., Mahajan, D. A., & Dari, S. S. (2024). Smart big data collection for intelligent supply chain improvement. In AI and Machine Learning Impacts in Intelligent Supply Chain (pp. 180-195). IGI Global Scientific Publishing.

Kennedy, G. W., Sunday, S. E., Pandey, D., Kabari, A. D., Pandey, B. K., George, A. S., & Dadheech, P. (2024). Building Information Modeling: Harnessing Innovations for Professional Proficiency. In Emerging Engineering Technologies and Industrial Applications (pp. 305-331). IGI Global.

Khadka, M., Sah, M., Chaudhary, R., Sahani, S. K., Sahani, K., Pandey, B. K., & Pandey, D. (2025). Spectroscopic, quantum chemical, and topological calculations of the phenylephrine molecule using density functional theory. *Scientific Reports*, *15*(1), 208. DOI: 10.1038/s41598-024-81633-2 PMID: 39747169

Konapure, C. G., Pandey, D., Shete, H., Thakar, C. M., Pandey, B. K., & George, A. S. (2025). Artificial Intelligence in Automated Concrete Mix Design Using Computerized Grading Curves. Interdisciplinary Approaches to AI, Internet of Everything, and Machine Learning, 567-586.

Kumar, B., Pandey, D., Pandey, B. K., & George, A. S. (2024). Higher Education in the Last Four Decades: A Review of Paradigm Shifts in Policy Frameworks. Design and Implementation of Higher Education Learners' Learning Outcomes (HELLO), 333-348.

Kumar, M. S., Prasanna, P. L., Lalitha, M., Joy, M., Jha, S. S., & Pandey, B. K. (2025). Utilizing the Internet of Everything and Artificial Intelligence for Real-Time Workforce Management. In Role of Internet of Everything (IOE), VLSI Architecture, and AI in Real-Time Systems (pp. 153-168). IGI Global Scientific Publishing.

Kumarganesh, S., & Malathi Murugesan, C. (2024). Hybrid plasmonic biosensors with deep learning for colorectal cancer detection. *Plasmonics*, •••, 1–15. DOI: 10.1007/s11468-024-02568-y

Lakshmi, K. V. N., Rajan, R., Pandey, D., & Pandey, B. K. (2024). Circular economy: A catalyst for economic growth-an empirical study. *Circular Economy and Sustainability*, •••, 1–22.

Maheshwari, R., Kumarganesh, S., K v M, S., Gopalakrishnan, A., Selvi, K., Paulchamy, B., Rishabavarthani, P., Sagayam, K. M., Pandey, B. K., & Pandey, D. (2024). Advanced plasmonic resonance-enhanced biosensor for comprehensive real-time detection and analysis of deepfake content. *Plasmonics*, •••, 1–18. DOI: 10.1007/s11468-024-02407-0

Maheshwari, R. U., Paulchamy, B., Pandey, B. K., & Pandey, D. (2024). Enhancing sensing and imaging capabilities through surface plasmon resonance for deepfake image detection. *Plasmonics*, •••, 1–20. DOI: 10.1007/s11468-024-02492-1

Muralidhar, L. B., Lakshmi, K. V. N., Swapna, H. R., Rupani, J., Nethravathi, K., Pandey, B. K., & Pandey, D. (2024). Impact of Organizational Culture on The Level of Corporate Social Responsibility Investments: An Exploratory Study. *Circular Economy and Sustainability*, *4*(3), 1–19. DOI: 10.1007/s43615-024-00371-9

Palaniappan, S. V. R., & David, B. (2022). Prediction of epidemic disease dynamics on the infection risk using machine learning algorithms. *SN Computer Science*, *3*(1), 47. DOI: 10.1007/s42979-021-00902-3 PMID: 34755116

Pandey, B. K., Kanike, U. K., George, A. S., & Pandey, D. (Eds.). (2024d). *AI and machine learning impacts in intelligent supply chain*. IGI Global. DOI: 10.4018/979-8-3693-1347-3

Pandey, B. K., Nassa, V. K., Mukundan, A. P., Mahajan, D. A., Pandey, D., George, A. S., & Dadheech, P. (2024c). An Industry-Focused Traffic System Utilising Internet of Things. In *Emerging Engineering Technologies and Industrial Applications* (pp. 200–213). IGI Global. DOI: 10.4018/979-8-3693-1335-0.ch009

Pandey, B. K., & Pandey, D. (2023). Parametric optimization and prediction of enhanced thermoelectric performance in co-doped CaMnO3 using response surface methodology and neural network. *Journal of Materials Science Materials in Electronics*, *34*(21), 1589. DOI: 10.1007/s10854-023-10954-1

Pandey, B. K., & Pandey, D. (2025). Securing healthcare medical image information using advance morphological component analysis, information hiding systems, and hybrid convolutional neural networks on IoMT. *Computers in Biology and Medicine*, *185*, 109499. DOI: 10.1016/j.compbiomed.2024.109499 PMID: 39642698

Pandey, B. K., Pandey, D., & Lelisho, M. E. (2024a). Face mask identification with enhanced cuckoo optimization and deep learning-based faster regional neural network. *Scientific Reports*, *14*(1), 29719. DOI: 10.1038/s41598-024-78746-z PMID: 39613761

Pandey, B. K., Pandey, D., & Sahani, S. K. (2024b). Autopilot control unmanned aerial vehicle system for sewage defect detection using deep learning. *Engineering Reports*, •••, 12852.

Pandey, B. K., Paramashivan, M. A., Pandey, D., George, A. S., Agarwal, A., Mahajan, D. A., . . . Pramanik, S. (2024e). Future Directions of Digital Twin Architectures for 6G Communication Networks. In Security Issues and Solutions in 6G Communications and Beyond (pp. 197-211). IGI Global.

Pandey, D., Nassa, V. K., Pandey, B. K., Thankachan, B., Dadheech, P., Mahajan, D. A., & George, A. S. (2024a). Artificial Intelligence and Machine Learning and Its Application in the Field of Computational Visual Analysis. In Emerging Engineering Technologies and Industrial Applications (pp. 36-57). IGI Global. DOI: 10.4018/979-8-3693-1335-0.ch003

Pandey, D., & Pandey, B. K. (2022). An efficient deep neural network with adaptive galactic swarm optimization for complex image text extraction. In *Process Mining Techniques for Pattern Recognition* (pp. 121–137). CRC Press. DOI: 10.1201/9781003169550-10

Pandey, D., Pandey, B. K., Nassa, V. K., Mahajan, D. A., George, A. S., & Dadheech, P. (2024c). Optimized Throughput-Based Broadcasting for Next Generation Wireless Networks. In Emerging Engineering Technologies and Industrial Applications (pp. 355-368). IGI Global. DOI: 10.4018/979-8-3693-1335-0.ch018

Pandey, D., Pandey, B. K., Paramashivan, M. A., Mahajan, D. A., Dadheech, P. D., George, A. S., & Hameed, A. S. (2024b). Advanced Digital Data Processing Using Cloud Cryptography: Industrial Applications. In Emerging Engineering Technologies and Industrial Applications (pp. 255-268). IGI Global.

Provenzano, S., Santangelo, O. E., Giordano, D., Alagna, E., Piazza, D., Genovese, D., & Firenze, A. (2019). Predicting disease outbreaks: Evaluating measles infection with Wikipedia Trends. *Recenti Progressi in Medicina*, *110*(6), 292–296. PMID: 31282485

Roy, S., Biswas, P., & Ghosh, P. (2021). Spatiotemporal tracing of pandemic spread from infection data. *Scientific Reports*, *11*(1), 17689.

Rai, P. K., Pandey, D., & Pandey, B. K. (2024). The future of enterprise and innovation is compute as a commodity, or CaaC. *Partners Universal International Research Journal*, *3*(2), 89–94.

Roth, J. A., Battegay, M., Juchler, F., Vogt, J. E., & Widmer, A. F. (2018). Introduction to machine learning in digital healthcare epidemiology. *Infection Control and Hospital Epidemiology*, *39*(12), 1457–1462. DOI: 10.1017/ice.2018.265 PMID: 30394238

Saravanakumar, R., TamilSelvi, T., Pandey, D., Pandey, B. K., Mahajan, D. A., & Lelisho, M. E. (2024). Big data processing using hybrid Gaussian mixture model with salp swarm algorithm. *Journal of Big Data*, *11*(1), 167. DOI: 10.1186/s40537-024-01015-3

Satheesh, N., Gopisankar, N., Kumarganesh, S., Anthoniraj, S., Saravanakumar, S., & Martin Sagayam, K. (2025). Advanced AI-driven emergency response systems for enhanced vehicle and human safety. *Iran Journal of Computer Science*, •••, 1–16. DOI: 10.1007/s42044-025-00228-w

Saxena, A., Agarwal, A., Pandey, B. K., & Pandey, D. (2024). Examination of the Criticality of Customer Segmentation Using Unsupervised Learning Methods. *Circular Economy and Sustainability*, *4*(2), 1–14. DOI: 10.1007/s43615-023-00336-4

Shahul, A., Muniandi, B., Paramashivan, M. A., Pandey, D., Pandey, B. K., Dadheech, P., & George, H. (2024). An Analysis of Algorithms and Methods Based on Image Processing for Medical Applications. In *Emerging Engineering Technologies and Industrial Applications* (pp. 173–186). IGI Global. DOI: 10.4018/979-8-3693-1335-0.ch007

Sheela, M. S., Kumarganesh, S., Pandey, B. K., & Lelisho, M. E. (2025). Integration of silver nanostructures in wireless sensor networks for enhanced biochemical sensing. *Discover Nano*, *20*(1), 7. DOI: 10.1186/s11671-024-04159-6 PMID: 39804434

Singh, S., Madaan, G., Swapna, H. R., Singh, A., Pandey, D., George, A. S., & Pandey, B. K. (2025a). Empowering Connectivity: Exploring the Internet of Things. In Interdisciplinary Approaches to AI, Internet of Everything, and Machine Learning (pp. 89-116). IGI Global Scientific Publishing.

Singh, S., Madaan, G., Swapna, H. R., Singh, A., Pandey, B. K., George, A. S., & Pandey, D. (2025b). Unleashing the Power of AI and Data Analysis: Transforming Insights into Action. In Interdisciplinary Approaches to AI, Internet of Everything, and Machine Learning (pp. 1-24). IGI Global Scientific Publishing.

Stewart, L. A., Clarke, M., Rovers, M., Riley, R. D., Simmonds, M., Stewart, G., & Tierney, J. F. (2015). Preferred reporting items for a systematic review and meta-analysis of individual participant data: The PRISMA-IPD statement. *Journal of the American Medical Association*, *313*(16), 1657–1665. DOI: 10.1001/jama.2015.3656 PMID: 25919529

Chapter 9

IoT-Driven Secure Data Sharing in Telemedicine Systems

Megha Mudholkar
https://orcid.org/0009-0005-3472-8037
Department of Computer Engineering, Marwadi University, India

Pankaj Mudholkar
https://orcid.org/0000-0003-1639-0704
Faculty of Computer Applications, Marwadi University, India

S. Prince Chelladurai
https://orcid.org/0000-0003-3432-0515
Faculty of Engineering and Technology, SRM Institute of Science and Technology, Kattankulathur, India

Krishna Murthy Inumula
https://orcid.org/0000-0002-4556-549X
Symbiosis Institute of International Business, Symbiosis International University, Pune, India

M. Selvi
Department of Computer Science and Engineering, Sathyabama Institute of Science and Technology, Chennai, India

Joshuva Arockia Dhanraj
https://orcid.org/0000-0001-5048-7775
Dayananda Sagar University, India

A. S. Hovan George
Tbilisi State Medical University, Georgia

ABSTRACT

The crucial part that connected devices play in the process of transforming the delivery of healthcare through telemedicine, with an emphasis on the potential of these devices to improve patient care, increase access to services, and make it easier to monitor health conditions in real time. The need for robust security measures to protect sensitive patient data has emerged as a primary concern as the integration of these technologies in healthcare facilities becomes increasingly widespread. There

DOI: 10.4018/979-8-3693-9821-0.ch009

is an immediate need for ongoing research and development in the field of secure telemedicine systems. As the state of technology continues to advance, healthcare organizations are required to remain one step ahead of new dangers by continuously enhancing their security protocols and compliance measures.

INTRODUCTION

The integration of smart devices, sensors, and networks to gather and transfer real-time data is transforming the healthcare industry through the Internet of Things (IoT) (Lakshmi, K. V. N. et al., 2024), opening up new opportunities for patient care and medical services. IoT enables medical professionals to provide more individualized care, better manage chronic illnesses, and remotely monitor patients. The trend toward data-driven healthcare (Kumarganesh, S. et al., 2024) is decreasing the need for frequent in-person consultations and increasing the effectiveness of treatment, especially for patients with chronic illnesses. Remote patient monitoring is among the Internet of Things' most significant uses in the medical field. Vital signs like blood pressure, oxygen saturation, heart rate, and glucose levels can be monitored by gadgets like wearable sensors, smartwatches, and home health monitors. Healthcare practitioners are able to monitor a patient's condition in real time thanks to the constant flow of this information. For example, patients with diabetes can send regular blood sugar readings to their doctors via Internet of Things glucose monitors, enabling timely treatment plan adjustments. (Khadka, M. et al., 2025). The management of chronic diseases is another important application of IoT, especially for patients with long-term conditions like diabetes, asthma, or heart disease. IoT devices monitor health metrics and have the ability to notify medical professionals if a patient's condition deteriorates. For example, an asthma patient's connected inhaler can monitor usage patterns and notify physicians when usage rises, enabling early intervention. Physicians can take action prior to a serious cardiac event by using wearable heart monitors, which can also transmit alerts about abnormal heart activity. Hospital management systems are improved by IoT as well. Medical equipment tracking, inventory level monitoring, and timely maintenance are all made possible by connected hospital devices. By streamlining hospital workflows and cutting down on delays, this increases operational efficiency, lowers costs, and ultimately improves patient care.

Safeguarded Data Exchange in Telemedicine

In telemedicine, secure data transmission (Pandey, B. K., & Pandey, D., 2025) is essential to maintain the privacy and confidentiality of patient information. Securing the transmission of medical data, including diagnostic images, medical records, and real-time health metrics, is crucial to avert data breaches, unauthorized access, and cyberattacks. A fundamental element of secure data sharing in telemedicine is encryption. Encrypting sensitive data renders (Saravanakumar, R. et al., 2024) it incomprehensible to unauthorized individuals, thereby safeguarding the confidentiality and integrity of the information during transmission. Symmetric and asymmetric encryption methods are extensively employed to safeguard communication channels (Sheela, M. S. et al., 2025).) between healthcare providers and patients. End-to-end encryption guarantees that only the designated recipient can decrypt and access the shared medical information, protecting it from possible interception. Besides encryption, secure communication protocols (Pandey, D. et al., 2025) are crucial in telemedicine systems. Protocols like Transport Layer Security (TLS) and Message Queuing Telemetry Transport (MQTT) guarantee the confidentiality and integrity of data exchanged between IoT devices and healthcare platforms (Muralidhar, L. B. et al., 2024). These protocols offer authentication mechanisms to validate the identity of devices and users, thereby mitigating unauthorized access to sensitive patient information. Verification of data integrity is an essential component of secure data sharing. Methods such as hashing and digital signatures are frequently utilized to guarantee that the data remains unaltered during transmission (Satheesh, N. et al., 2025). This ensures that the medical information obtained by healthcare providers is precise and credible, allowing them to make informed decisions based on dependable data. Stringent access control protocols are vital for safeguarding data in telemedicine. Authentication mechanisms, such as multi-factor authentication (MFA), guarantee that only authorized individuals can access medical information. Access control policies restrict the ability to view, modify, or disseminate patient data, thereby mitigating the risk of data exposure (Vyas, S. et al., 2023).

Advancements in IoT Security Technologies

The protection of Internet of Things networks has emerged as a top priority in light of the rapid proliferation of Internet of Things devices in the healthcare industry and other fields. Growing concerns regarding data breaches, unauthorized access (Kumar, M. S. et al., 2025), and device vulnerabilities are being addressed by advancements in Internet of Things (IoT) security technologies are as shown in the figure 1.

- *AI and ML in Security*: Artificial intelligence (AI) (Singh, S. et al., 2025a) and machine learning (ML) are pivotal in augmenting security for interconnected systems. These technologies can scrutinize extensive datasets produced by devices, detecting patterns and anomalies that may indicate a cyber threat. AI-driven solutions can independently identify vulnerabilities and react to potential breaches instantaneously, enhancing the capacity to avert attacks prior to their occurrence. AI and ML algorithms can progress over time, acquiring knowledge from new data and adapting to advanced attack techniques. This dynamic strategy guarantees that security measures stay ahead of emerging threats, fostering a more resilient and adaptive defense system (Pandey, B. K. et al., 2024a). Through predictive analytics, AI can anticipate potential vulnerabilities, facilitating proactive measures prior to the emergence of a problem.
- Blockchain in Device Networks: Blockchain technology provides a decentralized method for securing interconnected systems. This method employs a distributed ledger to maintain data integrity and prevent unauthorized modifications. The decentralized architecture of blockchain eliminates single points of failure, thereby enhancing data security against tampering or hacking attempts (Konapure, C. G. et al., 2025). The implementation of smart contracts within blockchain technology can facilitate the automation of secure procedures such as device authentication and access control. These contracts guarantee that device interactions adhere to established security protocols without intermediaries, thereby minimizing the potential for human error or external interference. The transparency of blockchain provides an additional layer of security, as all transactions are publicly verifiable (Shamshad, F. et al., 2023).
- Zero Trust Security Framework: Zero trust architecture is progressively being implemented to safeguard interconnected systems. This security model operates under the premise of no intrinsic trust within the network, persistently validating each access request through stringent authentication and authorization protocols. By discarding the presumption that internal devices or users are secure, the system markedly diminishes the risk of internal and external threats (Pandey, B. K. et al., 2024b). This containment strategy guarantees that if one segment of the network is breached, it will not propagate to other regions. Ongoing surveillance and instantaneous analytics augment security, guaranteeing that any anomalous activity is promptly identified and rectified.
- Quantum Cryptography: With the progression of quantum computing, quantum cryptography arises as a promising security technology. Quantum key distribution (QKD) facilitates the generation of encryption keys that are impervious to interception without detection, providing exceptional security for data transmission. Quantum-resistant algorithms (Maheshwari, R. U. et al.,

2024) are being devised to safeguard against the computational capabilities of forthcoming quantum machines, which could readily compromise existing encryption techniques. The implementation of quantum-safe cryptographic protocols guarantees the security of sensitive communications and data against quantum threats, rendering it a crucial element in future-proofing security systems.

- *Hardware-Centric Security Solutions*: Hardware-level security technologies, including Trusted Platform Modules (TPMs) and Hardware Security Modules (HSMs), are progressively incorporated into connected devices. These specialized security chips protect cryptographic keys and establish secure environments for essential processes, guaranteeing strong defense against software-based threats (Maheshwari, R. Uma. et al., 2024). Integrating hardware-based security solutions enables the system to execute essential functions such as encryption, authentication, and secure booting in a controlled environment. This markedly diminishes the risk of compromise from external malware or hacking endeavors. Hhardware-level defenses exhibit greater resistance to tampering as they are integrated directly into the device, providing enhanced assurance for sensitive applications (Dwivedi, R. et al., 2022).
- *Secure Over-the-Air (OTA) Updates*: To mitigate device vulnerabilities, secure over-the-air (OTA) updates are evolving in sophistication. These updates enable manufacturers to rectify and enhance software remotely, thereby ensuring devices maintain security post-deployment. The secure OTA process depends on authenticating updates via digital signatures and encryption, thereby obstructing the installation of unauthorized software (Saxena, A. et al., 2024). Consistent updates guarantee that systems are safeguarded against emerging threats, while rollback mechanisms enable devices to revert to a prior version in the event of complications during an update, thereby minimizing downtime and mitigating risks associated with potential defects in new software releases.

Figure 1. Advancements in IoT security technologies

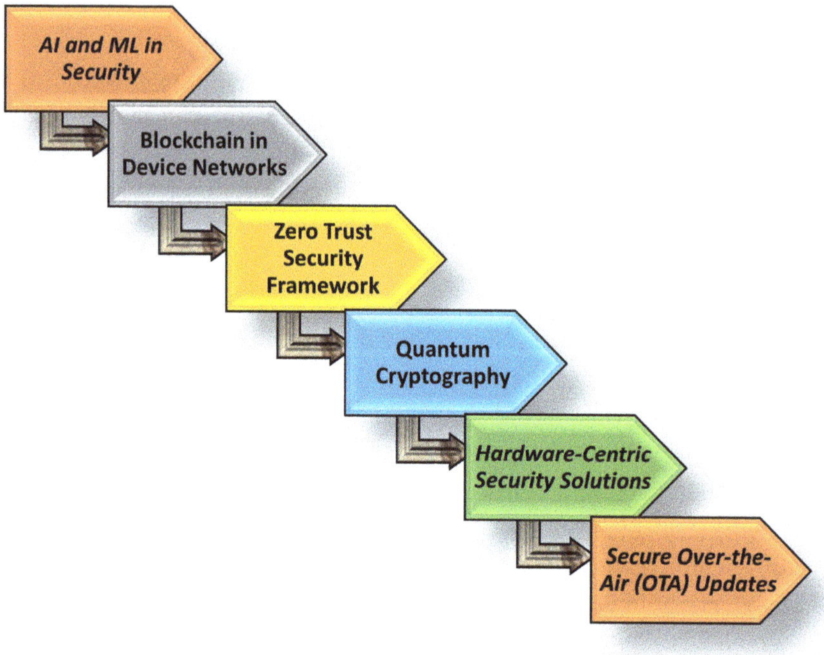

TELEMEDICINE SYSTEMS AND IOT INTEGRATION

IoT Enhancements for Telemedicine

Real-time, remote, data-driven telemedicine has revolutionized healthcare with IoT. Telemedicine is more efficient and personalized thanks to connected devices, improving patient outcomes and access to medical services. IoT improves telemedicine by improving real-time monitoring, personalized treatment, seamless integration with healthcare systems, and access to care. One of the biggest benefits of connected devices in telemedicine is real-time health data collection and transmission (Rai, P. K. et al., 2024). Smartwatches, fitness trackers, and health sensors continuously monitor heart rate, blood pressure, and oxygen levels. Telemedicine platforms send this data directly to doctors, allowing real-time patient monitoring. Real-time monitoring allows early detection of health issues and timely interventions to prevent worsening. A patient's blood pressure can spike, alerting the doctor, who can adjust treatment remotely. Medical professionals can make data-driven decisions faster with immediate access to health metrics, improving patient care. Chronically ill patients benefit from remote patient management via connected health devices. Diabetes, heart disease, and respiratory patients can remotely manage their health with home-based medical devices. Medical professionals receive continuous updates from these devices. Diabetes patients can use a connected glucose monitor to track their blood sugar levels and send their doctor real-time updates. Continuous oversight allows proactive treatment plan adjustments, reducing complications and hospital visits. IoT devices improve patient engagement in health management and reduce healthcare facility workload by providing continuous, at-home care. Another area where IoT has improved telemedicine is personalized healthcare. The massive amounts of data collected by connected devices can help healthcare providers understand individual health patterns. This data helps doctors customize treatments, improving accuracy and efficacy. Wearable devices that track sleep, diet, and exercise can give doctors a complete picture of a patient's lifestyle. This data lets doctors give personalized advice and adjust treatments based on patient behavior. Customization improves health outcomes by providing more relevant and precise care. Telemedicine services are more efficient because IoT integrates well with healthcare systems (Ge, H. et al., 2022). Device data can be stored in EHRs or cloud platforms to help healthcare providers review patient histories. This integration improves medical team coordination by connecting telemedicine platforms and healthcare databases. In addition, AI and machine learning algorithms can find patterns and trends in connected devices' massive data sets. Healthcare providers can adjust treatments proactively using predictive analytics to predict future health risks. IoT-enabled telemedicine improves healthcare access, especially for remote or underserved areas. Rural patients who have trouble getting to a clinic or hospital can use connected health devices to receive care remotely. These devices allow virtual consultations and real-time monitoring, reducing in-person visits. Seniors and those with mobility issues can get quality healthcare without traveling, which is important. IoT reduces healthcare access barriers so more people can use telemedicine regardless of location (Usak, M. et al., 2020).

IoT Devices Used in Telemedicine

Internet of Things (IoT) devices have become a crucial component of telemedicine, improving remote healthcare services by facilitating data collection, real-time monitoring, and easy communication between patients and medical professionals. These gadgets, which range from wearable health trackers to cutting-edge medical equipment, are all intended to enhance patient outcomes and lessen the need for in-person consultations. Among the IoT devices most frequently used in telemedicine are wearable health devices, like smartwatches, fitness trackers, and biosensors. Vital signs such as blood pressure, oxygen saturation, heart rate, and physical activity are tracked by these wearables. They gather health data continuously and send it to telemedicine platforms so medical professionals can monitor patients' conditions in real time. A patient with a cardiac ailment, for instance, might wear a smartwatch that has an ECG sensor built into it, which tracks heart rhythms and notifies the wearer if abnormalities are found. By taking a proactive stance, the likelihood of complications is decreased and prompt medical interventions are made possible. In telemedicine, remote patient monitoring tools including blood pressure cuffs, pulse oximeters, and linked glucose monitors are frequently utilized. Patients with long-term medical conditions like diabetes or hypertension can benefit most from these devices. Patients can avoid making repeated trips to the hospital by monitoring important health metrics from home, and healthcare providers can use the continuous data to modify treatment plans as necessary. For example, real-time adjustments to insulin dosage are made possible by a connected glucose monitor that automatically transmits a patient's blood sugar readings to their physician (Calegari, L. P., & Fettermann, D. C., 2022).

DATA SHARING IN TELEMEDICINE

Types of Medical Data Shared

In remote medical services, diverse data types are exchanged to enable accurate diagnosis, treatment, and continuous care. These data types encompass images, patient records, and real-time information, each significantly contributing to the improvement of service delivery quality. By disseminating various forms of medical data, remote services promote thorough, patient-centered care that is prompt, efficient, and effective. The incorporation of advanced technologies which are shown in Figure 2, guarantees that providers obtain the necessary information to deliver superior care while enhancing the overall experience for individuals seeking medical assistance.

- *Medical Imaging*: Medical imaging is an essential element of remote consultations, enabling professionals to diagnose and monitor conditions without necessitating in-person visits. Prevalent categories of medical imaging disseminated encompass X-rays, MRIs, CT scans, and ultrasounds. These visuals offer comprehensive insights into an individual's anatomical structure and function, facilitating evaluations of injuries, diseases, and other health concerns. Advancements in telecommunication technologies enable the secure and rapid transmission of images to specialists for review and interpretation, thereby facilitating prompt consultations and treatment recommendations.

Remote platforms frequently employ sophisticated imaging technologies that facilitate image enhancement and manipulation, allowing providers to examine visuals with increased detail. Radiologists can execute image segmentation or 3D reconstructions that facilitate the accurate assessment of tumors or fractures. This capability enhances diagnostic accuracy and facilitates improved communication of findings among teams and individuals, thereby augmenting overall comprehension and treatment outcomes.

- *Patient Records*: Electronic Health Records (EHRs) are extensive digital documents encompassing an individual's medical history, treatment protocols, pharmaceuticals, allergies, and laboratory findings. Exchanging electronic health records among professionals facilitates a comprehensive understanding of an individual's health condition. This collaborative access improves communication among healthcare professionals, facilitates coordinated care, and diminishes the probability of errors. The system facilitates secure access to records, allowing providers to make informed decisions based on a comprehensive understanding of an individual's medical history, thereby enhancing the quality of care. EHR systems frequently incorporate decision-support tools that aid healthcare professionals in clinical decision-making. Alerts regarding potential drug interactions or reminders for preventive screenings can markedly improve safety. By incorporating these tools into remote care, providers can guarantee that individuals receive both timely and suitable treatment, thus fostering a more holistic and systematic approach to health management.
- *Real-Time Data*: Real-time data denotes the incessant flow of health information gathered from diverse monitoring devices and wearables. This information encompasses vital signs such as heart rate, blood pressure, blood glucose levels, and oxygen saturation, all of which are essential for the management of chronic conditions and acute medical scenarios. A connected blood pressure monitor can transmit readings directly to a provider, facilitating prompt modifications to treatment plans if required. This data-sharing promotes proactive healthcare, allowing for timely interventions and improved health management beyond conventional clinical environments. The incorporation of artificial intelligence and machine learning algorithms into real-time data analysis can improve the predictive abilities of remote monitoring. These technologies can detect trends and patterns in an individual's vital signs over time, notifying medical professionals of potential health risks before they intensify. By utilizing these advanced analytics, providers can execute tailored interventions that enhance outcomes and guarantee ongoing, high-quality care.

- *Laboratory Results*: Laboratory test results constitute a crucial category of data disseminated in remote services. These results furnish essential information regarding an individual's health, encompassing blood tests, urinalysis, and microbiological cultures. Through the electronic dissemination of laboratory results, professionals can promptly evaluate conditions, detect anomalies, and formulate suitable treatment strategies. The swift dissemination of information expedites the diagnostic process and improves care, especially for conditions necessitating immediate attention. Numerous platforms now integrate automated systems for the generation and dissemination of lab reports, which can considerably decrease turnaround times. Individuals may receive notifications upon the readiness of their results, facilitating discussions of findings during virtual consultations. This not only optimizes the process but also enables individuals to actively participate in their health journey, promoting a collaborative management approach.
- *Medication Information*: Medication information, encompassing prescriptions and medication history, constitutes another vital data type exchanged in remote services. This information guarantees that providers are informed of the medications an individual is currently using, thereby mitigating potential drug interactions and ensuring the safety and efficacy of treatment plans. Utilizing secure messaging platforms and EHR systems, physicians can efficiently convey prescription modifications and furnish individuals with essential instructions, thereby improving adherence to medication protocols. Certain platforms offer functionalities for medication tracking and reminders, which can greatly enhance adherence. For instance, individuals may receive notifications on their mobile devices to prompt them to take their medications or replenish prescriptions. This degree of support facilitates adherence to prescribed treatment regimens, potentially resulting in improved health outcomes and diminished hospital readmissions. These systems utilize technology to oversee and regulate medication usage, thereby significantly enhancing safety and facilitating effective chronic disease management.

Figure 2. Types of medical imaging data

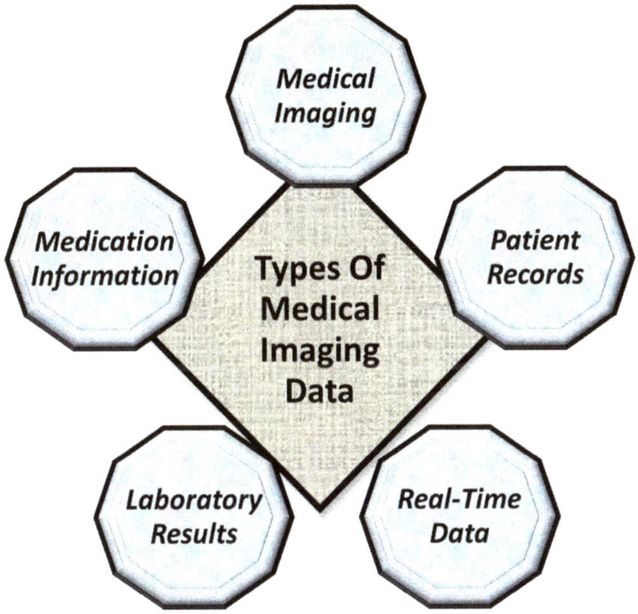

Data Management and Sharing

Medical data management and sharing in remote care systems can affect service quality and efficiency. The volume of data from medical devices, EHRs, and patient monitoring systems is a problem. More healthcare organizations are using digital solutions and connected devices, which has exponentially increased data collection. This massive volume makes data storage, processing, and analysis difficult. Data storage management can be difficult and require significant infrastructure investments to handle the influx of information (Pandey, D. et al., 2024c). As data volume increases, maintaining security and privacy while ensuring access becomes more difficult. Latency is another major data management and sharing issue. Remote healthcare relies on timely information for decision-making and patient safety. Transmission delays can result from network congestion, bandwidth issues, or poor data processing. High latency can prevent real-time monitoring and communication between providers and patients, missing treatment opportunities (Pandey, D., & Pandey, B. K., 2022). A healthcare provider may miss critical patient changes if wearable device vital sign data takes too long to arrive. Interoperability of data is another issue. Many electronic health record systems and medical devices use different standards and protocols, making data sharing between platforms difficult.

Lack of interoperability can fragment care because providers may not have a complete medical history. While data formats and protocols are being standardized, seamless integration across diverse systems remains a challenge (Ahathiyan, G. S. et al., 2025). Data security and privacy are crucial but difficult, especially in an age of cyberattacks. Multiple platforms share sensitive medical data, increasing the risk of data breaches and unauthorized access. To comply with HIPAA, organizations must use encryption and secure access protocols to protect patient data. Balancing accessibility with strict security requirements is difficult and requires specialized expertise and resources. Staff training and technology adaptation can hinder data management and sharing. Medical and administrative staff must be proficient in digital tools and understand data accuracy and integrity. Insufficient training can cause data entry errors, miscommunication, and inefficient workflows, lowering care quality. To ensure staff can handle modern data management, organisations must invest in comprehensive training and support.

IOT-DRIVEN SECURITY FRAMEWORKS

Secure Data Transmission in IoT Networks

Data transmission must be secure in Internet of Things (IoT) networks to protect sensitive data and device communications. Security architectures with different features and methods have been developed to address these issues. Edge computing reduces latency and bandwidth by processing data closer to the source. Instead of sending IoT data to a cloud server, edge nodes process it locally. Edge nodes encrypt and control access to sensitive data before sending it over the network. This architecture increases security and reduces data breaches by minimizing data transmission and sending only relevant data to the central server. For applications like health monitoring and industrial automation (Pandey, B. K. et al., 2024c) that require real-time analysis, processing data locally is beneficial. Cloud-based architecture, which manages IoT data storage and processing using centralized cloud services, is another popular framework. In this architecture, the cloud service provider's encryption, multi-factor authentication, and security audits are crucial. In transit and at rest, IoT data to the cloud is encrypted to prevent unauthorized access. Scalable and flexible, this architecture supports more connected devices and data streams (Pandey, B. K. et al., 2024d). Since cloud breaches can affect all connected devices, organizations must carefully choose cloud service providers that meet strict security standards and regulatory requirements. Blockchain architecture helps IoT networks secure data transmission decentralized. This architecture uses a distributed ledger to guarantee data integrity and security by recording all transactions. Every IoT device can validate transactions and contribute to the blockchain consensus mechanism. Cryptography protects and verifies data shared between devices. For trust and verification applications like supply chain management and financial transactions, this architecture prevents data tampering and improves device accountability (Elarmathi, S. et al., 2024). To balance secure data transmission, hybrid architectures combine edge and cloud-based approaches. This model processes data at the edge for immediate analysis and sends only relevant data to the cloud for storage and advanced analytics (Pandey, B. K. et al., 2024e). By filtering and pre-processing sensitive data locally, this hybrid approach improves performance and security by reducing cloud data transmission. Keeping critical data at the edge allows organizations to use cloud services scalability while protecting data sovereignty and privacy. In the hierarchical architecture, security controls are applied at various IoT network levels. Each device, communication, and application layer in this architecture has its own security mechanisms. For example, devices may use lightweight encryption algorithms for data transmission, while the communication layer uses more secure protocols like TLS. Application layer policies may control access and detect anomalies. Multi-layered security ensures that even if one layer is compromised, the others remain protected (George, W. K. et al., 2024).

Authentication and Access Control Mechanisms

Mechanisms for authentication and access control are essential components in the process of securing Internet of Things networks and ensuring that sensitive data is kept secure. An individual, a device, or an application that is attempting to gain access to a system is said to be authenticated when the process of verifying their identity is carried out (Abdullahi, M. et al., 2024). Password-based authentication, biometric verification (such as fingerprints or facial recognition), and multifactor authentication (MFA), which combines two or more verification methods to increase security, are all examples of common methods of authentication. Through the implementation of these measures, unauthorized access can be prevented, and it is ensured that only authorized users can interact with devices and data. The permissions that are granted to authenticated users or devices are determined by access control mechanisms, which in turn define the actions that these individuals or devices are able to carry out within the system. There are a few different models of access control, such as role-based access control (RBAC), in which permissions are assigned to users based on their roles within an organization, and attribute-based access control (ABAC), which takes into consideration a variety of attributes (such as the location of the user and the time of access) when making decisions regarding access. Through the implementation of strong authentication and access control mechanisms, organizations are able to safeguard sensitive information from being accessed by unauthorized individuals, as well as preserve the integrity and confidentiality of data that is transmitted across Internet of Things networks (Kumar, B. et al., 2024). The implementation of these security measures is absolutely necessary in order to establish trust in Internet of Things applications, particularly in sectors such as healthcare, finance, and smart home automation.

IoT Security Frameworks in Healthcare

A number of security frameworks have been developed in response to the growing integration of connected devices in healthcare (Shahul, A. et al., 2024) in order to safeguard private patient information and maintain the integrity of medical systems. The NIST Cybersecurity Framework, created by the National Institute of Standards and Technology, is one well-known framework. This framework offers a thorough method for handling cybersecurity risks in a number of industries, including medicine. Identify, Protect, Detect, Respond, and Recover are its five main tasks. Healthcare companies can use this framework to evaluate their cybersecurity posture, put in place the required controls, and handle security incidents with efficiency. Adopting it can help organizations protect patient data transmitted by connected devices and strengthen their defenses against cyberattacks. The Health Information Trust Alliance (HITRUST) CSF is an additional illustration, as it integrates multiple security and privacy standards, such as HIPAA, ISO, and NIST, into a unified framework customized for the healthcare sector. In order to help organizations implement efficient security controls for connected devices and other digital assets, the HITRUST CSF provides a prescriptive approach to risk management (Pandey, D. et al., 2024a). Healthcare organizations can guarantee the security of patient information in an increasingly connected environment by utilizing this framework, which highlights the significance of data protection, risk assessment, and continuous compliance. The IoT Security Foundation (IoTSF) offers frameworks and guidelines aimed at securing devices in a number of industries, including the medical field. Organizations can use the best practices provided by their security compliance framework to reduce the risks related to connected devices. Encouraging end-to-end security across the device lifecycle, it contains guidelines for secure device design, communication protocols, and operational procedures. Healthcare companies can improve the security of their ecosystems and safeguard sensitive patient data by adhering to these recommendations (Pandey, D. et al., 2024b). Another important framework that offers a methodical approach to managing sensitive information security is the ISO/IEC 27001 standard. This standard, which offers a comprehensive set of requirements for setting up, implementing, maintaining, and continuously improving an information security management system (ISMS), is widely applicable in healthcare settings even though it is not specifically focused on connected devices. Healthcare organizations can ensure regulatory compliance and effectively manage risks associated with connected devices by aligning their security practices with ISO/IEC 27001. A security framework that describes best practices for safeguarding connected devices across multiple industries, including healthcare, has been developed by the Industrial Internet Consortium (IIC). This framework offers guidance on risk assessment, threat modelling, (Kennedy, G. W. et al., 2024) and the application of security controls that are suited to the particular requirements of these environments. It highlights the significance of putting in place a risk-based approach to security. Healthcare organizations can better understand and manage the security risks associated with connected devices and systems by implementing this framework.

CONCLUSION

The incorporation of connected devices in healthcare has profoundly altered the provision of medical services, facilitating remote monitoring, real-time data acquisition, and enhanced patient outcomes. These advancements facilitate improved management of chronic conditions, prompt interventions, and enhanced communication between healthcare professionals and patients. Nevertheless, the advantages of these technologies entail significant risks, rendering it imperative to prioritize security. Security frameworks like the NIST Cybersecurity Framework, HITRUST CSF, and ISO/IEC 27001 are essential for protecting sensitive patient information and maintaining system integrity. These frameworks offer protocols for evaluating risks, instituting requisite controls, and addressing security incidents, enabling organizations to bolster their resilience against cyber threats. The implementation of best practices for authentication, access control, and data management is crucial for ensuring security in an increasingly interconnected environment. Efficient authentication methods, including multifactor authentication, and stringent access control policies mitigate unauthorized access to sensitive information. Effective data management practices guarantee that sensitive information is encrypted and transmitted securely, thereby reducing the likelihood of data breaches. As technology advances and devices become increasingly interconnected, the risk of cyber threats will escalate. It is imperative to innovate and enhance security measures through continuous advancements in protocols, risk management strategies, and compliance standards to safeguard patient information. By emphasizing security, the healthcare sector can establish trust with users and cultivate a secure environment for providing medical care, ultimately resulting in improved health outcomes and enhanced quality of life for patients. Investing in security will guarantee the realization of the full potential of connected healthcare technologies while protecting the sensitive data that underpins these innovations.

REFERENCES

Abdullahi, M., Ahmad, A., Pandey, B. K., & Pandey, D. (2024). Digital Currency Adoption: A Comparative Analysis of Global Trends and the Nigerian eNaira Digital Currency. *SN Computer Science*, *5*(5), 1–11. DOI: 10.1007/s42979-024-02882-6

Ahathiyan, G. S., Du John, H. V., Moni, D. J., Sagayam, K. M., Pandey, B. K., Pandey, D., & Lelisho, M. E. (2025). Design and simulation of a highly efficient eco-friendly, non-toxic perovskite solar cell. *Discover Nano*, *20*(1), 32. DOI: 10.1186/s11671-025-04190-1 PMID: 39937384

Calegari, L. P., & Fettermann, D. C. (2022). A review of e-health technologies applications. *International Journal of Bioinformatics Research and Applications*, *18*(4), 318–357. DOI: 10.1504/IJBRA.2022.126742

Dwivedi, R., Mehrotra, D., & Chandra, S. (2022). Potential of Internet of Medical Things (IoMT) applications in building a smart healthcare system: A systematic review. *Journal of Oral Biology and Craniofacial Research*, *12*(2), 302–318. DOI: 10.1016/j.jobcr.2021.11.010 PMID: 34926140

Elarmathi, S., Rishabavarthani, P., Sindhuja, M., Elayaraja, P., & Malathi Murugesan, S. (2024). Novel manufacturing systems for cancer diagnosis using ultra-sensitive photonic crystal fiber biosensor with dual-functionalized aptamer-nanocavity. *Microsystem Technologies*, •••, 1–20. DOI: 10.1007/s00542-024-05820-x

Ge, H., Li, L., Zhang, D., & Ma, F. (2022). Applications of digital Medicine in oncology: Prospects and challenges. *Cancer Innovation*, *1*(4), 285–292. DOI: 10.1002/cai2.37 PMID: 38089082

George, W. K., Silas, E. I., Pandey, D., & Pandey, B. K. (2024). Utilization of Industry 4.0 Technologies in Nigerian Technical and Vocational Education: A Conundrum for Educators. In *Examining the Rapid Advance of Digital Technology in Africa* (pp. 270–293). IGI Global. DOI: 10.4018/978-1-6684-9962-7.ch014

JayaLakshmi. G., Pandey, D., Pandey, B. K., Kaur, P., Mahajan, D. A., & Dari, S. S. (2024). Smart big data collection for intelligent supply chain improvement. In AI and Machine Learning Impacts in Intelligent Supply Chain (pp. 180-195). IGI Global.

Kennedy, G. W., Sunday, S. E., Pandey, D., Kabari, A. D., Pandey, B. K., George, A. S., & Dadheech, P. (2024). Building Information Modeling: Harnessing Innovations for Professional Proficiency. In Emerging Engineering Technologies and Industrial Applications (pp. 305-331). IGI Global.

Khadka, M., Sah, M., Chaudhary, R., Sahani, S. K., Sahani, K., Pandey, B. K., & Pandey, D. (2025). Spectroscopic, quantum chemical, and topological calculations of the phenylephrine molecule using density functional theory. *Scientific Reports*, *15*(1), 208. DOI: 10.1038/s41598-024-81633-2 PMID: 39747169

Konapure, C. G., Pandey, D., Shete, H., Thakar, C. M., Pandey, B. K., & George, A. S. (2025). Artificial Intelligence in Automated Concrete Mix Design Using Computerized Grading Curves. Interdisciplinary Approaches to AI, Internet of Everything, and Machine Learning, 567-586.

Kumar, B., Pandey, D., Pandey, B. K., & George, A. S. (2024). Higher Education in the Last Four Decades: A Review of Paradigm Shifts in Policy Frameworks. Design and Implementation of Higher Education Learners' Learning Outcomes (HELLO), 333-348.

Kumar, M. S., Prasanna, P. L., Lalitha, M., Joy, M., Jha, S. S., & Pandey, B. K. (2025). Utilizing the Internet of Everything and Artificial Intelligence for Real-Time Workforce Management. In Role of Internet of Everything (IOE), VLSI Architecture, and AI in Real-Time Systems (pp. 153-168). IGI Global Scientific Publishing.

Kumarganesh, S., & Malathi Murugesan, C. (2024). Hybrid plasmonic biosensors with deep learning for colorectal cancer detection. *Plasmonics*, •••, 1–15. DOI: 10.1007/s11468-024-02568-y

Lakshmi, K. V. N., Rajan, R., Pandey, D., & Pandey, B. K. (2024). Circular economy: A catalyst for economic growth-an empirical study. *Circular Economy and Sustainability*, •••, 1–22.

Maheshwari, R., Kumarganesh, S., K v M, S., Gopalakrishnan, A., Selvi, K., Paulchamy, B., Rishabavarthani, P., Sagayam, K. M., Pandey, B. K., & Pandey, D. (2024). Advanced plasmonic resonance-enhanced biosensor for comprehensive real-time detection and analysis of deepfake content. *Plasmonics*, •••, 1–18. DOI: 10.1007/s11468-024-02407-0

Maheshwari, R. U., Paulchamy, B., Pandey, B. K., & Pandey, D. (2024). Enhancing sensing and imaging capabilities through surface plasmon resonance for deepfake image detection. *Plasmonics*, •••, 1–20. DOI: 10.1007/s11468-024-02492-1

Muralidhar, L. B., Lakshmi, K. V. N., Swapna, H. R., Rupani, J., Nethravathi, K., Pandey, B. K., & Pandey, D. (2024). Impact of Organizational Culture on The Level of Corporate Social Responsibility Investments: An Exploratory Study. *Circular Economy and Sustainability*, *4*(3), 1–19. DOI: 10.1007/s43615-024-00371-9

Pandey, B. K., Kanike, U. K., George, A. S., & Pandey, D. (Eds.). (2024d). *AI and machine learning impacts in intelligent supply chain*. IGI Global. DOI: 10.4018/979-8-3693-1347-3

Pandey, B. K., Nassa, V. K., Mukundan, A. P., Mahajan, D. A., Pandey, D., George, A. S., & Dadheech, P. (2024c). An Industry-Focused Traffic System Utilising Internet of Things. In *Emerging Engineering Technologies and Industrial Applications* (pp. 200–213). IGI Global. DOI: 10.4018/979-8-3693-1335-0.ch009

Pandey, B. K., & Pandey, D. (2023). Parametric optimization and prediction of enhanced thermoelectric performance in co-doped CaMnO3 using response surface methodology and neural network. *Journal of Materials Science Materials in Electronics*, *34*(21), 1589. DOI: 10.1007/s10854-023-10954-1

Pandey, B. K., & Pandey, D. (2025). Securing healthcare medical image information using advance morphological component analysis, information hiding systems, and hybrid convolutional neural networks on IoMT. *Computers in Biology and Medicine*, *185*, 109499. DOI: 10.1016/j.compbiomed.2024.109499 PMID: 39642698

Pandey, B. K., Pandey, D., & Lelisho, M. E. (2024a). Face mask identification with enhanced cuckoo optimization and deep learning-based faster regional neural network. *Scientific Reports*, *14*(1), 29719. DOI: 10.1038/s41598-024-78746-z PMID: 39613761

Pandey, B. K., Pandey, D., & Sahani, S. K. (2024b). Autopilot control unmanned aerial vehicle system for sewage defect detection using deep learning. *Engineering Reports*, •••, 12852.

Pandey, B. K., Paramashivan, M. A., Pandey, D., George, A. S., Agarwal, A., Mahajan, D. A., . . . Pramanik, S. (2024e). Future Directions of Digital Twin Architectures for 6G Communication Networks. In Security Issues and Solutions in 6G Communications and Beyond (pp. 197-211). IGI Global.

Pandey, D., Nassa, V. K., Pandey, B. K., Thankachan, B., Dadheech, P., Mahajan, D. A., & George, A. S. (2024a). Artificial Intelligence and Machine Learning and Its Application in the Field of Computational Visual Analysis. In Emerging Engineering Technologies and Industrial Applications (pp. 36-57). IGI Global. DOI: 10.4018/979-8-3693-1335-0.ch003

Pandey, D., & Pandey, B. K. (2022). An efficient deep neural network with adaptive galactic swarm optimization for complex image text extraction. In *Process Mining Techniques for Pattern Recognition* (pp. 121–137). CRC Press. DOI: 10.1201/9781003169550-10

Pandey, D., Pandey, B. K., Nassa, V. K., Mahajan, D. A., George, A. S., & Dadheech, P. (2024c). Optimized Throughput-Based Broadcasting for Next Generation Wireless Networks. In Emerging Engineering Technologies and Industrial Applications (pp. 355-368). IGI Global. DOI: 10.4018/979-8-3693-1335-0.ch018

Pandey, D., Pandey, B. K., Paramashivan, M. A., Mahajan, D. A., Dadheech, P. D., George, A. S., & Hameed, A. S. (2024b). Advanced Digital Data Processing Using Cloud Cryptography: Industrial Applications. In Emerging Engineering Technologies and Industrial Applications (pp. 255-268). IGI Global.

Pandey, D., Sharma, M., Talwar, R., & Pandey, B. K. (2025). A compact quintuple band miniaturized elliptical planar monopole antenna for 5G/6G wireless systems. *Analog Integrated Circuits and Signal Processing*, *122*(3), 1–16. DOI: 10.1007/s10470-025-02310-6

Rai, P. K., Pandey, D., & Pandey, B. K. (2024). The future of enterprise and innovation is compute as a commodity, or CaaC. *Partners Universal International Research Journal*, *3*(2), 89–94.

Saravanakumar, R., TamilSelvi, T., Pandey, D., Pandey, B. K., Mahajan, D. A., & Lelisho, M. E. (2024). Big data processing using hybrid Gaussian mixture model with salp swarm algorithm. *Journal of Big Data*, *11*(1), 167. DOI: 10.1186/s40537-024-01015-3

Satheesh, N., Gopisankar, N., Kumarganesh, S., Anthoniraj, S., Saravanakumar, S., & Martin Sagayam, K. (2025). Advanced AI-driven emergency response systems for enhanced vehicle and human safety. *Iran Journal of Computer Science*, •••, 1–16. DOI: 10.1007/s42044-025-00228-w

Saxena, A., Agarwal, A., Pandey, B. K., & Pandey, D. (2024). Examination of the Criticality of Customer Segmentation Using Unsupervised Learning Methods. *Circular Economy and Sustainability*, *4*(2), 1–14. DOI: 10.1007/s43615-023-00336-4

Shahul, A., Muniandi, B., Paramashivan, M. A., Pandey, D., Pandey, B. K., Dadheech, P., & George, H. (2024). An Analysis of Algorithms and Methods Based on Image Processing for Medical Applications. In *Emerging Engineering Technologies and Industrial Applications* (pp. 173–186). IGI Global. DOI: 10.4018/979-8-3693-1335-0.ch007

Shamshad, F., Khan, S., Zamir, S. W., Khan, M. H., Hayat, M., Khan, F. S., & Fu, H. (2023). Transformers in medical imaging: A survey. *Medical Image Analysis*, *88*, 102802. DOI: 10.1016/j.media.2023.102802 PMID: 37315483

Sheela, M. S., Kumarganesh, S., Pandey, B. K., & Lelisho, M. E. (2025). Integration of silver nanostructures in wireless sensor networks for enhanced biochemical sensing. *Discover Nano*, *20*(1), 7. DOI: 10.1186/s11671-024-04159-6 PMID: 39804434

Singh, S., Madaan, G., Swapna, H. R., Singh, A., Pandey, B. K., George, A. S., & Pandey, D. (2025b). Unleashing the Power of AI and Data Analysis: Transforming Insights into Action. In Interdisciplinary Approaches to AI, Internet of Everything, and Machine Learning (pp. 1-24). IGI Global Scientific Publishing.

Singh, S., Madaan, G., Swapna, H. R., Singh, A., Pandey, D., George, A. S., & Pandey, B. K. (2025a). Empowering Connectivity: Exploring the Internet of Things. In Interdisciplinary Approaches to AI, Internet of Everything, and Machine Learning (pp. 89-116). IGI Global Scientific Publishing.

Usak, M., Kubiatko, M., Shabbir, M. S., Viktorovna Dudnik, O., Jermsittiparsert, K., & Rajabion, L. (2020). Health care service delivery based on the Internet of things: A systematic and comprehensive study. *International Journal of Communication Systems*, *33*(2), e4179. DOI: 10.1002/dac.4179

Vyas, S., Bhargava, D., & Khan, S. (2023). Healthcare 4.0: A systematic review and its impact over conventional healthcare system. Artificial Intelligence for Health 4.0: Challenges and Applications, 1-17.

Chapter 10
Telemedicine IoT Networks and Secure Image Transmission

A. S. Arvind
https://orcid.org/0009-0005-3472-8037
Department of Politics and Public Administration, University of Madras, Chennai, India

Niladri Maiti
Central Asian University, Tashkent, Uzbekistan

Riddhi Chawla
School of Dentistry, Central Asian University, Tashkent, Uzbekistan

Simmi Madaan
Faculty of Engineering and Technology, SGT University, Gurugram, India

P. Sheela Rani
Department of Information Technology, Panimalar Engineering College, Chennai, India

Mukundan Appadurai Paramashivan
https://orcid.org/0009-0009-5608-4788
Champions Group, Singapore

ABSTRACT

The integration of Internet of Things (IoT) networks and secure image transmission in telemedicine is investigated in this chapter, with the purpose of highlighting the significance of these two concepts in the delivery of contemporary medical care. The Internet of Things (IoT) is utilized by telemedicine in order to facilitate remote patient monitoring, improve accessibility to medical services, and enhance the efficiency of healthcare systems. Considering the growing reliance on medical imaging for accurate diagnosis, the need for secure transmission methods is of the utmost importance in order to protect sensitive patient data from being accessed by unauthorized parties and being exposed to cyber threats.

DOI: 10.4018/979-8-3693-9821-0.ch010

INTRODUCTION

The practice of providing medical care remotely via telecommunications technology is known as telemedicine. It makes communication between patients and medical professionals possible even when they are not in the same place. A variety of services, including consultations, diagnosis, treatments, and follow-up care, can be provided through telemedicine. These services can be facilitated by phone calls, video conferences, messaging apps, or specialized medical software. The idea of telemedicine was developed to overcome the logistical and geographic obstacles that frequently impede access to healthcare, especially in underserved or rural areas. Patients no longer need to travel great distances or make in-person appointments with doctors and specialists thanks to the use of telecommunications. This can be especially helpful for managing mental health consultations, post-surgical follow-ups, and chronic diseases. Thanks to technological advancements such as wearables, high-speed internet, smartphones, and Internet of Things (IoT) sensors, telemedicine has experienced significant growth. Real-time monitoring of patients' health data by healthcare providers is made possible by these tools, which promote ongoing care and the early identification of possible health problems. Wearable technology, for instance, can monitor vital signs like blood pressure, heart rate, and glucose levels and send the information for analysis to medical specialists. The COVID-19 pandemic hastened the adoption of telemedicine by offering a secure and effective means of delivering healthcare while reducing the need for in-person contact and infection risk. Telemedicine has become an essential tool in pandemic response as many healthcare systems have expanded their services to handle the surge of patients remotely.

Role of IoT in Healthcare

Real-time data collection, transmission, and analysis are all made possible by the Internet of Things (IoT), which plays a transformative role in the healthcare industry by connecting various devices, sensors, and operating systems. With the help of smart devices and advanced communication technologies, the Internet of Things (IoT) in the healthcare industry makes it possible to provide better patient care, improve diagnostics, and streamline medical workflows. Through the use of this interconnected network of devices, medical professionals are able to remotely monitor the health of their patients, assist in the management of chronic conditions, and implement timely interventions. Remote patient monitoring is one of the most important parts of the Internet of Things in the healthcare industry. This data is automatically transmitted to healthcare professionals, which enables them to monitor the conditions of patients without the need for them to visit the hospital. Not only does this lessen the workload of healthcare facilities, but it also makes it possible to identify abnormalities at an earlier stage, which ultimately leads to better outcomes for patients. A significant part of the Internet of Things is also played by personalized medicine. IoT devices enable healthcare providers to tailor treatments based on specific patient profiles by collecting vast amounts of health data from individuals. This data can be collected from these individuals. Specifically, Internet of Things (IoT)-enabled insulin pumps have the capability to automatically adjust dosage based on real-time blood glucose levels, thereby ensuring that diabetes patients receive accurate treatment. In healthcare facilities, Internet of Things devices contribute to the streamlining of inventory management and medical asset tracking. It is possible for smart sensors to monitor the location of medical equipment, medications, and even staff, which can improve the efficiency of hospitals and reduce the costs associated with their operations. This ensures that essential resources are available at the appropriate time and reduces the amount of time that patients have to wait for care. The Internet of Things improves medication management by making it possible to have smart pill dispensers that remind patients to take their medication at the appropriate time and alert caregivers if a dose is missed (Moore, M., 1999).

Secure Image Transmission in Telemedicine

The growing dependence of telemedicine on digital communication for patient diagnosis and treatment necessitates secure image transmission. Because telemedicine entails the sharing of private medical images via digital platforms such as MRIs, ultrasounds, and X-rays ensuring the security of these transmissions is essential to protecting patient privacy and data integrity (Konapure, C. G. et al., 2025). Protection against cyberattacks is a key motivation for secure image transmission. Cybercriminals find healthcare data, particularly medical images, to be highly valuable targets due to the sensitive personal and medical information they contain. These pictures could be used for identity theft, blackmail, or sold on the dark web if they are intercepted during transmission. Secure communication protocols and strong encryption guard against unwanted access and guarantee the safe delivery of these image (Singh, S. et al., 2025). Secure image transmission improves healthcare practitioners ability to collaborate. In order to make well-informed decisions, telemedicine frequently involves consultations between a numbers of specialists, who depend on the timely and accurate sharing of medical images. Better clinical collaboration and quicker decision-making are made possible by secure transmission protocols, which guarantee timely delivery of images free from tampering or loss (Sharma, M. et al., 2025). These qualities can be especially important in emergency situations. Image quality preservation is an additional factor. To maintain their diagnostic clarity during transmission, medical images used for diagnosis must either remain uncompressed or undergo minimal alteration. By ensuring that high-quality images are shared amongst healthcare providers, secure transmission techniques lessen the possibility of misinterpretation due to poor image quality (Pandey, B. K. et al., 2024a). In underserved or rural areas, secure transmission supports remote health-care services. The ability to safely transfer medical images from nearby healthcare facilities to specialists in urban areas enhances access to high-quality care, even in remote areas, where patients might not have easy access to sophisticated medical facilities. Wider use of telemedicine services is encouraged by ensuring the security of these transmissions (Pandian, P. S. et al., 2007).

TELEMEDICINE IOT NETWORKS

Components of IoT Networks in Healthcare

A system wherein networked devices and sensors exchange data with one another to gather, send, and evaluate health-related data via the internet is known as an IoT (Internet of Things) network in the healthcare industry. Patient care and operational efficiency (Pandey, B. K. et al., 2024b) within healthcare systems are enhanced by these networks capacity for remote control, data sharing, and continuous monitoring of medical equipment. IoT networks are used in the healthcare industry to link sensors, wearables, and diagnostic equipment to a central system (Basha, A. J. et al., 2024). Medical professionals can obtain vital patient information remotely, in real-time, and without physical contact thanks to this networked systems data analytics, real-time monitoring (KVM, S. et al., 2024), and remote access features. Applications such as remote monitoring, early health issue detection, and better chronic disease management are made possible by IoT networks in the healthcare industry.

Figure 1. Elements of IoT networks in healthcare

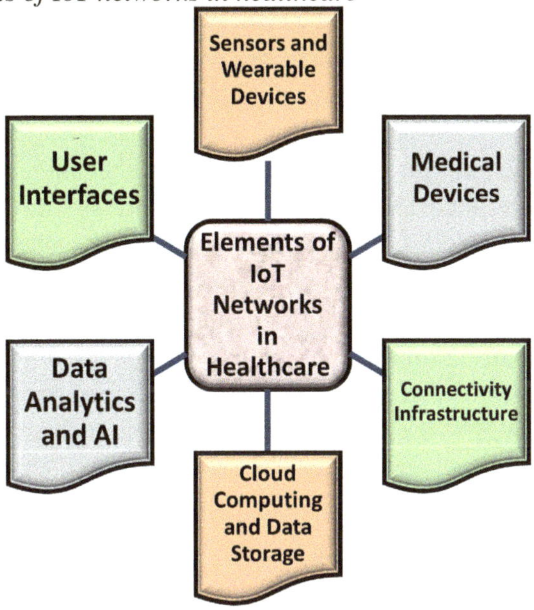

- *Sensors and Wearable Devices*: Sensors and wearable devices are essential for collecting real-time health data directly from patients. These devices can be worn continuously, facilitating the continuous monitoring of vital signs including heart rate, oxygen saturation, glucose concentration, temperature, and physical activity (Lakshmi, K. V. N. et al., 2024). Certain advanced sensors can detect specific conditions such as sleep apnea or arrhythmias. These devices enable healthcare providers to monitor patient health trends over time, facilitating early identification of potential issues before they develop into serious conditions (Saravanakumar, R. et al., 2024). Ongoing monitoring enables proactive care, minimizing hospital visits and permitting patients to receive treatment at home.
- *Medical Devices*: The Internet of Things (IoT) encompasses an array of medical devices, including insulin pumps, pacemakers, and connected inhalers, which autonomously modify treatment in accordance with the patient's real-time health data. Smart insulin pumps can deliver insulin according to real-time glucose levels, enhancing diabetes management. Likewise, IoT-enabled pacemakers can monitor cardiac rhythms and notify healthcare providers upon detecting irregularities, thereby averting emergencies. These devices can remotely transmit data to healthcare providers, facilitating treatment adjustments without necessitating a patient visit to a clinic or hospital. This

instantaneous data exchange can be crucial in scenarios requiring prompt intervention (Devaraj, S. J., & Ezra, K., 2011).

- *Connectivity Infrastructure*: The connectivity infrastructure constitutes the foundation of the IoT network, facilitating uninterrupted communication among devices, healthcare providers, and cloud-based systems. Technologies such as 5G are vital for IoT networks, offering the high-speed, low-latency connections essential for real-time data transmission and remote diagnostics (Kumarganesh, S. et al., 2024). Dependable connectivity guarantees the prompt delivery of critical data, which is vital for timely interventions, particularly in emergencies. Furthermore, this infrastructure must guarantee secure data transmission to avert breaches, given the highly sensitive nature of healthcare data. The selection of communication protocols (e.g., Wi-Fi, Zigbee, LoRaWAN) is contingent upon variables such as range, data capacity, and security specifications (Muralidhar, L. B. et al., 2024).
- *Cloud Computing and Data Storage*: The substantial quantity of data produced by IoT devices in healthcare necessitates a scalable and secure cloud infrastructure for storage and processing. Cloud platforms not only store data but also enable sophisticated data analytics, offering insights into patient health trends, forecasting potential health issues, and recommending personalized treatment plans. Cloud computing facilitates remote data access for authorized healthcare professionals, permitting real-time consultations and specialist second opinions. Cloud systems must adhere to stringent data security standards (Pandey, B. K. et al., 2024c), such as HIPAA, to safeguard patient privacy and guarantee that data is encrypted during transmission and storage.
- *Data Analytics and AI*: Data analytics, augmented by artificial neural network (Pandey, B. K., & Pandey, D., 2023), analyzes the raw data obtained from IoT devices to yield actionable insights. AI algorithms can identify patterns and trends in patient data, forecast health decline, and suggest preventive strategies. Predictive analytics can identify patients at risk of chronic conditions such as diabetes or heart disease by analyzing their lifestyle and historical data (Pandey, B. K., & Pandey, D., 2025). Artificial intelligence can also automate administrative functions, such as scheduling follow-up appointments or notifying physicians of anomalies in the data. As additional data is collected, AI systems evolve and refine, thereby augmenting the precision of diagnoses and treatment strategies over time.
- *User Interfaces* (Mobile Applications/Software): User interfaces, including mobile applications and specialized healthcare software, serve as the conduit between patients, healthcare providers, and the IoT system. Patients can access their real-time health data, monitor medication compliance, and receive

alerts concerning their condition or forthcoming medical appointments via these applications (Elarmathi, S. et al., 2024). Healthcare professionals can oversee patient dashboards, retrieve medical records, and react to alerts produced by the IoT system. These interfaces must be intuitive and accessible to facilitate seamless interaction between patients and medical personnel with the system. Mobile applications frequently incorporate communication functionalities that facilitate direct messaging or video calls between patients and physicians for remote consultations (Chakraborty, C. et al., 2013).

The IoT networks in healthcare comprise various components, including sensors, wearable devices, medical imaging apparatus, and cloud-based platforms, as illustrated in Figure 1. These components collaboratively gather, transmit, and analyze patient data in real-time, facilitating remote monitoring, individualized treatment, and enhanced patient outcomes. Device interoperability (Khadka, M. et al., 2025) is crucial for efficient data exchange.

Data Collection and Transfer in Telemedicine IoT

In telemedicine IoT networks, data collection and transmission are essential procedures that enable remote patient monitoring, diagnosis, and healthcare delivery. These procedures guarantee that healthcare professionals have timely access to accurate health information, facilitating efficient decision-making and patient management. Data collection in telemedicine IoT networks involves using a variety of tools and sensors to collect patient health-related data (Pandey, B. K. et al., 2024d). Vital signs like heart rate, blood pressure, glucose levels, and activity levels are continuously monitored by wearable technology, such as smart watches and fitness trackers. These gadgets can also gather information about general fitness levels and sleep habits, giving doctors a complete picture of their patients health. Certain health metrics are easier to gather with in-home medical devices like blood glucose monitors and smart thermometers. These gadgets frequently have sensors built in that take readings automatically (George, W. K. et al., 2024), reducing human error and guaranteeing data accuracy. A lot of telemedicine platforms incorporate patient-reported outcomes and questionnaires, allowing patients to submit qualitative information about their symptoms, way of life, and compliance with treatment regimens. This comprehensive method of gathering data guarantees that medical professionals have access to an accurate and comprehensive picture of a patients health. Data Transmission (Abdullahi, M. et al., 2024) in IoT-Based Telemedicine Networks: Safe data transmission to healthcare providers is crucial after it has been gathered. IoT networks for telemedicine make use of a variety of communication protocols and technologies to guarantee secure and dependable data transmission (Kumar, B.

et al., 2024). Wi-Fi, Bluetooth, Zigbee, and cellular networks (such as 4G and 5G) are examples of common transmission methods. Each is chosen based on various criteria, including device compatibility, bandwidth requirements, and distance. An essential part of this transmission process is data encryption. Encryption protocols like TLS (Transport Layer Security) and AES (Advanced Encryption Standard) are used to protect sensitive health information during transfer from unauthorized access. To add an additional degree of security, secure channels like virtual private networks (VPNs) can be set up (Pandey, D. et al., 2024). After transmission, the data is frequently transferred to databases for healthcare or cloud-based systems so that it can be processed, stored, and examined. Healthcare providers can access patient data from any location with this centralized storage, enabling real-time monitoring and speedy responses to any health issues. By processing the transferred data, data analytics tools can produce reports, alerts, and insights that support treatment planning and patient management (Alenoghena, C. O. et al., 2022).

SECURE IMAGE TRANSMISSION IN TELEMEDICINE

Significance of Medical Image Security

Medical image security is crucial to patient privacy and healthcare system integrity. Medical images like X-rays, MRIs, CT scans, and ultrasounds contain sensitive data that can affect patient care and treatment. Unauthorized access to these images can expose patients health conditions and treatments. HIPAA requires medical image security to protect patient confidentiality and privacy (Shahul, A. et al., 2024). Healthcare organizations are prime targets for cybercriminals because medical data is valuable. Medical image breaches can cause significant financial losses, legal issues, and brand damage. Healthcare providers can prevent data breaches and cyberattacks that compromise medical images by using encryption, secure access controls, and regular audits. In addition to financial losses, such breaches can damage patient trust and healthcare institutions' credibility (Muniandi, B. et al., 2024) . Accurate diagnosis and treatment depend on medical image integrity. Images that are altered during transmission or storage can cause misinterpretations that harm patient care. Safely transmitting and storing medical images helps healthcare professionals make informed decisions based on unaltered data (Sheela, M. S. et al., 2025). In time-sensitive situations where prompt diagnosis can improve patient outcomes, reliability is essential. Healthcare organizations must follow patient data regulations, including medical image handling. Non-compliance can lead to fines, lawsuits, and accreditation loss. Strong medical image security is essential for patient data protection, legal and regulatory compliance, and healthcare providers' credibility and operational integrity. Healthcare data law changes frequently, so organizations must stay informed and compliant. As telemedicine grows, secure medical image transmission is essential (Satheesh, N. et al., 2025). Patients must trust that medical images and other sensitive health data are protected. By protecting medical images, healthcare providers can build trust and increase telemedicine use, improving access to care. Secure telemedicine benefits patients and improves healthcare providers' operational efficiency by reducing data breaches (Kumar, M. S. et al., 2025). Healthcare professionals often share medical images for collaboration and second opinions. These images must be secure to build practitioner trust. Secure sharing mechanisms protect data, enabling patient care communication and collaboration without compromise. Multiple specialists can share insights based on secure data, improving patient outcomes and care (Campbell, I. M. et al., 2022).

COMMON THREATS: TAMPERING, EAVESDROPPING, UNAUTHORIZED ACCESS

The protection of medical data, particularly sensitive images, is of utmost importance in the context of telemedicine and Internet of Things networks. This is because there are numerous common threats that threaten the availability, integrity (Singh, S. et al., 2025), and confidentiality of healthcare services. "Data tampering," which occurs when unauthorized changes are made to medical images or data related to them while they are being transmitted or stored, is one of the most significant threats. It is possible for even minute changes to medical images to lead to incorrect diagnoses and treatments, which can have potentially life-threatening consequences. Due to the fact that medical imagery plays an essential part in the diagnostic process, it is essential to guarantee the accuracy of this data. Both the detection of unauthorized changes and the maintenance of the information's accuracy are frequently accomplished through the utilization of methods such as digital signatures and sophisticated cryptographic hashing algorithms (Vinodhini, V. et al., 2022). The practice of eavesdropping, which involves the act of intercepting data while it is being transmitted, is another significant threat. Unsecured or unencrypted communication channels have the potential to expose sensitive medical images to individuals or groups that are not authorized to view them. Theft of identity, insurance fraud, and even ransomware attacks are all examples of malicious activities that can be carried out by attackers using data that has been intercepted. In order to protect against this danger, it is necessary to implement strong encryption protocols such as Transport Layer Security (TLS) and end-to-end encryption software. The confidentiality of patient information is protected by these security measures, which ensure that even if data is intercepted, it will continue to be inaccessible without the appropriate decryption key (Rai, P. K. et al., 2024). Another significant risk is unauthorized access, which occurs when unauthorised individuals gain access to medical images that have been stored without the appropriate credentials. This has the potential to result in widespread data breaches, which could expose the medical histories of patients, diagnostic images, and other details that are considered sensitive. These kinds of breaches can have severe repercussions for healthcare providers, both financially and legally, and they can also erode the trust that patients have in healthcare institutions. To prevent unauthorized individuals from gaining access to sensitive information, it is essential to implement stringent access controls. Some examples of these controls include multi-factor authentication (MFA), role-based access control (RBAC), and regular auditing of access logs. The critical security challenges that are faced in telemedicine Internet of Things networks are demonstrated by these threats, which include data tampering, eavesdropping, and unauthorized access. When it comes to protecting sensitive medical images and ensuring the privacy and trustworthiness of healthcare services, it is absolutely necessary to implement a combination of techniques that include authentication, monitoring, and encryption (Brian Brenner, M. D. et al., 2022).

BLOCKCHAIN FOR SECURE IMAGE TRANSMISSION

Blockchain as a Distributed Ledger for Image Security

The blockchain technology provides a novel approach to the protection of medical images by utilizing its decentralized framework to ensure the safety of data. The application of this technology in the field of healthcare guarantees that medical images, once they have been saved, are safeguarded against unauthorized modifications and data manipulation. Since the data is distributed across multiple nodes, each of which contains a copy of the ledger, the decentralized aspect means that rather than relying on a single central authority, the data is distributed across multiple nodes. Considering that this distribution ensures that any attempt to modify the data would require control over the majority of the nodes, tampering is extremely impractical because of this distribution. Blockchain technology offers audit trails that are completely transparent, which enables administrators and healthcare professionals to monitor each and every transaction or access to a medical image (Kumar Pandey, B. et al.,, 2021). This feature is especially helpful for ensuring accountability and complying with regulatory requirements. By recording each access or update as a time-stamped entry on the blockchain, healthcare providers are able to track the flow of sensitive information and identify any irregularities or unauthorized actions that may have occurred. The consensus mechanisms of blockchain technology improve security. A new transaction, such as the transmission or modification of an image, must be validated by the majority of the network participants before it can be accepted into the blockchain. If it is not validated, the transaction will not be accepted. Due to the fact that the system is based on collective agreement rather than a single point of authority, the risk of data fraud or manipulation is decreased as a result. The incorporation of smart contracts can automate processes such as the granting of access to medical images, thereby ensuring that only authorized parties are able to retrieve or view sensitive information. Blockchain technology provides an additional layer of security in the field of telemedicine, which involves the transmission of images on a regular basis and across multiple networks. This can be accomplished by verifying the origin of the images as well as their authenticity. Together, patients and healthcare providers can have a higher level of confidence that the data that is being shared is accurate and has not been altered, which will ultimately lead to an increase in trust and an improvement in the security framework of telemedicine systems.

Benefits of Blockchain in Data Integrity and Transparency

In the healthcare industry, where protecting sensitive data like medical images is essential, blockchain technology offers major advantages are as shown in Figure 2, in terms of guaranteeing data integrity and transparency. Its ability to maintain data integrity through the use of an immutable, decentralized ledger is one of its main advantages. A medical image or associated patient data added to the blockchain cannot be removed without the network as a whole agreeing to do so. This guarantees the integrity and consistency of medical data, giving medical professionals accurate and dependable information for diagnosis and treatment.

Figure 2. Blockchain benefits for data integrity and transparency

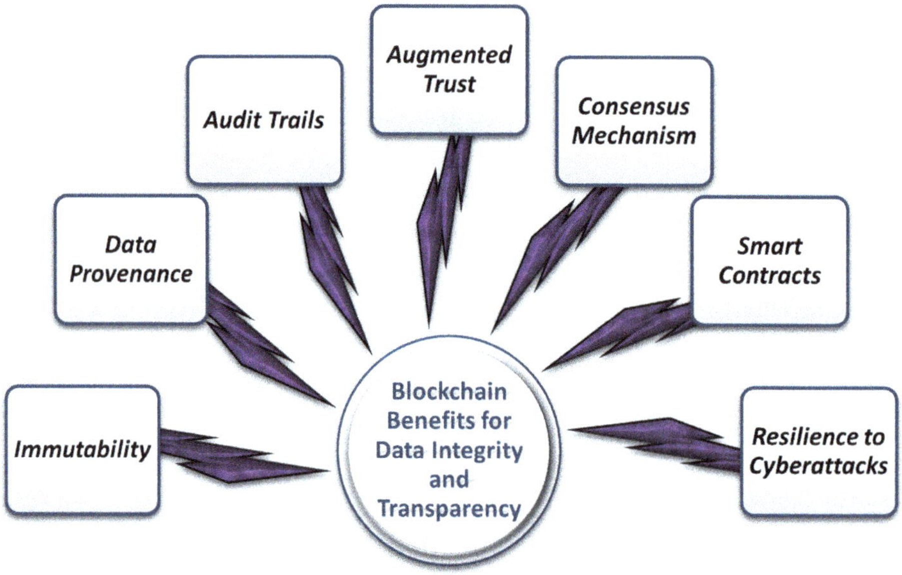

- *Immutability*: A fundamental characteristic of blockchain is its immutability, guaranteeing that data, once inscribed, cannot be modified or erased. In the realm of healthcare, this signifies that medical records, images, and other patient-related data remain immutable from the instant they are entered into the system. This is crucial as even slight modifications to medical data can significantly impact patient treatment and care. The immutability of blockchain is ensured by cryptographic hashing, which connects each data block to its predecessor. This chain structure guarantees that any modification to a record would compromise the entire chain, rendering it instantly identifiable. This characteristic ensures the integrity of diagnostic data in medical image security, guaranteeing that physicians and healthcare providers utilize accurate and reliable information. Regardless of whether these images are disseminated across various healthcare networks or preserved for extended periods, immutability guarantees that the original data remains unaltered and secure from manipulation. This is particularly vital in legal or compliance contexts, where the veracity of medical records must be established.
- *Data Provenance*: Blockchain offers a comprehensive record of every data entry, encompassing its creation and all subsequent modifications or accesses. This concept is referred to as data provenance, which is particularly beneficial in the healthcare sector, where monitoring the lifecycle of medical

data, including images, is essential. Blockchain enables healthcare providers to ascertain the precise time and individual responsible for capturing, transmitting, or viewing a medical image, thereby guaranteeing that the complete history of the image remains transparent and traceable. This functionality is especially beneficial in multi-specialist contexts where various physicians or technicians require access to and analysis of identical medical data. Blockchain guarantees that every access point is documented, establishing a dependable audit trail. This also inhibits unauthorized modifications or inadvertent alterations by ensuring that every interaction with the data is recorded and can be readily traced to its origin.

- *Audit Trails*: The transparency of blockchain facilitates the maintenance of thorough audit trails, as every transaction or data access is documented on the distributed ledger. This feature is essential for maintaining accountability in healthcare. For example, when medical images are disseminated or examined, the blockchain ledger offers an immutable record of who accessed the data, the timing of access, and the actions undertaken. Traceability is crucial for legal compliance, especially concerning regulations like HIPAA in the U.S. and GDPR in Europe, which require stringent supervision of patient data management. Audit trails enhance trust among healthcare providers, patients, and regulators. Blockchain guarantees the provision of clear, traceable records of all actions performed on sensitive medical data, facilitating the prompt identification and resolution of any anomalies or unauthorized access attempts. This additional layer of transparency fosters enhanced accountability among healthcare professionals and guarantees the responsible management of patient data.
- *Augmented Trust*: Blockchains capacity to furnish a verifiable and transparent ledger of all transactions cultivates trust among all participants in the healthcare system. Patients, healthcare providers, and regulatory authorities can depend on the accuracy, tamper-resistance, and transparent management of data stored in a blockchain. This is particularly crucial in telemedicine, where sensitive information, including medical images, is transmitted across networks. The immutable characteristics of blockchain guarantee that patients can rely on telemedicine platforms to safeguard their confidential information. This trust is augmented by the cryptographic security protocols of blockchain technology. All transactions are encrypted, and access is regulated via cryptographic keys, rendering unauthorized data access nearly impossible. Blockchain enhances the reliability and credibility of telemedicine and other healthcare technologies by promoting a secure and transparent data-sharing environment.

- *Consensus Mechanism*: A fundamental principle of blockchain is its consensus mechanism, necessitating the agreement of the majority of network participants on the legitimacy of any new data entry. This guarantees that no individual entity can independently modify or append data without network consent, significantly mitigating the risk of fraudulent actions or unauthorized alterations. This feature is especially advantageous in medical data management, where the precision and veracity of patient records are crucial. In telemedicine, where sensitive data such as medical images is transmitted across various platforms, the consensus mechanism ensures that all transactions involving patient data are accurately validated prior to their acceptance into the blockchain. This adds an extra layer of security and deters malicious entities from injecting false or misleading data into the system, guaranteeing that all parties have access to reliable and verified medical information.
- *Smart Contracts*: Smart contracts are autonomous agreements with the stipulations encoded directly into programming language. In the realm of healthcare, they can facilitate the automation of processes including data sharing and access permissions. A smart contract can autonomously provide access to a medical image for an authorized physician upon the fulfillment of specific prerequisites, such as patient consent or validation of a legitimate request. This automation diminishes the necessity for manual intervention, thereby reducing the likelihood of human error and guaranteeing that only authorized personnel can access sensitive medical images. Smart contracts can augment security by ensuring adherence to data protection regulations, as they can be programmed to record every action involving a patient's medical data, thereby guaranteeing that the entire process is secure, transparent, and accountable.
- *Resilience to Cyberattacks*: Blockchains decentralized architecture renders it exceptionally resistant to cyberattacks. Conventional centralized databases are susceptible to attacks, as a breach of the central authority grants the hacker access to all data. Conversely, blockchain disseminates data across numerous nodes, significantly increasing the difficulty for attackers to breach the system. To manipulate blockchain data, a hacker must acquire control of a majority of the nodes, a task that is exceedingly challenging and expensive to accomplish. This resilience is particularly crucial in healthcare, where data breaches can result in significant repercussions. Cyberattacks on healthcare institutions may lead to the compromise of confidential medical data, financial detriment, and harm to the organization's reputation. Utilizing blockchain for the storage and management of medical images and patient data enables healthcare providers to substantially mitigate the risk of cyberattacks, thereby safeguarding their data against advanced threats.

IMAGE COMPRESSION AND TRANSMISSION EFFICIENCY

Balancing Compression and Image Quality

Telemedicine requires balancing compression and image quality to transmit medical images over IoT networks for timely diagnosis and treatment. Medical images like CT scans, MRIs, and X-rays are large due to their high resolution, which helps detect subtle anomalies and provide accurate medical assessments. Transferring large files over bandwidth-constrained networks can slow transmission speeds, increase latency, and raise storage costs. Thus, image compression is used to reduce file sizes, but balancing compression and diagnostic image quality is essential. This challenge has been addressed by advanced compression techniques. Some methods use adaptive compression algorithms that analyze image content and apply different compression levels to regions of interest. Image areas with critical diagnostic information are preserved at a higher resolution, while less important regions are compressed to save bandwidth. Medical professionals can still use the images key diagnostic features while reducing file size for faster transmission with selective compression. AI and ML are also improving compression algorithms. AI-based systems can optimize compression without compromising image quality using massive medical image data. These systems intelligently predict which image parts will affect diagnosis and adjust compression parameters. Integrating AI into telemedicine systems allows healthcare providers to maintain medical image integrity while reducing transmission and storage time, improving remote healthcare efficiency. Telemedicine compression and image quality depend on the use case and network infrastructure. Diagnostic images must retain detail for accurate medical decisions, but high-compression methods may be suitable for non-critical data or archiving. As telemedicine grows, sophisticated compression technologies will help deliver high-quality healthcare over IoT networks without compromising quality.

Optimizing Transmission in IoT Networks

Telemedicine requires fast and secure transmission of large amounts of data, including high-resolution medical images, over IoT networks. Sensors, diagnostic equipment, and imaging systems generate and transmit data in healthcare IoT networks. Telemedicine requires efficient medical image transfer through these networks for real-time diagnostics, remote consultations, and continuous monitoring. To optimize transmission efficiency, IoT networks use compression and data prioritization. Over low-bandwidth networks, JPEG 2000 or wavelet-based compression algorithms reduce medical image size without affecting quality, enabling faster data transfer. In IoT networks, 5G and edge computing can boost transmission speed and reduce latency. Instead of using cloud servers, edge computing processes data at the network edge. Faster response times and more efficient data transmission result from reduced main network load. IoT networks can optimize transmission by prioritizing data type, compression, and advanced protocols. Real-time vital signs and emergency images must be transmitted quickly in healthcare. While less urgent data can be transmitted later or compressed, network algorithms can prioritize this critical information and deliver it to healthcare providers quickly. This data prioritisation efficiently handles time-sensitive data in congested or low-bandwidth networks. IoT devices, especially remote patient monitors, must also use less energy for efficient transmission. To maintain data flow and battery life, wearable health sensors must be energy-efficient. IoT systems use energy-saving protocols like data aggregation and selective transmission to send only relevant or abnormal data in real time and less routine or unchanged data. This improves data transmission and device lifespans by reducing network and device strain. Security must be strong without compromising performance for IoT transmission. Medical images and sensitive patient data are secured using lightweight encryption to avoid slowing data transfer. Telemedicine must protect patient privacy and data while balancing security and transmission speed.

CONCLUSION

The incorporation of IoT networks into telemedicine signifies a noteworthy progression in the provision of healthcare, augmenting the effectiveness and availability of medical services. Internet of Things technology is to the gathering, sharing, and safe storage of medical image data. It is impossible to exaggerate how crucial secure image transmission is because it has an immediate impact on patient outcomes and care. Protecting sensitive medical data requires putting strong encryption techniques into practice, using blockchain technology to ensure data integrity, and making sure that transmission strategies are effective. In terms of future developments, secure image transmission in telemedicine appears ready for more advancements. Faster and more secure data transfer will improve the telemedicine experience for patients and healthcare providers as technological innovations like artificial intelligence and 5G connectivity continue to develop. These technologies promise to strengthen the security frameworks required to safeguard patient data from new cyber threats in addition to enhancing the speed and dependability of medical image transmission. In addition, continuous research and development in real-time data processing and compression methods will guarantee that medical images are efficiently transmitted without sacrificing quality. IoT networks have a significant impact on the transformation of healthcare. They make it easier to monitor patients remotely, improve access to specialized care, and make timely decisions when things get urgent. Creating safe, effective, and dependable systems will be critical to maintaining the accessibility and efficacy of healthcare as telemedicine grows. The effective integration of these technologies is critical to the future of telemedicine as it will open the door to a more responsive and interconnected healthcare system that places a premium on patient safety and care quality.

REFERENCES

Abdullahi, M., Ahmad, A., Pandey, B. K., & Pandey, D. (2024). Digital Currency Adoption: A Comparative Analysis of Global Trends and the Nigerian eNaira Digital Currency. *SN Computer Science*, *5*(5), 1–11. DOI: 10.1007/s42979-024-02882-6

Alenoghena, C. O., Onumanyi, A. J., Ohize, H. O., Adejo, A. O., Oligbi, M., Ali, S. I., & Okoh, S. A. (2022). eHealth: A survey of architectures, developments in mHealth, security concerns and solutions. *International Journal of Environmental Research and Public Health*, *19*(20), 13071. DOI: 10.3390/ijerph192013071 PMID: 36293656

Basha, A. J., Maheshwari, R. U., Pandey, B. K., & Pandey, D. (2024). Ultra-sensitive photonic crystal fiber–based SPR sensor for cancer detection utilizing hybrid nanocomposite layers. *Plasmonics*, •••, 1–15. DOI: 10.1007/s11468-024-02584-y

Brian Brenner, M. D., Scott Brancolini, M. D., Yashar Eshraghi, M. D., Maged Guirguis, M. D., Shravani Durbhakula, M. D., David Provenzano, M. D., & Kevin Vorenkamp, M. D. (2022). Telemedicine implementation in pain medicine: A survey evaluation of pain medicine practices in spring 2020. *Pain Physician*, *25*, 387–390. PMID: 35901479

Campbell, I. M., Crowley, T. B., Keena, B., Donoghue, S., McManus, M. L., & Zackai, E. H. (2022). The experience of one pediatric geneticist with telemedicine-based clinical diagnosis. *American Journal of Medical Genetics. Part A*, *188*(12), 3416–3422. DOI: 10.1002/ajmg.a.62920 PMID: 35906847

Chakraborty, C., Gupta, B., & Ghosh, S. K. (2013). A review on telemedicine-based WBAN framework for patient monitoring. *Telemedicine Journal and e-Health*, *19*(8), 619–626. DOI: 10.1089/tmj.2012.0215 PMID: 23841489

Devaraj, S. J., & Ezra, K. (2011, April). Current trends and future challenges in wireless telemedicine system. In *2011 3rd International Conference on Electronics Computer Technology* (Vol. 4, pp. 417-421). IEEE. DOI: 10.1109/ICECTECH.2011.5941933

Elarmathi, S., Rishabavarthani, P., Sindhuja, M., Elayaraja, P., & Malathi Murugesan, S. (2024). Novel manufacturing systems for cancer diagnosis using ultra-sensitive photonic crystal fiber biosensor with dual-functionalized aptamer-nanocavity. *Microsystem Technologies*, •••, 1–20. DOI: 10.1007/s00542-024-05820-x

George, W. K., Silas, E. I., Pandey, D., & Pandey, B. K. (2024). Utilization of Industry 4.0 Technologies in Nigerian Technical and Vocational Education: A Conundrum for Educators. In *Examining the Rapid Advance of Digital Technology in Africa* (pp. 270–293). IGI Global. DOI: 10.4018/978-1-6684-9962-7.ch014

Khadka, M., Sah, M., Chaudhary, R., Sahani, S. K., Sahani, K., Pandey, B. K., & Pandey, D. (2025). Spectroscopic, quantum chemical, and topological calculations of the phenylephrine molecule using density functional theory. *Scientific Reports*, *15*(1), 208. DOI: 10.1038/s41598-024-81633-2 PMID: 39747169

Konapure, C. G., Pandey, D., Shete, H., Thakar, C. M., Pandey, B. K., & George, A. S. (2025). Artificial Intelligence in Automated Concrete Mix Design Using Computerized Grading Curves. Interdisciplinary Approaches to AI, Internet of Everything, and Machine Learning, 567-586.

Kumar, B., Pandey, D., Pandey, B. K., & George, A. S. (2024). Higher Education in the Last Four Decades: A Review of Paradigm Shifts in Policy Frameworks. Design and Implementation of Higher Education Learners' Learning Outcomes (HELLO), 333-348.

Kumar, M. S., Prasanna, P. L., Lalitha, M., Joy, M., Jha, S. S., & Pandey, B. K. (2025). Utilizing the Internet of Everything and Artificial Intelligence for Real-Time Workforce Management. In Role of Internet of Everything (IOE), VLSI Architecture, and AI in Real-Time Systems (pp. 153-168). IGI Global Scientific Publishing.

Kumar Pandey, B., Pandey, D., Nassa, V. K., Ahmad, T., Singh, C., George, A. S., & Wakchaure, M. A. (2021). Encryption and steganography-based text extraction in IoT using the EWCTS optimizer. *Imaging Science Journal*, *69*(1-4), 38–56. DOI: 10.1080/13682199.2022.2146885

Kumarganesh, S., & Malathi Murugesan, C. (2024). Hybrid plasmonic biosensors with deep learning for colorectal cancer detection. *Plasmonics*, •••, 1–15. DOI: 10.1007/s11468-024-02568-y

KVM, S., Pandey, B. K., & Pandey, D. (2024). Design of Surface Plasmon Resonance (SPR) Sensors for Highly Sensitive Biomolecular Detection in Cancer Diagnostics. *Plasmonics*, •••, 1–13.

Lakshmi, K. V. N., Rajan, R., Pandey, D., & Pandey, B. K. (2024). Circular economy: A catalyst for economic growth-an empirical study. *Circular Economy and Sustainability*, •••, 1–22.

Moore, M. (1999). The evolution of telemedicine. *Future Generation Computer Systems*, *15*(2), 245–254. DOI: 10.1016/S0167-739X(98)00067-3

Muniandi, B., Nassa, V. K., Pandey, D., Pandey, B. K., Dadheech, P., & George, A. S. (2024). Pattern Analysis for Feature Extraction in Complex Images. In Using Machine Learning to Detect Emotions and Predict Human Psychology (pp. 145-167). IGI Global. DOI: 10.4018/979-8-3693-1910-9.ch007

Muralidhar, L. B., Lakshmi, K. V. N., Swapna, H. R., Rupani, J., Nethravathi, K., Pandey, B. K., & Pandey, D. (2024). Impact of Organizational Culture on The Level of Corporate Social Responsibility Investments: An Exploratory Study. *Circular Economy and Sustainability*, *4*(3), 1–19. DOI: 10.1007/s43615-024-00371-9

Pandey, B. K., Nassa, V. K., Mukundan, A. P., Mahajan, D. A., Pandey, D., George, A. S., & Dadheech, P. (2024c). An Industry-Focused Traffic System Utilising Internet of Things. In *Emerging Engineering Technologies and Industrial Applications* (pp. 200–213). IGI Global. DOI: 10.4018/979-8-3693-1335-0.ch009

Pandey, B. K., & Pandey, D. (2023). Parametric optimization and prediction of enhanced thermoelectric performance in co-doped CaMnO3 using response surface methodology and neural network. *Journal of Materials Science Materials in Electronics*, *34*(21), 1589. DOI: 10.1007/s10854-023-10954-1

Pandey, B. K., & Pandey, D. (2025). Securing healthcare medical image information using advance morphological component analysis, information hiding systems, and hybrid convolutional neural networks on IoMT. *Computers in Biology and Medicine*, *185*, 109499. DOI: 10.1016/j.compbiomed.2024.109499 PMID: 39642698

Pandey, B. K., Pandey, D., & Lelisho, M. E. (2024a). Face mask identification with enhanced cuckoo optimization and deep learning-based faster regional neural network. *Scientific Reports*, *14*(1), 29719. DOI: 10.1038/s41598-024-78746-z PMID: 39613761

Pandey, B. K., Pandey, D., & Sahani, S. K. (2024b). Autopilot control unmanned aerial vehicle system for sewage defect detection using deep learning. *Engineering Reports*, •••, 12852.

Pandey, B. K., Paramashivan, M. A., Pandey, D., George, A. S., Agarwal, A., Mahajan, D. A., . . . Pramanik, S. (2024d). Future Directions of Digital Twin Architectures for 6G Communication Networks. In Security Issues and Solutions in 6G Communications and Beyond (pp. 197-211). IGI Global.

Pandey, D., Nassa, V. K., Pandey, B. K., Mahajan, D. A., Patidar, P. K., Dadheech, P., & George, A. S. (2024). An Analysis of Internet-of-Things-Based Fire Detection and Alert Systems. In *Emerging Engineering Technologies and Industrial Applications* (pp. 295–304). IGI Global. DOI: 10.4018/979-8-3693-1335-0.ch014

Pandian, P. S., Safeer, K. P., Shakunthala, D. T. I., Gopal, P., & Padaki, V. C. (2007). Store and Forward Applications in Telemedicine for Wireless IP Based Networks. *J. Networks*, *2*(6), 58–65. DOI: 10.4304/jnw.2.6.58-65

Rai, P. K., Pandey, D., & Pandey, B. K. (2024). The future of enterprise and innovation is compute as a commodity, or CaaC. *Partners Universal International Research Journal, 3*(2), 89–94.

Saravanakumar, R., TamilSelvi, T., Pandey, D., Pandey, B. K., Mahajan, D. A., & Lelisho, M. E. (2024). Big data processing using hybrid Gaussian mixture model with salp swarm algorithm. *Journal of Big Data, 11*(1), 167. DOI: 10.1186/s40537-024-01015-3

Satheesh, N., Gopisankar, N., Kumarganesh, S., Anthoniraj, S., Saravanakumar, S., & Martin Sagayam, K. (2025). Advanced AI-driven emergency response systems for enhanced vehicle and human safety. *Iran Journal of Computer Science*, •••, 1–16. DOI: 10.1007/s42044-025-00228-w

Shahul, A., Muniandi, B., Paramashivan, M. A., Pandey, D., Pandey, B. K., Dadheech, P., & George, H. (2024). An Analysis of Algorithms and Methods Based on Image Processing for Medical Applications. In *Emerging Engineering Technologies and Industrial Applications* (pp. 173–186). IGI Global. DOI: 10.4018/979-8-3693-1335-0.ch007

Sharma, M., Talwar, R., Nassa, V. K., Binay, K., & Pandey, D. (2025). Design and performance analysis of a multiband vivaldi antenna for wireless broadband communication in 3-5.6 GHz spectrum. In *Artificial Intelligence and Information Technologies* (pp. 86–91). CRC Press.

Sheela, M. S., Kumarganesh, S., Pandey, B. K., & Lelisho, M. E. (2025). Integration of silver nanostructures in wireless sensor networks for enhanced biochemical sensing. *Discover Nano, 20*(1), 7. DOI: 10.1186/s11671-024-04159-6 PMID: 39804434

Singh, S., Madaan, G., Swapna, H. R., Singh, A., Pandey, D., George, A. S., & Pandey, B. K. (2025). Empowering Connectivity: Exploring the Internet of Things. In Interdisciplinary Approaches to AI, Internet of Everything, and Machine Learning (pp. 89-116). IGI Global Scientific Publishing.

Singh, S., Madaan, G., Swapna, H. R., Singh, A., Pandey, D., George, A. S., & Pandey, B. K. (2025). Empowering Connectivity: Exploring the Internet of Things. In Interdisciplinary Approaches to AI, Internet of Everything, and Machine Learning (pp. 89-116). IGI Global Scientific Publishing.

Vinodhini, V., Kumar, M. S., Sankar, S., Pandey, D., Pandey, B. K., & Nassa, V. K. (2022). IoT-based early forest fire detection using MLP and AROC method. *International Journal of Global Warming, 27*(1), 55–70. DOI: 10.1504/IJGW.2022.122794

Chapter 11
Role of IoT in Enhancing Secure Medical Image Transfers

C. Saravanakumar
https://orcid.org/0009-0005-3472-8037
Department of Electronics and Communication Engineering, SRM Valliammai Engineering College, India

Niladri Maiti
School of Dentistry, Central Asian University, Tashkent, Uzbekistan

Babacar Toure
Faculty of Dental Medicine, College of Health Sciences, International University of Rabat, Morocco

B. Vidhya
https://orcid.org/0000-0003-1771-3595
Department of Computational Intelligence, SRM Institute of Science and Technology, India

G. M. Karpura Dheepan
Department of Computer Science and Engineering, Sathyabama Institute of Science and Technology, Chennai, India

Joshuva Arockia Dhanraj
https://orcid.org/0000-0001-5048-7775
University Centre for Research and Development, Chandigarh University, Mohali, India

Aakifa Shahul
SRM Medical College, Kattankulathur, India

ABSTRACT

The secure transmission of medical images is one area where the Internet of Things (IoT) is transforming the healthcare industry. The importance of IoT in improving the privacy, accuracy, and usability of medical imaging data is examined in this chapter. Healthcare providers can use IoT technologies to enable the real-time

DOI: 10.4018/979-8-3693-9821-0.ch011

transmission of sensitive medical images while reducing the risks of unauthorized access and data breaches, thanks to the proliferation of connected devices. Effective data transfer is made possible by IoT through the use of secure and lightweight communication protocols like MQTT and CoAP.

INTRODUCTION

Securing medical image transfers is a vital component of telemedicine, and the Internet of Things (IoT) has a revolutionary effect on this. Imaging data collection, analysis (Pandey, B. K., & Pandey, D., 2025).), and transmission have become more efficient with the widespread use of IoT devices in the healthcare industry. Still, given the sensitive nature of medical images, worries regarding security and privacy are also heightened by this increase in data transmission. Medical images are safely transferred from the source to the intended recipient to the integration of cutting-edge security measures like end-to-end encryption that IoT technology offers. Medical data is shielded from unauthorized access and manipulation by encryption, which also maintains its integrity and confidentiality. Authentication mechanisms enabled by IoT also guarantee that patient data is only accessible by authorized personnel, lowering the possibility of data breaches. Its capacity to enable edge computing is another important part of IoT's role in secure image transfer. Sensitive medical images are exposed to fewer vulnerabilities during transmission thanks to this model's data processing that takes place closer to the device level (Satheesh, N. et al., 2025). Attackers will find it more difficult to intercept and alter medical data with this method since it eliminates the need for centralized cloud-based storage. Transparency and traceability can be ensured by integrating cutting-edge technologies like blockchain with Internet of Things systems to create immutable records of medical image transfers. The security and portability of medical image transfers in telemedicine applications are further improved by IoT protocols like MQTT and CoAP.

Medical Image Transmission in Telemedicine

The transmission of medical images is an essential component of telemedicine, as it enables remote diagnosis, treatment planning, and patient monitoring. Regardless of the patient's physical location, medical professionals are able to provide timely and accurate medical interventions thanks to the capability of transmitting images in real time (Kumar, M. S. et al., 2025). These images include X-rays, CT scans, MRIs, and ultrasounds. This is especially helpful in areas that are underserved or rural, either of which may have limited access to specialists. When it comes to diagnosing conditions, tracking the progression of diseases, and determining the efficacy of treatments, medical images are frequently indispensable. The capability of securely transmitting these images enables specialists to work together with primary care providers in the field of telemedicine, which ultimately results in improved patient outcomes through the utilization of expert consultations. It makes follow-up care easier to provide by enabling continuous monitoring of patients' conditions without the requirement of frequent visits in person. The incorporation of medical image transmission into telemedicine results in a reduction in both the amount of time and money required to provide care to patients. It is no longer necessary for patients to travel significant distances in order to receive consultations from specialists, and medical professionals are able to streamline their workflow by reviewing images remotely. When it comes to providing medical care, this efficiency not only enhances the overall patient experience but also maximizes the utilization of available medical resources (Lee, D., & Yoon, S. N., 2021).

IoT in Healthcare and Telemedicine

The Internet of Things (IoT) has profoundly altered healthcare and telemedicine by establishing an interconnected network of medical devices, healthcare systems, and patients, facilitating effortless data exchange and remote care (Konapure, C. G. et al., 2025) In healthcare, the Internet of Things (IoT) is predominantly utilized for patient surveillance via wearable devices, intelligent sensors, and diagnostic instruments. These devices incessantly gather data on vital signs, physical activity, and health metrics including heart rate, blood pressure, glucose levels, and oxygen saturation. This information is relayed instantaneously to healthcare professionals, allowing them to oversee patients from a distance, detect potential health concerns promptly, and administer timely interventions. For patients with chronic conditions such as diabetes or heart disease, IoT devices are essential for health management. Wearable devices can notify healthcare professionals upon detecting abnormalities, thereby diminishing the necessity for frequent hospital visits. This ongoing surveillance facilitates tailored, preemptive healthcare, addressing issues prior to their escalation into critical conditions. In emergencies, IoT devices can activate alerts for both patients and healthcare providers, facilitating swift responses and potentially preserving lives. In the domain of telemedicine, IoT improves healthcare service delivery by facilitating remote consultations, diagnostics, and follow-up care (Tortorella, G. L. et al., 2021).

IoT devices can convey medical data, such as vital signs, test results, and images, enabling healthcare professionals to evaluate patient conditions without requiring in-person consultations. This capability is particularly crucial in remote or underserved regions where access to specialized healthcare is restricted. IoT enhances telemedicine platforms, allowing healthcare providers to consult, diagnose, and treat patients remotely. The Internet of Things enhances the operational efficiency of healthcare institutions. Automated data collection from IoT-enabled devices diminishes the necessity for manual data entry, thereby reducing human errors and optimizing workflow processes (Singh, S. et al., 2025a). Healthcare providers can obtain patient data instantaneously, enhancing decision-making and treatment precision. The Internet of Things facilitates predictive maintenance of medical apparatus, guaranteeing their operational readiness (Khadka, M. et al., 2025) and availability when required. This minimizes downtime and improves the quality of care delivered. Security is a paramount concern in the implementation of IoT within healthcare and telemedicine. Due to the transmission of sensitive medical data across networks, IoT systems incorporate encryption, authentication protocols, and secure communication channels to safeguard patient information from unauthorized access. Edge computing, which involves local data processing on the device instead of in the cloud, improves security by reducing vulnerability to cyber threats (Aceto, G. et al., 2020).

IoT in Healthcare

IoT Applications in Healthcare

IoT applications in healthcare are revolutionizing the collection, transmission, and analysis of patient data, resulting in more efficient, personalized, and accessible healthcare solutions (Singh, S. et al., 2025b). The Internet of Things (IoT) is enhancing health outcomes and optimizing healthcare systems through advancements in remote monitoring, telemedicine, smart hospitals, and diagnostics. The Internet of Things (IoT) has transformed healthcare by facilitating diverse applications are as shown in the figure 1, that enhance patient care, operational efficiency, and data-informed decision-making. These applications utilize interconnected devices, sensors, and data analytics to develop more responsive, personalized, and efficient healthcare systems (Pandey, B. K. et al., 2024a).

- *Remote Patient Monitoring*: IoT devices, including wearable sensors, smartwatches, and health trackers, facilitate the continuous monitoring of vital signs such as heart rate, blood pressure, and glucose levels. These devices relay real-time data to healthcare providers, facilitating proactive management of chronic conditions such as diabetes and hypertension. By enabling the early identification of anomalous health metrics, healthcare providers can intervene swiftly, averting complications and diminishing emergency hospital admissions. This real-time monitoring enhances care quality by facilitating more personalized and data-informed decisions. Alongside real-time health monitoring, remote patient monitoring via IoT markedly diminishes the necessity for frequent hospital or clinic visits. Patients with chronic conditions can remain at home while being monitored by their physicians. This improves patient comfort and convenience while reducing healthcare expenses. IoT systems can transmit alerts to healthcare providers or caregivers during critical health events, guaranteeing that patients receive prompt interventions prior to the escalation of symptoms.

- *Telemedicine and Remote Consultations*: The Internet of Things (IoT) is an essential facilitator of telemedicine, allowing for virtual consultations through remote data collection and transmission. IoT devices, including smart stethoscopes, otoscopes, and vital sign monitors, enable healthcare providers to collect essential patient data remotely (Pandey, B. K. et al., 2024b). These devices relay real-time data, providing physicians with precise information to evaluate and diagnose patients remotely, thereby enhancing the accuracy and efficacy of telemedicine consultations. This is especially advantageous in rural or underserved regions where access to specialized medical care is restricted. IoT-enabled telemedicine systems provide patients the convenience of receiving care at home, thereby minimizing travel expenses and wait times (Maheshwari, R. U. et al., 2024). Individuals with restricted mobility or residing in isolated areas can access virtual consultations and obtain prompt medical care. The Internet of Things facilitates the secure transmission of medical data and images, thereby improving collaboration among healthcare professionals and specialists during virtual consultations, which enhances the overall quality of care (Dhanvijay, M. M., & Patil, S. C., 2019).
- *Intelligent Healthcare Facilities*: IoT applications are crucial for developing smart hospitals by enhancing operational efficiency. IoT systems facilitate the tracking and monitoring of medical equipment, allowing hospital personnel to swiftly locate devices such as wheelchairs, ventilators, or IV pumps, thereby minimizing time spent searching for critical tools. IoT-enabled hospital inventory management guarantees that medications, supplies, and equipment are adequately stocked and operational, enhancing efficiency (Maheshwari, R. Uma. et al., 2024) and averting delays in patient care. IoT can anticipate equipment malfunctions by analyzing usage patterns, facilitating prompt maintenance and minimizing downtime. Operational enhancements, IoT improves patient safety and comfort by utilizing environmental monitoring systems that control air quality, temperature, and lighting. Hospitals utilizing IoT technology can oversee patient rooms and modify environmental variables to establish ideal healing conditions. Real-time data analytics (Saxena, A. et al., 2024) enhance the efficient utilization of hospital resources, mitigating

overcrowding and elevating the overall patient experience (Alsubaei, F. et al., 2019).

- *Pharmaceutical Oversight*: IoT-enabled smart pill bottles and dispensers are revolutionizing patient medication management. These devices prompt patients to administer their medications punctually and in the appropriate dosage, thereby mitigating the risk of missed doses and medication errors. This is especially crucial for elderly patients or individuals with chronic conditions who depend on various medications. Through the automation of medication management, IoT facilitates patient compliance with prescribed treatment regimens, thereby mitigating the risk of complications arising from missed or erroneous dosages. Besides enhancing patient adherence, IoT in medication management enables healthcare providers to remotely oversee a patient's medication consumption. In the event of a missed dose, the system can notify the healthcare provider, facilitating prompt follow-up and ensuring that potential concerns are swiftly addressed (Rai, P. K. et al., 2024). This form of monitoring is particularly beneficial for patients necessitating regular medication, such as individuals with cardiovascular diseases or diabetes, enhancing treatment efficacy and decreasing hospital readmissions.
- *Emergency Response Enhanced by IoT*: The Internet of Things (IoT) technology is essential in emergency response systems, especially for high-risk patients, including the elderly and individuals with chronic illnesses. Wearable devices with emergency response functionalities such as panic buttons or fall detection sensors enable patients to promptly notify emergency services or caregivers in the event of a fall or medical crisis. These devices can autonomously transmit notifications to designated contacts or healthcare professionals, facilitating prompt intervention and potentially preserving lives. IoT-enabled emergency response systems can interface with healthcare databases, enabling first responders to retrieve essential patient information prior to their arrival at the scene. This encompasses medical histories, allergies, and current medications, facilitating more informed and effective care during emergencies. These systems can evaluate real-time data (Lakshmi, K. V. N. et al., 2024) to forecast potential emergencies based on a patient's health trends, thereby offering an additional layer of safety and support.
- *Internet of Things in Diagnostics*: IoT-enabled diagnostic devices are transforming medical testing by delivering real-time results (Saravanakumar, R. et al., 2024), optimizing the diagnostic procedure, and minimizing patient wait times for results. Connected portable imaging devices and laboratory equipment can directly transmit test results to healthcare providers, enhancing the speed and precision of diagnosis. For instance, IoT-enabled ultrasound or MRI machines can promptly transmit images to radiologists, facil-

itating expedited interpretation and diagnosis, which is vital in emergency care scenarios. Besides optimizing diagnostics, IoT enhances accessibility to diagnostic instruments in remote regions. Portable IoT-enabled devices can be utilized in rural clinics or by mobile health units (Kumarganesh, S. et al., 2024), enabling healthcare providers to conduct tests and transmit data to specialists in real-time. The decentralization of diagnostic capabilities is especially beneficial in low-resource environments, as prompt access to diagnostic information can enhance treatment outcomes and minimize patient travel for specialized care (Muralidhar, L. B. et al., 2024).

Figure 1. Healthcare applications of IoT

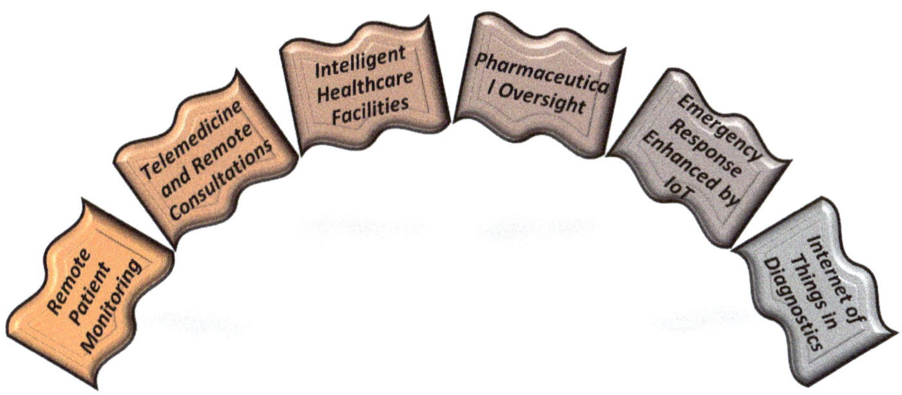

Integration of IoT in Telemedicine

Healthcare service delivery is changing as a result of the Internet of Things (IoT) integration with telemedicine platforms. This is because patient-centered, efficient, and easily accessible healthcare is now available to all. Personalized care, real-time data collection, and remote patient monitoring are all made possible by healthcare providers connecting telemedicine systems to a variety of medical devices, wearables, and diagnostic tools. The capacity to enable ongoing patient monitoring is one of the main benefits of telemedicine's integration of IoT (Pandey, B. K. et al., 2024c). Vital health metrics like blood pressure, oxygen saturation, and heart rate can be gathered by wearable technology like smartwatches and health trackers. By sending this data straight to telemedicine platforms, medical professionals can examine patterns and see possible health problems before they become serious ones (Pandey, B. K. et al., 2024d). Clinicians are therefore able to take proactive measures, which improve patient outcomes and decrease hospital stays. IoT also improves telemedicine by enabling medical professionals to conduct virtual consultations with patients utilizing real-time data (Elarmathi, S. et al., 2024). For example, medical professionals can conduct remote examinations using gadgets like digital otoscopes and smart stethoscopes, which send audio and visual data during virtual visits. Better communication between patients and healthcare providers is promoted by this integration, which also increases diagnostic accuracy. The administrative procedures in telemedicine platforms are also made more efficient by the integration of IoT. Automated data collection increases the effectiveness of electronic health records (EHRs) by reducing errors caused by human input. Healthcare providers can access comprehensive patient profiles through IoT devices, which facilitates seamless data collection and transmission, improving decision-making and treatment planning. Integrating IoT devices securely is crucial, and in order to safeguard patient data, telemedicine platforms need to use strong authentication and encryption procedures. Healthcare providers can confidently use IoT technology while protecting sensitive data by guaranteeing secure communication channels (Sheela, M. S. et al., 2025).

MEDICAL IMAGE TRANSMISSION REQUIREMENTS

The need for secure, real-time, and reliable image transfer is of the utmost importance. Medical image transmission in telemedicine is essential for effective remote diagnosis and treatment, which is why it takes precedence. Images used in medicine, such as X-rays, magnetic resonance imaging (MRI), and computed tomography (CT) scans, are typically large files that need to be transmitted as quickly as possible without compromising their quality or integrity. Particularly in emergency situations, where delays could potentially have a negative impact on patient outcomes, these images are essential for making decisions immediately in many instances. Using cutting-edge network technologies that enable the transfer of large amounts of data with minimal latency is necessary for telemedicine systems in order to fulfill these requirements. It is possible to ensure that the images are delivered to healthcare providers in a timely manner and in their original form by utilizing compression algorithms and optimizing (Ahathiyan, G. S. et al., 2025) the process. This helps to maintain the accuracy that is necessary for clinical diagnosis.

The principles of confidentiality, integrity, and availability (CIA) play a significant role in protecting sensitive patient data, which is another important factor in the transmission of medical images. Security is another necessary component of the process. In order to protect patient information from being accessed by unauthorized parties or being compromised, confidentiality ensures that only authorized personnel are able to view the images that are been transmitted. For the purpose of ensuring that the images are not corrupted or altered while in transit, integrity protects the accuracy of the images while they are being transferred (Pandey, B. K. et al., 2024e). Any manipulation of the data could result in incorrect diagnoses, so this is an extremely important consideration. In order to avoid delays in patient care caused by technical issues, availability ensures that the images are accessible whenever they are required. Encryption, secure transmission protocols, and redundancy mechanisms are utilized by telemedicine systems in order to uphold these CIA principles. This safeguards medical data while it is being transmitted, providing an additional layer of protection. During the process of transmitting medical images, it is also extremely important to ensure that compliance with medical data standards is maintained. These standards include the Health Insurance Portability and Accountability Act (HIPAA) in the United States and the General Data Protection Regulation (GDPR) in Europe. These regulations establish stringent guidelines for the management of patient data, including the manner in which it is handled, stored, accessed, and distributed (JayaLakshmi, G. et al., 2024). A patient's right to privacy is safeguarded by compliance, and it guarantees that healthcare providers are employing safe and legitimate means of data transmission. By implementing encryption, secure authentication, and audit trails to monitor and document data access (George, W. K. et al., 2024), telemedicine systems are required to comply with these standards in order to demonstrate compliance. In addition to protecting patient information, ensuring compliance with these requirements helps healthcare institutions avoid the legal and financial repercussions that can result from data breaches or non-compliance with regulations.

MEDICAL IMAGE TRANSFER SECURITY OBSTACLES

Data Breaches and Unauthorized Access

Risks associated with data breaches and unauthorized access in the healthcare industry are substantial, especially when it comes to private patient data (Abdullahi, M. et al., 2024). Cybercriminals find medical records which contain patient histories, diagnostic images, and personal identification information to be extremely valuable targets. Identity theft, financial fraud, and the unauthorized sale of personal health data can result from a data breach that exposes this private information to malevolent parties. When patients' privacy is violated and their personal information is used for insurance fraud, the consequences of such breaches can be disastrous for them and damage their trust in medical facilities. Serious clinical repercussions may also result from unauthorized access to medical systems and data. Medical records can be altered or manipulated by an attacker, endangering patient health and safety by causing incorrect diagnoses, ineffective treatments, or delays in care. Unauthorized access can also impair the availability and integrity of medical information systems, which can cause disruptions to healthcare services. Attacks using ransomware, for instance, can prevent hospitals from operating, postpone the delivery of essential medical care, and force them to use antiquated, ineffective manual procedures. In addition to seriously harming patient care, this also costs a lot of money. Healthcare organizations are required by law to protect patient data; otherwise, they risk significant fines, legal action, and harm to their reputation. It is imperative to adhere to regulations such as the GDPR in Europe and HIPAA in the United States, which impose stringent guidelines on patient privacy and data security. Data breaches can have long-term financial and operational consequences for the institutions involved, including regulatory fines and a decline in patient trust. Maintaining the integrity, trust, and functionality of healthcare systems in a digital healthcare environment requires protecting patient data.

Network Vulnerabilities in IoT Systems

IoT network vulnerabilities pose security risks, especially in healthcare, where sensitive patient data is transmitted across interconnected devices. IoT networks use many devices, sensors, and communication channels (Pandey, D. et al., 2025).) on different platforms with different security protocols. Cybercriminals can exploit multiple vulnerabilities due to complexity. If these vulnerabilities are not addressed (Kumar, B. et al., 2024), attackers can intercept data, manipulate medical devices, or disrupt critical healthcare services, endangering patient safety and system integrity. Weak or outdated encryption protocols are a major IoT network vulnerability (Pandey, D. et al., 2024a). Many IoT devices, especially those with limited computational resources, use lightweight encryption, which may not protect against sophisticated attacks. This can expose medical records and real-time patient monitoring data to unauthorized access. Insecure communication protocols between IoT devices and central networks can also help hackers launch man-in-the-middle attacks, which intercept and alter data. Healthcare providers may receive false medical information from such breaches, leading to incorrect diagnoses or treatment plans. Insufficient device authentication and authorization create another vulnerability (Pandey, D. et al., 2024b). Healthcare IoT devices often lack strong authentication, making it easier for unauthorized users to access the system. Attackers can move laterally through the network to compromise critical systems and other devices. Insecure software and firmware on IoT devices can be used to take control or disrupt services. Healthcare facilities where compromised medical devices could kill patients are especially at risk.

IOT IN ENHANCING SECURITY

The Internet of Things (IoT) is playing an increasingly important role in improving security, particularly in industries like healthcare where system dependability and data protection are vital. IoT networks and devices can be used to strengthen security protocols and safeguard sensitive data and critical infrastructure from attacks, in addition to enhancing healthcare operations. Organizations can better monitor, detect, and respond to possible vulnerabilities and breaches in real-time by integrating IoT with cutting-edge security technologies (Kennedy, G. W. et al., 2024). By enhancing these security features which are shown in the figure 2, IoT fosters more resilient and adaptive security frameworks, protecting both digital and physical assets from various threats.

- *Continuous Monitoring and Surveillance*: Internet of Things (IoT) devices, including sensors and cameras, facilitate real-time surveillance of both physical and digital environments. These devices continuously gather data on system performance, network activity, and environmental conditions, enabling organizations to monitor potential security threats as they arise. The automation enabled by IoT permits security teams to oversee extensive operations without necessitating human supervision for each device (Shahul, A. et al., 2024). In addition to real-time alerts, IoT systems can archive and analyze historical data to discern patterns or trends that may signify an emerging security concern. This longitudinal data monitoring enables organizations to proactively mitigate potential vulnerabilities and consistently enhance their overall security stance.
- *Enhanced Device Authentication*: IoT systems facilitate multi-factor authentication (MFA) and biometric authentication to augment device security. By necessitating additional authentication methods beyond a password, such as biometric scans (e.g., fingerprint or facial recognition) or a one-time password (OTP), IoT mitigates the risk of unauthorized access to sensitive information or essential systems. This is particularly crucial for safeguarding medical devices and systems that manage sensitive patient information. IoT devices can implement role-based access control (RBAC), guaranteeing that only authorized individuals with appropriate credentials can engage with

particular devices or systems. This stratified security methodology enhances safeguards against insider threats and mitigates the risk of inadvertent data breaches (Pandey, D. et al., 2024c).

- *Data Encryption*: IoT devices may employ end-to-end encryption protocols to safeguard data transmitted over networks. Encryption guarantees that intercepted data during transmission remains inaccessible to unauthorized individuals. In healthcare, safeguarding sensitive patient information, including medical records, diagnostic images, and treatment plans, is essential. IoT systems can employ advanced encryption standards (AES) and transport layer security (TLS) to safeguard data during transmission (Pandey, D., & Pandey, B. K., 2022). Moreover, encryption can be utilized on stored data, protecting it from breaches or alterations even if a device or server is compromised. This ensures that sensitive information is safeguarded throughout its entire lifecycle, from collection to storage.
- *Anomaly Detection and Threat Mitigation*: IoT networks employ sophisticated algorithms and artificial neural network (Pandey, B. K., & Pandey, D., 2023) to identify anomalous patterns in device behavior. Through the continuous analysis of extensive data sets, these systems can rapidly detect anomalies that may signify security breaches, malware attacks, or device malfunctions. The capacity for real-time response allows organizations to alleviate threats prior to inflicting substantial damage. Machine learning models can be developed to differentiate between normal and suspicious activity, enhancing their precision over time. This self-learning capability enables IoT systems to remain proactive against emerging cyber threats and autonomously adjust to novel attack patterns, thereby reducing the likelihood of false positives or missed incidents.
- *Automated System Updates*: IoT devices can be configured for automatic firmware and software updates to rectify vulnerabilities and address security gaps. Numerous cyberattacks leverage obsolete software devoid of recent security updates; thus, it is imperative to ensure that all devices are current to uphold strong defenses. Automated updates obviate the necessity for manual intervention, guaranteeing continuous system protection without interruption. Furthermore, automatic updates alleviate the workload on IT teams, enabling them to concentrate on additional security responsibilities. IoT systems can be configured to execute updates during off-peak hours to reduce operational disruption, thereby ensuring the implementation of the latest security features.
- *Augmented Physical Security*: IoT systems can amalgamate with access control technologies, including smart locks and facial recognition, to safeguard physical environments. These systems can oversee and regulate access to

sensitive locations such as server rooms, research laboratories, or healthcare facilities, permitting entry solely to authorized individuals. Organizations can enhance security at their physical locations by utilizing IoT, thereby preventing unauthorized access and interference with essential infrastructure. Furthermore, IoT-enabled access control systems can generate comprehensive logs of individuals who accessed specific areas and the corresponding timestamps, facilitating investigations in the event of security breaches. The integration of real-time alerts facilitates prompt responses to unauthorized access attempts, thereby augmenting the safety and security of the facility.

- *Network Segmentation*: The Internet of Things facilitates network segmentation, thereby isolating critical data flows from general traffic. This network isolation mitigates the risk of inter-network attacks, including the dissemination of malware across different segments of the system. Segmentation also aids in containing any breach within a specific segment, thereby minimizing the potential impact on the entire network. IoT-based segmentation facilitates the formation of micro-segments, wherein individual devices or small clusters of devices are segregated. This degree of control mitigates the risk of lateral movement by intruders within the network, as they cannot access other devices or systems beyond their micro-segment. This detailed methodology for network security substantially enhances an organizations protection against cyber threats.

Figure 2. IoT's role in security enhancement

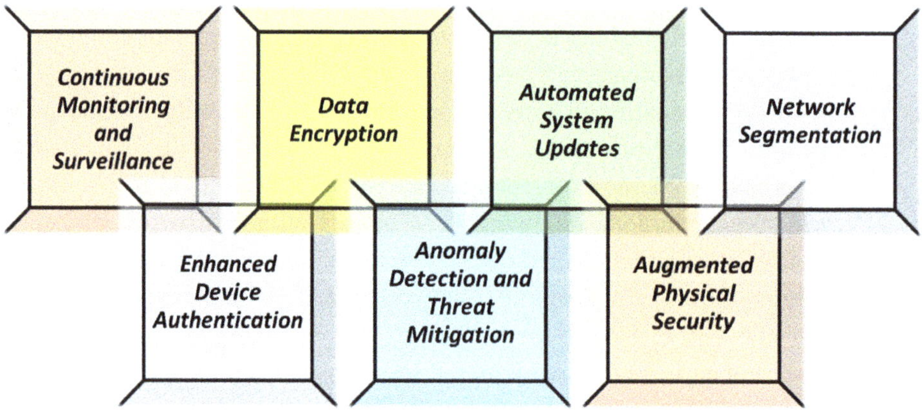

PROTOCOLS FOR SECURE IMAGE TRANSFER

Secure IoT Communication Protocols

IoT data confidentiality, integrity, and availability require secure communication protocols. IoT devices communicate over diverse networks and handle sensitive data like healthcare data and industrial control signals, so secure protocols prevent unauthorized access, data breaches, and cyberattacks. These protocols ensure efficient and secure data transmission while accommodating IoT device constraints like limited processing power and bandwidth. MQTT is a popular IoT protocol. Resources-constrained devices like sensors, wearables, and smart home systems benefit from MQTT's low-bandwidth, power-efficient IoT communication. In a publish/subscribe model, devices send data to a central broker, which distributes it to subscribed devices. MQTT uses Transport Layer Security (TLS) to encrypt data, preventing message tampering. MQTT can also use username-password pairs or digital certificates to verify device identities before allowing communication. Constrained Application Protocol (CoAP) is another important protocol for low-power, low-bandwidth device communication. CoAP is popular in smart energy grids and remote monitoring. IoT-friendly CoAP uses request/response communication like HTTP but is lighter. CoAP uses Datagram Transport Layer Security (DTLS) to secure data from malicious manipulation during transmission. DTLS provides encryption, message integrity, and anti-replay protection. IoT devices and web servers need HTTPS to communicate securely. HTTPS encrypts internet data using TLS, protecting login credentials, financial data, and medical records. To prevent data eavesdropping, IoT devices often use this protocol to communicate with cloud services or remote databases. IoT networks also use AMQP for secure message transmission. It supports encryption and message delivery guarantees, making it suitable for critical IoT applications like financial services and healthcare that require data accuracy and timeliness. Secure communication protocols help protect IoT ecosystems from cyberattacks. These protocols protect IoT devices' massive data sets with encryption, authentication, and integrity checks, ensuring security and efficiency in various applications.

IoT Protocols for Secure Transmission

Employing lightweight IoT protocols provides multiple advantages for secure and efficient data transmission in resource-limited settings. A key advantage is their capacity to reduce bandwidth consumption, which is essential for devices functioning in environments with restricted network capacity. Lightweight protocols are engineered to convey solely critical data, minimizing the overhead linked with conventional communication techniques. This efficiency enhances network performance and guarantees that devices function seamlessly without exhausting their finite resources. Besides bandwidth efficiency, lightweight IoT protocols improve energy conservation, which is essential for battery-powered devices. Numerous IoT applications, including remote sensors and wearables, depend on batteries for energy and possess a finite lifespan. By employing lightweight protocols, these devices can diminish the frequency and duration of their network connections, resulting in extended battery life. This feature is especially advantageous in applications necessitating continuous monitoring, as it enables devices to transmit essential data without the need for frequent recharging or replacement. The lightweight IoT protocols offer substantial security advantages. Although designed to be minimalistic, many of these protocols still integrate fundamental security features, including encryption and authentication mechanisms. Protocols such as MQTT and CoAP can utilize Transport Layer Security (TLS) or Datagram Transport Layer Security (DTLS) to safeguard data during transmission. These protocols protect sensitive information from unauthorized access and cyber threats by ensuring data encryption and device authentication prior to communication. Lightweight protocols enhance data transmission speed by minimizing overhead. This is especially crucial in time-sensitive applications, such as healthcare monitoring or industrial automation, where prompt data delivery can profoundly affect outcomes. Lightweight protocols facilitate expedited interactions between devices and servers by reducing data packet size and optimizing the communication process, thereby ensuring the prompt transmission of essential information without superfluous delays. The implementation of lightweight IoT protocols can enhance interoperability among diverse devices and platforms. Numerous protocols are engineered for simplicity, facilitating manufacturers integration into diverse applications. This adaptability fosters collaboration among diverse IoT ecosystems, enabling devices from multiple vendors to interact efficiently and securely. As the Internet of Things proliferates, the capacity to seamlessly integrate various devices will be crucial for developing cohesive and efficient systems.

CONCLUSION

The Internet of Things (IoT) is crucial for improving the secure transmission of medical images, tackling the specific challenges presented by the healthcare industry. By utilizing IoT devices and protocols, healthcare providers can guarantee the real-time transmission of medical images while upholding optimal security standards. The implementation of secure communication protocols, including MQTT and CoAP, enhances the safeguarding of sensitive data from unauthorized access and cyber threats. The utilization of lightweight IoT protocols facilitates efficient data transmission, guaranteeing prompt access to essential medical information while conserving bandwidth and power, which is especially crucial in remote or underserved regions. Various trends and prospective domains of advancement are expected to influence the evolution of IoT in secure medical image transmission. A significant trend is the growing implementation of artificial intelligence and machine learning technologies to improve data analytics and anomaly detection in IoT networks. These technologies can enhance the detection of security threats and optimize the management of medical data, facilitating proactive measures against potential breaches. The proliferation of 5G networks is anticipated to enhance data transmission speed and reliability, thereby enabling more advanced telemedicine applications and real-time monitoring. As regulatory standards concerning data privacy and security advance, there will be an increasing focus on adherence to frameworks such as HIPAA and GDPR within IoT systems. This will propel the advancement of sophisticated encryption techniques and enhanced authentication methods, guaranteeing the security of medical images and patient data. The ongoing advancement of IoT technology offers promising prospects for augmenting the security and efficiency of medical image transmission, thereby enhancing patient care and outcomes in the healthcare sector.

REFERENCES

Abdullahi, M., Ahmad, A., Pandey, B. K., & Pandey, D. (2024). Digital Currency Adoption: A Comparative Analysis of Global Trends and the Nigerian eNaira Digital Currency. *SN Computer Science*, *5*(5), 1–11. DOI: 10.1007/s42979-024-02882-6

Aceto, G., Persico, V., & Pescapé, A. (2020). Industry 4.0 and health: Internet of things, big data, and cloud computing for healthcare 4.0. *Journal of Industrial Information Integration*, *18*, 100129. DOI: 10.1016/j.jii.2020.100129

Ahathiyan, G. S., Du John, H. V., Moni, D. J., Sagayam, K. M., Pandey, B. K., Pandey, D., & Lelisho, M. E. (2025). Design and simulation of a highly efficient eco-friendly, non-toxic perovskite solar cell. *Discover Nano*, *20*(1), 32. DOI: 10.1186/s11671-025-04190-1 PMID: 39937384

Alsubaei, F., Abuhussein, A., Shandilya, V., & Shiva, S. (2019). IoMT-SAF: Internet of medical things security assessment framework. *Internet of Things : Engineering Cyber Physical Human Systems*, *8*, 100123. DOI: 10.1016/j.iot.2019.100123

Dhanvijay, M. M., & Patil, S. C. (2019). Internet of Things: A survey of enabling technologies in healthcare and its applications. *Computer Networks*, *153*, 113–131. DOI: 10.1016/j.comnet.2019.03.006

Elarmathi, S., Rishabavarthani, P., Sindhuja, M., Elayaraja, P., & Malathi Murugesan, S. (2024). Novel manufacturing systems for cancer diagnosis using ultra-sensitive photonic crystal fiber biosensor with dual-functionalized aptamer-nanocavity. *Microsystem Technologies*, •••, 1–20. DOI: 10.1007/s00542-024-05820-x

George, W. K., Silas, E. I., Pandey, D., & Pandey, B. K. (2024). Utilization of Industry 4.0 Technologies in Nigerian Technical and Vocational Education: A Conundrum for Educators. In *Examining the Rapid Advance of Digital Technology in Africa* (pp. 270–293). IGI Global. DOI: 10.4018/978-1-6684-9962-7.ch014

JayaLakshmi. G., Pandey, D., Pandey, B. K., Kaur, P., Mahajan, D. A., & Dari, S. S. (2024). Smart big data collection for intelligent supply chain improvement. In AI and Machine Learning Impacts in Intelligent Supply Chain (pp. 180-195). IGI Global.

Kennedy, G. W., Sunday, S. E., Pandey, D., Kabari, A. D., Pandey, B. K., George, A. S., & Dadheech, P. (2024). Building Information Modeling: Harnessing Innovations for Professional Proficiency. In Emerging Engineering Technologies and Industrial Applications (pp. 305-331). IGI Global.

Khadka, M., Sah, M., Chaudhary, R., Sahani, S. K., Sahani, K., Pandey, B. K., & Pandey, D. (2025). Spectroscopic, quantum chemical, and topological calculations of the phenylephrine molecule using density functional theory. *Scientific Reports*, *15*(1), 208. DOI: 10.1038/s41598-024-81633-2 PMID: 39747169

Konapure, C. G., Pandey, D., Shete, H., Thakar, C. M., Pandey, B. K., & George, A. S. (2025). Artificial Intelligence in Automated Concrete Mix Design Using Computerized Grading Curves. Interdisciplinary Approaches to AI, Internet of Everything, and Machine Learning, 567-586.

Kumar, B., Pandey, D., Pandey, B. K., & George, A. S. (2024). Higher Education in the Last Four Decades: A Review of Paradigm Shifts in Policy Frameworks. Design and Implementation of Higher Education Learners' Learning Outcomes (HELLO), 333-348.

Kumar, M. S., Prasanna, P. L., Lalitha, M., Joy, M., Jha, S. S., & Pandey, B. K. (2025). Utilizing the Internet of Everything and Artificial Intelligence for Real-Time Workforce Management. In Role of Internet of Everything (IOE), VLSI Architecture, and AI in Real-Time Systems (pp. 153-168). IGI Global Scientific Publishing.

Kumarganesh, S., & Malathi Murugesan, C. (2024). Hybrid plasmonic biosensors with deep learning for colorectal cancer detection. *Plasmonics*, •••, 1–15. DOI: 10.1007/s11468-024-02568-y

Lakshmi, K. V. N., Rajan, R., Pandey, D., & Pandey, B. K. (2024). Circular economy: A catalyst for economic growth-an empirical study. *Circular Economy and Sustainability*, •••, 1–22.

Lee, D., & Yoon, S. N. (2021). Application of artificial intelligence-based technologies in the healthcare industry: Opportunities and challenges. *International Journal of Environmental Research and Public Health*, *18*(1), 271. DOI: 10.3390/ijerph18010271 PMID: 33401373

Maheshwari, R., Kumarganesh, S., K v M, S., Gopalakrishnan, A., Selvi, K., Paulchamy, B., Rishabavarthani, P., Sagayam, K. M., Pandey, B. K., & Pandey, D. (2024). Advanced plasmonic resonance-enhanced biosensor for comprehensive real-time detection and analysis of deepfake content. *Plasmonics*, •••, 1–18. DOI: 10.1007/s11468-024-02407-0

Maheshwari, R. U., Paulchamy, B., Pandey, B. K., & Pandey, D. (2024). Enhancing sensing and imaging capabilities through surface plasmon resonance for deepfake image detection. *Plasmonics*, •••, 1–20. DOI: 10.1007/s11468-024-02492-1

Muralidhar, L. B., Lakshmi, K. V. N., Swapna, H. R., Rupani, J., Nethravathi, K., Pandey, B. K., & Pandey, D. (2024). Impact of Organizational Culture on The Level of Corporate Social Responsibility Investments: An Exploratory Study. *Circular Economy and Sustainability*, *4*(3), 1–19. DOI: 10.1007/s43615-024-00371-9

Pandey, B. K., Kanike, U. K., George, A. S., & Pandey, D. (Eds.). (2024d). *AI and machine learning impacts in intelligent supply chain*. IGI Global. DOI: 10.4018/979-8-3693-1347-3

Pandey, B. K., Nassa, V. K., Mukundan, A. P., Mahajan, D. A., Pandey, D., George, A. S., & Dadheech, P. (2024c). An Industry-Focused Traffic System Utilising Internet of Things. In *Emerging Engineering Technologies and Industrial Applications* (pp. 200–213). IGI Global. DOI: 10.4018/979-8-3693-1335-0.ch009

Pandey, B. K., & Pandey, D. (2023). Parametric optimization and prediction of enhanced thermoelectric performance in co-doped CaMnO3 using response surface methodology and neural network. *Journal of Materials Science Materials in Electronics*, *34*(21), 1589. DOI: 10.1007/s10854-023-10954-1

Pandey, B. K., & Pandey, D. (2025). Securing healthcare medical image information using advance morphological component analysis, information hiding systems, and hybrid convolutional neural networks on IoMT. *Computers in Biology and Medicine*, *185*, 109499. DOI: 10.1016/j.compbiomed.2024.109499 PMID: 39642698

Pandey, B. K., Pandey, D., & Lelisho, M. E. (2024a). Face mask identification with enhanced cuckoo optimization and deep learning-based faster regional neural network. *Scientific Reports*, *14*(1), 29719. DOI: 10.1038/s41598-024-78746-z PMID: 39613761

Pandey, B. K., Pandey, D., & Sahani, S. K. (2024b). Autopilot control unmanned aerial vehicle system for sewage defect detection using deep learning. *Engineering Reports*, •••, 12852.

Pandey, B. K., Paramashivan, M. A., Pandey, D., George, A. S., Agarwal, A., Mahajan, D. A., . . . Pramanik, S. (2024e). Future Directions of Digital Twin Architectures for 6G Communication Networks. In Security Issues and Solutions in 6G Communications and Beyond (pp. 197-211). IGI Global.

Pandey, D., Nassa, V. K., Pandey, B. K., Thankachan, B., Dadheech, P., Mahajan, D. A., & George, A. S. (2024a). Artificial Intelligence and Machine Learning and Its Application in the Field of Computational Visual Analysis. In Emerging Engineering Technologies and Industrial Applications (pp. 36-57). IGI Global. DOI: 10.4018/979-8-3693-1335-0.ch003

Pandey, D., & Pandey, B. K. (2022). An efficient deep neural network with adaptive galactic swarm optimization for complex image text extraction. In *Process Mining Techniques for Pattern Recognition* (pp. 121–137). CRC Press. DOI: 10.1201/9781003169550-10

Pandey, D., Pandey, B. K., Nassa, V. K., Mahajan, D. A., George, A. S., & Dadheech, P. (2024c). Optimized Throughput-Based Broadcasting for Next Generation Wireless Networks. In Emerging Engineering Technologies and Industrial Applications (pp. 355-368). IGI Global. DOI: 10.4018/979-8-3693-1335-0.ch018

Pandey, D., Pandey, B. K., Paramashivan, M. A., Mahajan, D. A., Dadheech, P. D., George, A. S., & Hameed, A. S. (2024b). Advanced Digital Data Processing Using Cloud Cryptography: Industrial Applications. In Emerging Engineering Technologies and Industrial Applications (pp. 255-268). IGI Global.

Pandey, D., Sharma, M., Talwar, R., & Pandey, B. K. (2025). A compact quintuple band miniaturized elliptical planar monopole antenna for 5G/6G wireless systems. *Analog Integrated Circuits and Signal Processing*, *122*(3), 1–16. DOI: 10.1007/s10470-025-02310-6

Rai, P. K., Pandey, D., & Pandey, B. K. (2024). The future of enterprise and innovation is compute as a commodity, or CaaC. *Partners Universal International Research Journal*, *3*(2), 89–94.

Saravanakumar, R., TamilSelvi, T., Pandey, D., Pandey, B. K., Mahajan, D. A., & Lelisho, M. E. (2024). Big data processing using hybrid Gaussian mixture model with salp swarm algorithm. *Journal of Big Data*, *11*(1), 167. DOI: 10.1186/s40537-024-01015-3

Satheesh, N., Gopisankar, N., Kumarganesh, S., Anthoniraj, S., Saravanakumar, S., & Martin Sagayam, K. (2025). Advanced AI-driven emergency response systems for enhanced vehicle and human safety. *Iran Journal of Computer Science*, •••, 1–16. DOI: 10.1007/s42044-025-00228-w

Saxena, A., Agarwal, A., Pandey, B. K., & Pandey, D. (2024). Examination of the Criticality of Customer Segmentation Using Unsupervised Learning Methods. *Circular Economy and Sustainability*, *4*(2), 1–14. DOI: 10.1007/s43615-023-00336-4

Shahul, A., Muniandi, B., Paramashivan, M. A., Pandey, D., Pandey, B. K., Dadheech, P., & George, H. (2024). An Analysis of Algorithms and Methods Based on Image Processing for Medical Applications. In *Emerging Engineering Technologies and Industrial Applications* (pp. 173–186). IGI Global. DOI: 10.4018/979-8-3693-1335-0.ch007

Sheela, M. S., Kumarganesh, S., Pandey, B. K., & Lelisho, M. E. (2025). Integration of silver nanostructures in wireless sensor networks for enhanced biochemical sensing. *Discover Nano*, *20*(1), 7. DOI: 10.1186/s11671-024-04159-6 PMID: 39804434

Singh, S., Madaan, G., Swapna, H. R., Singh, A., Pandey, D., George, A. S., & Pandey, B. K. (2025a). Empowering Connectivity: Exploring the Internet of Things. In Interdisciplinary Approaches to AI, Internet of Everything, and Machine Learning (pp. 89-116). IGI Global Scientific Publishing.

Singh, S., Madaan, G., Swapna, H. R., Singh, A., Pandey, B. K., George, A. S., & Pandey, D. (2025b). Unleashing the Power of AI and Data Analysis: Transforming Insights into Action. In Interdisciplinary Approaches to AI, Internet of Everything, and Machine Learning (pp. 1-24). IGI Global Scientific Publishing.

Tortorella, G. L., Saurin, T. A., Fogliatto, F. S., Rosa, V. M., Tonetto, L. M., & Magrabi, F. (2021). Impacts of Healthcare 4.0 digital technologies on the resilience of hospitals. *Technological Forecasting and Social Change*, *166*, 120666. DOI: 10.1016/j.techfore.2021.120666

Chapter 12
Securing IoT Devices for Bio-Medical Image Sharing

Vinay Kumar Nassa
https://orcid.org/0009-0005-3472-8037
Ellenki College of Engineering and Technology, Hyderabad, India

Mukta Sharma
https://orcid.org/0000-0001-6784-3932
School of Life Science and Technology, IIMT University, Meerut, India

Sonia Duggal
https://orcid.org/0000-0003-0713-5904
School of Computer Applications, Manav Rachna International Institute of Research and Studies, India

Rohit Tripathi
Department of Electronics Engineering, J.C. Bose University of Science and Technology, YMCA, Faridabad, India

S. Prayla Shyry
Sathyabama Institute of Science and Technology, Chennai, India

Joshuva Arockia Dhanraj
https://orcid.org/0000-0001-5048-7775
Chandigarh University, India

Ashish Jolly
https://orcid.org/0000-0002-0849-8232
Department of Computer Science, Government PG College Ambala Cantt, India

ABSTRACT

Enhanced patient care and diagnostic capabilities have been made possible as a result of the rapid integration of Internet of Things (IoT) devices in the healthcare industry. This has resulted in a transformation in the sharing of biomedical images. Nevertheless, this technological advancement also presents significant security challenges that need to be addressed in order to protect sensitive patient data. The critical security priorities for the Internet of Things (IoT) in biomedical image shar-

DOI: 10.4018/979-8-3693-9821-0.ch012

ing are discussed in this chapter. Particular attention is paid to the importance of implementing robust authentication and authorization mechanisms, data encryption, and advanced anomaly detection techniques.

INTRODUCTION

Medical systems have been greatly impacted by the integration of smart devices, sensors (Dhanasekar, S. et al., 2023), and cutting-edge communication technologies, which has improved patient care and operational efficiency. The quality and delivery of services in medical environments can be enhanced by this technology, which makes it possible to collect, analyze, and transmit data in real-time (Pandey, B. K. et al., 2024a). Improvements in data sharing, remote patient monitoring, and general clinical setting management have resulted from it. Constant monitoring is a big advantage, especially for people with long-term illnesses. Important metrics like heart rate, blood pressure, and glucose levels can be monitored by devices (Du John. et al., 2022) like smart watches, fitness trackers, and specialized medical sensors (Shahul, A. et al., 2024).

Healthcare providers can instantly access this data, which makes it possible to identify possible health issues early and take appropriate action. By enabling personalized care and reducing the need for frequent hospital visits, remote monitoring improves patient outcomes while lowering overall costs (Pandey, D. et al., 2024). Connected medical imaging systems have also revolutionized diagnostics. Modern medical devices such as CT scanners, MRI machines, and X-ray machines make it possible to share images with medical specialists easily, leading to faster diagnosis and remote consultations. This feature improves patient care by speeding up treatment and increasing the effectiveness of diagnostic procedures (Pandey, B. K. et al., 2024b). Smart technologies help hospitals manage resources and equipment more effectively. Automated systems keep track of patient information, oversee medication inventories, and keep an eye on the availability and state of vital medical equipment. These solutions send out alerts for required maintenance and repairs, which helps to prevent equipment malfunctions(Pandey, B. K. et al., 2024c).. All things considered, automation streamlines hospital operations and guarantees that patients receive timely and effective care. Although there are many advantages to these innovations, there are security risks as well. The growing interconnectivity of systems and devices makes sensitive patient data more susceptible to cyberattacks. Strong encryption, safe authentication, and adherence to legal frameworks like HIPAA and GDPR are necessary to guarantee the security and privacy of this data (Swapna, H. R. et al., 2024a).

Bio-Medical Image Sharing in Medical Diagnostics

Information exchange in the field of biomedical imaging is an essential component of contemporary medical diagnostics. Medical professionals are able to collaborate (Pandey, B. K. et al., 2024d), consult, and diagnose patients more effectively when they have the ability to share diagnostic images across healthcare systems. Examples of diagnostic images include X-rays, MRIs, CT scans, and ultrasounds. The ability of specialists to access patient images remotely, which enables expert opinions to be gathered from a variety of geographical locations, contributes to an increase in both the speed and accuracy of diagnosis achieved through this exchange (Tareke, S. A. et al., 2022). It is possible that having timely access to diagnostic images could save lives in situations that are either urgent or complex. The rapid dissemination of information ensures that medical professionals and specialists are able to make well-informed decisions without any delays, which ultimately results in more expedient treatments and improved outcomes (Pandey, B. K. et al., 2024f). In the event of a stroke or other type of trauma, for instance, having immediate access to images is absolutely necessary in order to determine the most appropriate course of action. Sharing images also helps to reduce the number of redundant tests. Patients frequently have to undergo multiple imaging procedures, which not only wastes time and resources but also exposes them to radiation that is not necessary.

This occurs when proper sharing is not being done. The ability to easily access images once they have been captured is made possible by a sharing system that is both secure and efficient (Pandey, B. K. et al., 2024e). The sharing of biomedical images is something that is absolutely necessary for telemedicine and remote consultations. The capacity to transmit high-quality images enables patients to receive specialized care without having to travel long distances, which is especially beneficial in areas that are underserved or rural. Telehealth services are expanding. Patients all over the world will have better access to more advanced diagnostics as a result of specialists being able to examine images and lending their expertise. The final benefit of this sharing is that it improves the efficiency of medical workflows and the level of collaboration that exists between radiologists, technicians, and physicians. Through improved communication, it is possible to arrive at diagnoses more quickly and accurately, which ultimately results in higher-quality care for patients (Thomasian, N. M., & Adashi, E. Y., 2021).

IOT ARCHITECTURE IN BIO-MEDICAL IMAGE SHARING

Components of Biomedical Image Sharing

1. *Devices*: Diverse devices are essential to the biomedical image sharing process. Their functions encompass image capture, analysis, and display. Essential apparatus comprises
   i. *Imaging Equipment*: Employs magnetic fields and radio waves to generate intricate images of organs and tissues. Frequently utilized for imaging of the brain, spine, and joints. MRI is especially beneficial for assessing soft tissue, aiding in the diagnosis of conditions like tumors, neurological disorders, and joint abnormalities. Integrates numerous X-ray images to generate cross-sectional representations of bones, organs, and soft tissues. Beneficial in trauma situations and oncological diagnostics. The swift scanning capabilities of CT scanners render them indispensable in emergency scenarios, where prompt and precise evaluations are crucial. Conventional imaging apparatus that employs radiation to depict internal structures. Crucial for identifying fractures and infections. Advanced digital X-ray systems enhance image quality and minimize radiation exposure, thereby improving patient safety. Utilizes high-frequency sound waves to generate images of organs and tissues. Secure for overseeing gestations and assessing soft tissues. Moreover, ultrasound can facilitate minimally invasive procedures, such as biopsies, by offering real-time imaging of the targeted region (Pandey, B. K. et al., 2022).
   ii. *Wearable Devices*: Capable of monitoring heart rate, activity levels, and various vital signs. Certain models possess ECG characteristics for identifying arrhythmias. These devices facilitate continuous monitoring of health metrics, promoting proactive management of chronic conditions. Devices specifically engineered for the management of chronic diseases, such as continuous glucose monitors for individuals with diabetes. These monitors deliver real-time data, enabling patients and healthcare providers to make informed decisions about treatment modifications. Numerous wearable devices are now equipped with mobile applications that enable users to track their health data chronologically (Swapna, H. R. et al., 2024b). This integration can improve patient engagement and promote communication between patients and their healthcare providers.
   iii. *Workstations and Viewing Monitors*: Furnished with specialized software for image analysis, facilitating radiologists in the manipulation and interpretation of data efficiently. These workstations frequently incorporate sophisticated tools for image enhancement and comparison, thereby enhancing diagnostic

precision. Furnish precise, comprehensive visuals essential for accurate diagnosis. Monitors frequently adhere to DICOM standards to guarantee compatibility with medical imaging data. Dual-monitor configurations are prevalent, enabling radiologists to examine multiple images concurrently for thorough analysis. With the growing prevalence of telemedicine, workstations are progressively outfitted to enable remote consultations. Radiologists can disseminate their findings instantaneously to other healthcare professionals, facilitating collaborative care and prompt decision-making (Sadoughi, F. et al., 2020).

2. *Sensors*: Sensors are essential in the biomedical image-sharing ecosystem, serving a crucial function in data acquisition and transmission. Below are several fundamental categories of sensors:
   i. *Imaging Sensors*: These sensors, frequently utilized in digital imaging systems, transform light into electrical signals, thereby capturing high-resolution images. Charge-coupled devices (CCDs) are recognized for their sensitivity and image quality, rendering them appropriate for use in diagnostic imaging and research. CMOS sensors are increasingly utilized as an alternative to CCDs because of their reduced power consumption and enhanced processing speed (Swapna, H. R. et al., 2024c). They provide comparable image quality while frequently being more economical, thereby enhancing accessibility to advanced imaging technologies in healthcare (Annamalai, M., & Jesintha, D. X. M., 2021).
   ii. *Physiological Sensors*: These devices, embedded in smart apparel or accessories, incessantly track physiological metrics including heart rate, temperature, and respiration. They furnish essential data (Khan, B. et al., 2021) that can be integrated with imaging information to offer healthcare providers a comprehensive perspective of a patient's health. Handheld ultrasound probes and portable ECG monitors are engineered for application in various clinical environments. These sensors enable prompt data acquisition and dissemination, facilitating rapid decision-making in emergency and primary care contexts.
   iii. *Ecological Sensors*: These sensors assess the conditions in imaging rooms and equipment storage areas, guaranteeing that the environments are conducive to maintaining the quality of medical images and the functionality of equipment. Ensuring optimal conditions is essential for the precision of diagnostic outcomes. Crucial for assessing exposure levels in settings where imaging devices are utilized (Devasenapathy, D. et al., 2023). These sensors facilitate adherence to safety standards and regulations, safeguarding both patients and healthcare personnel from superfluous radiation exposure (Martin. R., 2015).

3. *Communication Protocols*: Efficient communication is crucial for the uninterrupted transfer of biomedical images. Diverse communication protocols enable this process:
   i. *DICOM (Digital Imaging and Communications in Medicine)*: This standard protocol guarantees interoperability among imaging devices, facilitating the sharing and storage of medical images and associated information. DICOM is essential for preserving image quality and metadata accuracy during transmission. It establishes a framework for uniform image formatting (Bhatt, D. et al., 2024), guaranteeing accessibility across various platforms and devices. DICOM accommodates a diverse array of imaging modalities and is perpetually updated to integrate emerging technologies. Its implementation enables healthcare institutions to optimize workflows and incorporate imaging data into electronic health records (EHRs), thereby improving patient management (Hester, R. J., 2020).
   ii. *HL7 (Health Level Seven)*: This collection of international standards enables the interchange of clinical and administrative data among various healthcare systems. Although not exclusively related to imaging, HL7 facilitates the integration of imaging data with other health information systems. This standardization facilitates the seamless transfer of essential patient information across departments, enhancing overall care coordination. HL7 enhances interoperability by allowing diverse healthcare applications (Abdulkarim, Yadgar I. et al., 2024) to communicate efficiently, thereby minimizing errors and augmenting data accuracy. As healthcare progresses towards more integrated systems, the significance of HL7 escalates.
   iii. *Secure Transmission Protocols*: Protocols (Pandey, B. K. et al., 2024g) such as HTTPS and SSL/TLS are crucial for guaranteeing the secure transmission of shared images across networks. These protocols safeguard sensitive patient information from unauthorized access during transmission. Implementing these secure protocols is essential, particularly as healthcare increasingly depends on remote access to images and data. Moreover, secure transmission methods are essential for complying with regulatory mandates regarding patient data protection (Pandey, B. K. et al., 2024h). Encryption during data transfer enhances security and cultivates patient trust in the healthcare system, safeguarding sensitive information from breaches. This partnership augments diagnostic precision and elevates patient care results. Modern medical systems depend on patient-to-provider data flow, especially for biomedical image sharing. Using imaging devices, wearable sensors, and health monitoring apps, patient data is collected. Patients may undergo X-rays, MRIs, or CT scans at a hospital. Advanced imaging equipment converts physical data into digital formats for analysis and sharing.

The data (Pandey, B. K., & Pandey, D., 2023) is processed and stored in a secure, centralized database called a Picture Archiving and Communication System after imaging. Authorized healthcare professionals can easily access medical images and information in PACS. The system secures images and organizes clinical imaging data. Integrating imaging data with EHR systems improves correlation with medical history, lab results, and treatment plans. The next step is sending images and data to healthcare professionals after data storage. Security protocols like DICOM (Digital Imaging and Communications in Medicine) standardize medical image transmission and ensure device and system compatibility. Radiologists and specialists can retrieve these images from their workstations or mobile devices for quick consultation and review (Pandey, B. K., & Pandey, D., 2025). Sharing and discussing images in real time helps healthcare professionals collaborate remotely. Multidisciplinary teams that must assess a patient from multiple angles should prioritize this. In emergencies like trauma, rapid imaging data (Saravanakumar, R. et al., 2024) can improve patient outcomes by enabling timely interventions and treatment decisions. Patients and healthcare professionals share images and integrate data to get a complete picture of a patient's health. This comprehensive approach improves clinical decision-making, diagnostic accuracy, and patient care. Healthcare systems can better use technology to improve efficiency and quality by streamlining data flow (Potter, L. et al., 2021).

SECURITY CHALLENGES IN IOT DEVICE

The interconnectedness of IoT devices in the healthcare industry, along with the sensitive data they manage, present a number of security challenges are as shown in Figure 1. One of the main risks is the possibility of unauthorized access to devices and networks due to inadequate authentication procedures. Data that is not sufficiently encrypted while it is in transit or at rest is more susceptible to breaches (Revathi, T. K. et al., 2022). Attackers may take advantage of device vulnerabilities like out-of-date software or unpatched security holes. Protection efforts are further complicated by the absence of standardized security protocols among various IoT devices. The growing number of devices only exacerbates these issues, so putting robust, flexible security measures in place is essential to protecting patient data.

Figure 1. Security risks in IoT devices

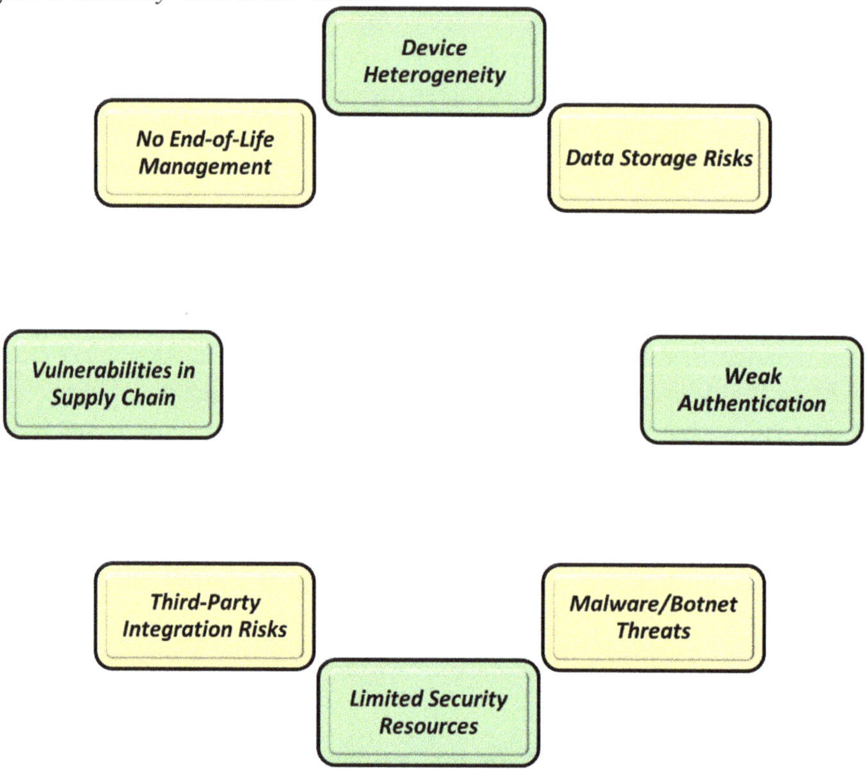

- *Device Heterogeneity*: IoT devices vary in type, manufacturer, and function. Devices may use different software and hardware architectures, making security protocols difficult to implement. Due to the sensitive data (Pandey, B. K. et al., 2023), it handles, a medical imaging device may need stricter security than a smart thermostat. Lack of uniformity makes it hard for organizations to enforce comprehensive security measures across all devices, resulting in inconsistent protection. Compatibility and security become even harder as new devices enter the market. Organizations may accidentally deploy insecure or out-of-date devices. Attackers may exploit these vulnerabilities to breach or disrupt service. To create effective security strategies for each IoT device, a cohesive approach that considers its diversity is needed.
- *Data Storage Risks*: Data stored locally or in cloud environments by IoT devices may not be secure. Hackers may target devices that collect and analyze sensitive personal data if their storage systems are not secure. Data breaches can lead to identity theft, fraud, and other crimes. Cloud storage risks are

increased by cloud service provider infrastructure vulnerabilities. Data on the provider's servers may be at risk if they don't implement strong security controls or comply with regulations. IoT data must be encrypted in transit and at rest, and organizations must implement strict access controls to limit who can view or manipulate it (Palmer, X. et al., 2021).

- *Weak Authentication*: Static passwords or no authentication are used by many IoT devices. Brute-force and social engineering attacks can easily exploit these weak mechanisms. An attacker can quickly gain access and remotely control a device with a widely known factory-set password. In environments where devices handle sensitive data, this weak authentication is dangerous. Managing multiple devices complicates authentication. Many users forget their passwords, so they reuse them across devices and services. One device breach can compromise others, making this behavior risky (Maheshwari, R. Uma. et al., 2024). To restrict IoT device access to authorized users, manufacturers should use multi-factor authentication, biometric verification, or device-specific credentials.
- *Malware/Botnet Threats*: Co-opting compromised IoT devices into botnets, which launch DDoS attacks, is easy. Using vulnerabilities, attackers can turn these devices into malicious agents without the owner's knowledge. High-profile DDoS attacks used large networks of compromised IoT devices to overwhelm targeted servers, disrupting services. These autonomous devices can launch attacks on command, making them dangerous. More connected IoT devices increase the potential for widespread impact. A single vulnerable device can let attackers into larger networks. Once inside, they can access sensitive data or launch more attacks. To prevent botnets, organizations must use regular software updates, intrusion detection systems, and anomaly detection technologies that can detect malware.
- *Limited Security Resources*: Many IoT devices, especially consumer ones, lack resources for comprehensive security. Complex security features are often not supported by devices because manufacturers prioritize cost and energy efficiency. Low-power sensors may not be able to run advanced encryption algorithms, making them more vulnerable to attacks. This resource shortage can damage devices and networks. Even basic security practices like updates and patch management may be impossible on these devices. Thus, manufacturers may make vulnerable devices throughout their lifespan. To address these issues, manufacturers should design devices with security in mind, balancing functionality with manageable security measures that don't overtax the device (Amiri, Shekarchizadeh, Esfahani, & Masoud, 2021).
- *Third-Party Integration Risks*: Integration of third-party apps and services with IoT devices can increase security risks. Third-party components can

compromise the IoT ecosystem if they lack security. Insecure third-party apps that interact with smart home devices could give attackers access to the home network. Assessing third-party integration security is crucial as organizations increasingly use them for enhanced functionality. Third-party services can also cause data sharing and compliance issues. If third-party apps mishandle data or violate GDPR or HIPAA, the organization may be liable for privacy breaches. Third-party vendors should be thoroughly vetted to ensure they meet the same security standards as their own systems to reduce these risks.

- *Vulnerabilities in Supply Chain*: The IoT supply chain is complex, introducing security vulnerabilities from manufacturing to deployment. Each supply chain vendor may have different security practices, causing inconsistencies and potential issues. An IoT device's component from a supplier with poor security could be a gateway for attackers. Maintaining IoT ecosystem integrity requires vendors to follow strong security standards. Lack of supply chain transparency can also hinder risk identification and mitigation. Organizations may not know their suppliers' security practices, making vulnerability assessments difficult. Implement strict vendor assessment processes that require suppliers to comply with security standards and regularly audit their security practices to address these issues.
- *No End-of-Life Management*: After their lifespan, IoT devices must be properly decommissioned to prevent unauthorized access to residual data. Lack of this crucial step leads to data leaks or unauthorized access to sensitive information in many organizations. A device that is disposed of without properly erasing its data could be recovered by malicious actors, resulting in serious privacy breaches. A clear end-of-life management plan is needed to securely wipe devices' data before retirement. Without a systematic decommissioning approach, outdated devices may not receive security updates. Legacy devices are more vulnerable to attacks, making them security risks. Organizations must create policies to properly decommission and mitigate security risks for their IoT devices.

SECURITY REQUIREMENTS FOR BIO-MEDICAL IMAGE SHARING

Patient Data Privacy Through Confidentiality

Confidentiality is essential in the healthcare sector, especially regarding the safeguarding of patient information. As healthcare practitioners increasingly depend on digital technologies for the storage and dissemination of sensitive information

(Kumarganesh, S. et al., 2024), the protection of patient privacy has become more complex yet imperative. Maintaining confidentiality necessitates the implementation of stringent measures to safeguard personal health information (PHI) against unauthorized access, breaches, or disclosures. Data encryption is one of the most effective methods for preserving confidentiality (Basha, A. J. et al., 2024). Data encryption guarantees that, even if intercepted or accessed without permission, it remains incomprehensible without the correct decryption key (Lakshmi, K. V. N. et al., 2024). This method is essential for transmitting medical data over networks or cloud services, where the likelihood of interception is elevated. Healthcare organizations must implement access controls to guarantee that only authorized individuals can view or alter patient data. Role-based access control (RBAC) systems can restrict access according to job responsibilities, thereby augmenting data security (Rai, P. K. et al., 2024). Consistent training and awareness initiatives for healthcare personnel are essential for upholding confidentiality. Employees must be informed about the significance of data privacy, potential threats like phishing attacks, and optimal practices for protecting patient information. Fostering a culture of security awareness promotes vigilance among employees, aiding in the prevention of inadvertent breaches. Organizations must routinely perform audits and evaluations to ensure adherence to these regulations, identifying and rectifying vulnerabilities in their data protection practices (Sahani, S. K. et al., 2024a). Healthcare providers can enhance patient trust and safeguard sensitive medical information by emphasizing confidentiality through technological solutions, employee education, and adherence to regulations.

Reliable Access for Authorized Users

Availability is a crucial element of healthcare data management, guaranteeing that authorized users can consistently access patient information as required. In a medical context, prompt access to data can profoundly influence patient outcomes, necessitating that healthcare providers uphold elevated levels of system availability (Kennedy, G. W. et al., 2024). Continuous access to medical records, diagnostic instruments, and treatment protocols allows healthcare professionals to make prompt, informed decisions, thereby improving the quality of care. Healthcare organizations must establish resilient infrastructure and redundancy protocols to guarantee availability. This entails employing redundant servers and backup systems to avert downtime resulting from hardware malfunctions or system overloads. Cloud-based solutions can improve availability by offering scalable resources and load balancing, which ensures that systems can accommodate fluctuating demands while remaining operational (Sahani, K. et al., 2024b). Consistent maintenance and updates are essential to guarantee that systems operate efficiently and securely, thereby reducing the likelihood of outages. Disaster recovery plans are essential for ensuring availability. Organizations must develop thorough strategies for data backup and recovery to guarantee the rapid restoration of critical information in the event of a cyber-attack, natural disaster, or hardware failure. Regularly testing these recovery plans enables organizations to pinpoint vulnerabilities and enhance their response strategies, thereby ensuring minimal service disruption. Implementing access control measures is crucial to avert unauthorized access that may jeopardize availability. Denial-of-service (DoS) attacks can inundate systems and obstruct access for authorized users. Consequently, the implementation of security protocols, including firewalls and intrusion detection systems, can alleviate these threats while guaranteeing that authorized personnel can access the necessary data at critical times.

Authentication and Authorization

Basic elements of protecting access to private patient information in healthcare settings are authentication and authorization (Kumar Pandey, B. et al., 2021). By combining these procedures, patients' privacy is safeguarded and data integrity is upheld, as only authorized individuals are able to view, alter, or share sensitive information. Verifying a user's identity when they try to access a system is called authentication. Something the user knows (like a password), something they have (like a smart card or security token), or something they are (like biometric data like fingerprints or facial recognition) are usually involved in this. In order to add an extra degree of security and make sure that unauthorized users cannot simply obtain access, multi-factor authentication, or MFA, is becoming more and more advised in the healthcare industry. For example, an employer in the healthcare industry might ask employees i9n workplace (Saxena, A. et al., 2021) to use a password to log in and then use a biometric scan to confirm who they are. The probability of illegal access brought about by phishing or stolen credentials is greatly decreased by using this method. Another way to improve security is to encourage staff to create strong, one-of-a-kind passwords and to update authentication procedures on a frequent basis. What an authenticated user is permitted to do within the system is determined by authorization, on the other hand. Only information pertinent to their roles is accessible to users thanks to this procedure. Users in the healthcare industry are frequently granted permissions according to their job functions through a technique called role-based access control, or RBAC. For instance, whereas administrative staff may only have access to billing data, nurses may have access to patient charts and medication records. By restricting access to sensitive information based on need-to-know principles, strict authorization protocols are implemented to help reduce the risk of data breaches. To guarantee adherence to these guidelines and to modify access privileges when staff members depart or take on new responsibilities, regular audits of access permissions are crucial. Ensuring the security of patient data in healthcare settings requires strong authentication and authorization protocols. Healthcare institutions can greatly lower the risk of unauthorized access and guarantee the confidentiality and integrity of sensitive patient information by implementing robust identity verification procedures and enforcing stringent access controls.

EMERGING SECURITY SOLUTIONS

Blockchain for Secure and Decentralized Data Sharing

Blockchain technology presents a viable solution for secure and decentralized data sharing, especially within the healthcare sector. Utilizing its fundamental attributes, including transparency, immutability, and decentralization, blockchain can resolve numerous issues related to conventional data sharing techniques, such as data breaches, interoperability deficiencies, and the requirement for patient consent. A key advantage of blockchain is its capacity to establish an immutable record of transactions. Every data element transmitted on the blockchain is encrypted and connected to the preceding block, creating a chain that is impervious to modifications. This immutability guarantees that once data is recorded, it cannot be altered or erased without the agreement of the network participants. This feature can improve the integrity of patient records in healthcare, mitigating the risk of fraud and ensuring that all stakeholders access accurate and current information. Blockchain facilitates secure and transparent data sharing among various parties without requiring a central authority.

This decentralized method alleviates the risks linked to data silos, wherein information is confined to isolated systems that are challenging to access and disseminate. Blockchain enables secure collaboration and data sharing among healthcare providers, patients, and researchers, facilitating enhanced care coordination, improved patient outcomes, and more efficient clinical trials. Smart contracts self-executing agreements encoded on the blockchain can enhance data sharing processes by automating tasks like consent management and data access permissions. Blockchain technology also enhances patient privacy and control. Patients may maintain ownership of their health data and possess the capacity to grant or revoke access to designated parties as required. This control not only empowers patients but also complies with regulatory mandates, such as HIPAA, which underscore the significance of patient consent in the management of personal health information.

AI and Machine Learning for Anomaly Detection

A number of industries, including healthcare, finance, and cybersecurity, are undergoing significant transformations as a result of the implementation of sophisticated algorithms for anomaly detection. During this process, patterns that significantly deviate from expected behavior are identified. These patterns can be indicative of critical issues such as fraud, network intrusions, or medical emergencies. The ability of organizations to detect these irregularities in a timely and accurate manner can be improved through the utilization of sophisticated techniques. Using these algorithms for anomaly detection allows for the analysis of massive amounts of data in real time, which is one of the most significant advantages of working with these algorithms. When applied in dynamic environments, where patterns are constantly evolving, traditional methods frequently rely on predefined rules and thresholds, which can be ineffective. On the other hand, contemporary methods are able to acquire knowledge from past events and modify their detection models in order to identify new irregularities through the absence of human intervention. As an illustration, models can be utilized in the field of healthcare to analyze patient information in order to recognize unusual patterns that may be indicative of deteriorating health conditions, thereby enabling timely interventions.

These cutting-edge methods have the potential to significantly cut down on false positives, which is a very common problem in anomaly detection. Conventional systems have the potential to identify insignificant variations as anomalies, which can result in unneeded alerts and the allocation of resources. More advanced algorithms are able to differentiate between normal and abnormal behavior with greater accuracy, which leads to increased precision and a reduction in the number of false alarms. It is especially useful in high-stakes environments, such as financial transactions, where accurate anomaly detection can prevent significant losses due to fraud. This capability is particularly valuable in these kinds of environments. Among the many significant applications of these methods in anomaly detection, predictive analytics is another important application. A combination of anomaly detection and predictive modeling allows organizations to identify current irregularities and anticipate potential future issues based on historical trends. This allows organizations to better manage their operations. Specifically, in the realm of network security, models have the capability to identify abnormal traffic patterns that may be indicative of a breach. These models can also predict future attack vectors based on these patterns, which enables proactive measures to be taken to strengthen defences.

Zero Trust Architecture for IoT Networks

IoT network security is becoming increasingly dependent on Zero Trust Architecture (ZTA), which emphasizes "never trust, always verify." Traditional perimeter-based security models no longer work in a world where devices are interconnected and threats can come from inside and outside. ZTA protects sensitive IoT data by moving from centralized security perimeters to user and device-centric ones. Zero Trust requires continuous network access verification of all users and devices. This requires strict authentication and authorization to restrict resource access to legitimate users and devices. Identity and access management solutions that use MFA and device-specific certificates to verify connections are needed for IoT networks. Organizations can reduce device and credential risks by rigorously verifying identities. In addition to verification, ZTA emphasizes least privilege, giving users and devices only the permissions they need.

This reduces attack surfaces and breach impact. In a smart healthcare environment, a wearable device that monitors patient vitals may only access relevant medical data, preventing it from interfering with other critical systems. This improves security and simplifies management by monitoring and controlling device access. Zero Trust Architecture also requires network segmentation. Companies can prevent breaches and limit lateral threat movement by dividing the network into smaller segments. IoT networks can segment devices by function or risk. Critical medical devices can be separated from general-purpose IoT devices to limit the organization's impact if one segment is compromised. Monitoring and analytics are crucial to Zero Trust Architecture. Organisations can detect security threats by continuously monitoring user and device behaviour. Analyzing access and usage patterns helps organizations set baselines for normal behavior and identify and address deviations. This proactive security approach protects organizations from evolving cyber threats.

CONCLUSION

Safeguarding the security of IoT devices in biomedical image sharing is crucial for protecting sensitive patient data and preserving trust in healthcare systems. Primary security priorities encompass the implementation of robust authentication and authorization protocols to regulate access to sensitive information, the application of encryption to protect data both in transit and at rest, and the deployment of sophisticated anomaly detection methods to proactively identify potential security threats. Furthermore, implementing a Zero Trust Architecture can strengthen security measures by authenticating every user and device seeking network access, consequently diminishing the likelihood of unauthorized entry and data breaches. As technology advances, future strategies for improving security in medical IoT systems must concentrate on several essential domains. The establishment of standardized security protocols and frameworks is essential for ensuring interoperability among various devices and systems. This will enhance collaboration among healthcare providers, manufacturers, and regulatory agencies to establish uniform security protocols. The incorporation of artificial intelligence and machine learning into security protocols will facilitate enhanced threat detection and response capabilities. These technologies facilitate the real-time identification of emerging threats, enabling organizations to swiftly adapt to new vulnerabilities and effectively mitigate risks. Cultivating a culture of security awareness among healthcare professionals is essential. Continuous training initiatives that underscore the significance of data privacy and security best practices will enable personnel to identify and address potential threats, thereby augmenting the overall security of medical IoT systems. By prioritizing these security measures and adopting innovative technologies, healthcare organizations can markedly enhance the safety and reliability of biomedical image sharing, ensuring the protection of patient information in an increasingly interconnected environment.

REFERENCES

Abdulkarim, Y. I., Awl, H. N., Muhammadsharif, F. F., Saeed, S. R., Sidiq, K. R., Khasraw, S. S., Dong, J., Pandey, B. K., & Pandey, D. (2024). Metamaterial-based sensors loaded corona-shaped resonator for COVID-19 detection by using microwave techniques. *Plasmonics*, *19*(2), 595–610. DOI: 10.1007/s11468-023-02007-4

Annamalai, M., & Jesintha, D. X. M. (2021). Smart iot system based patient monitoring and medicine reminder based on registry service selection scheme. *European Journal of Molecular and Clinical Medicine*, *7*, 2710–2721.

Basha, A. J., Maheshwari, R. U., Pandey, B. K., & Pandey, D. (2024). Ultra-Sensitive Photonic Crystal Fiber–Based SPR Sensor for Cancer Detection Utilizing Hybrid Nanocomposite Layers. *Plasmonics*, •••, 1–15. DOI: 10.1007/s11468-024-02584-y

Bhatt, D., Swapna, H. R., Madaan, G., Gayathri, D. K., Mahajan, D. A., Mahajan, R. D., & Paramashivan, M. A. (2024). From Theory to Practice: The Evolution of Artificial Intelligence in Business. In Utilization of AI Technology in Supply Chain Management (pp. 1-14). IGI Global.

Devasenapathy, D., Madhumathy, P., Umamaheshwari, R., Pandey, B. K., & Pandey, D. (2023). Transmission-efficient grid-based synchronized model for routing in wireless sensor networks using Bayesian compressive sensing. *SN Computer Science*, *5*(1), 128. DOI: 10.1007/s42979-023-02410-y

Dhanasekar, S., Martin Sagayam, K., Pandey, B. K., & Pandey, D. (2023). Refractive index sensing using metamaterial absorbing augmentation in elliptical graphene arrays. *Plasmonics*, •••, 1–11.

Du John, H. V., Jose, T., Jone, A. A. A., Sagayam, K. M., Pandey, B. K., & Pandey, D. (2022). Polarization insensitive circular ring resonator based perfect metamaterial absorber design and simulation on a silicon substrate. *Silicon*, *14*(14), 9009–9020. DOI: 10.1007/s12633-021-01645-9

Hester, R. J. (2020). Bioveillance: A techno-security infrastructure to preempt the dangers of informationalised biology. *Science as Culture*, *29*(1), 153–176. DOI: 10.1080/09505431.2019.1705270

Kennedy, G. W., Sunday, S. E., Pandey, D., Kabari, A. D., Pandey, B. K., George, A. S., & Dadheech, P. (2024). Building Information Modeling: Harnessing Innovations for Professional Proficiency. In *Emerging Engineering Technologies and Industrial Applications* (pp. 305-331). IGI Global.

Khan, B., Hasan, A., Pandey, D., Ventayen, R. J. M., Pandey, B. K., & Gowwrii, G. (2021). Fusion of datamining and artificial intelligence in prediction of hazardous road accidents. In *Machine learning and iot for intelligent systems and smart applications* (pp. 201–223). CRC Press. DOI: 10.1201/9781003194415-12

Kumar Pandey, B., Pandey, D., Nassa, V. K., Ahmad, T., Singh, C., George, A. S., & Wakchaure, M. A. (2021). Encryption and steganography-based text extraction in IoT using the EWCTS optimizer. *Imaging Science Journal*, *69*(1-4), 38–56. DOI: 10.1080/13682199.2022.2146885

Kumarganesh, S., & Malathi Murugesan, C. (2024). Hybrid Plasmonic Biosensors with Deep Learning for Colorectal Cancer Detection. *Plasmonics*, •••, 1–15. DOI: 10.1007/s11468-024-02568-y

Lakshmi, K. V. N., Rajan, R., Pandey, D., & Pandey, B. K. (2024). Circular Economy: A Catalyst for Economic Growth-An Empirical Study. *Circular Economy and Sustainability*, •••, 1–22.

Maheshwari, R., Kumarganesh, S., K v M, S., Gopalakrishnan, A., Selvi, K., Paulchamy, B., Rishabavarthani, P., Sagayam, K. M., Pandey, B. K., & Pandey, D. (2024). Advanced plasmonic resonance-enhanced biosensor for comprehensive real-time detection and analysis of deepfake content. *Plasmonics*, •••, 1–18. DOI: 10.1007/s11468-024-02407-0

Martin, R. (2015). The internet of things (iot)–removing the human element. *Infosec Writers*, *28*, 12.

Palmer, X., Potter, L. N., & Karahan, S. (2021). COVID-19 and biocybersecurity's increasing role on defending forward. [IJCWT]. *International Journal of Cyber Warfare & Terrorism*, *11*(3), 15–29. DOI: 10.4018/IJCWT.2021070102

Pandey, B. K., Mukundan, A. P., Nassa, V. K., Pandey, D., George, A. S., Hameed, A. S., & Dadheech, P. (2024f). Deployment of Load Balancing in Cloud Computing: Industrial Application and Benefits. In Emerging Engineering Technologies and Industrial Applications (pp. 342-354). IGI Global.

Pandey, B. K., Nassa, V. K., Mukundan, A. P., Mahajan, D. A., Pandey, D., George, A. S., & Dadheech, P. (2024d). An Industry-Focused Traffic System Utilising Internet of Things. In *Emerging Engineering Technologies and Industrial Applications* (pp. 200–213). IGI Global. DOI: 10.4018/979-8-3693-1335-0.ch009

Pandey, B. K., & Pandey, D. (2023). Parametric optimization and prediction of enhanced thermoelectric performance in co-doped CaMnO3 using response surface methodology and neural network. *Journal of Materials Science Materials in Electronics*, *34*(21), 1589. DOI: 10.1007/s10854-023-10954-1

Pandey, B. K., & Pandey, D. (2025). Securing healthcare medical image information using advance morphological component analysis, information hiding systems, and hybrid convolutional neural networks on IoMT. *Computers in Biology and Medicine*, *185*, 109499. DOI: 10.1016/j.compbiomed.2024.109499 PMID: 39642698

Pandey, B. K., Pandey, D., & Agarwal, A. (2022). Encrypted information transmission by enhanced steganography and image transformation. [IJDAI]. *International Journal of Distributed Artificial Intelligence*, *14*(1), 1–14. DOI: 10.4018/IJDAI.297110

Pandey, B. K., Pandey, D., Dadheech, P., Mahajan, D. A., George, A. S., & Hameed, A. S. (2023). Review on Smart Sewage Cleaning UAV Assistance for Sustainable Development. In *Handbook of Research on Safe Disposal Methods of Municipal Solid Wastes for a Sustainable Environment* (pp. 69–79). IGI Global. DOI: 10.4018/978-1-6684-8117-2.ch005

Pandey, B. K., Paramashivan, M. A., Hasan, A., Pramanik, S., Dadheech, P., Manaktala, S. S., & George, A. S. (2024a). Social Psychological Obstacles to the Implementation of Artificial Intelligence in Supply Chain Management. In AI and Machine Learning Impacts in Intelligent Supply Chain (pp. 17-24). IGI Global. DOI: 10.4018/979-8-3693-1347-3.ch002

Pandey, B. K., Paramashivan, M. A., Kanike, U. K., Mahajan, D. A., Mahajan, R., George, A. S., & Hameed, A. S. H. (2024b). Impacts of Artificial Intelligence and Machine Learning on Intelligent Supply Chains. In *AI and Machine Learning Impacts in Intelligent Supply Chain* (pp. 57–73). IGI Global. DOI: 10.4018/979-8-3693-1347-3.ch005

Pandey, B. K., Paramashivan, M. A., Mahajan, R., Mahajan, D. A., Behare, N., Gowwrii, G., & Pramanik, S. (2024c). Applications of Artificial Intelligence and Machine Learning in Supply Chain Management: An In-Depth Investigation. In *AI and Machine Learning Impacts in Intelligent Supply Chain* (pp. 74–90). IGI Global. DOI: 10.4018/979-8-3693-1347-3.ch006

Pandey, B. K., Paramashivan, M. A., Nassa, V. K., Mahajan, D. A., Dadheech, P., George, A. H., & George, A. S. (2024h). Blockchain's Potential Effect on the Healthcare Industry. In Emerging Engineering Technologies and Industrial Applications (pp. 214-232). IGI Global. DOI: 10.4018/979-8-3693-1335-0.ch010

. Pandey, B. K., Paramashivan, M. A., Pandey, D., George, A. S., Agarwal, A., Dadheech, P., & Mahajan, D. A. (2024g). A Recent Survey on 6G Vehicular Technology: Applications and Challenges. 6G Security Education and Multidisciplinary Implementation, 337-350.

Pandey, B. K., Paramashivan, M. A., Pandey, D., George, A. S., Agarwal, A., Mahajan, D. A., . . . Pramanik, S. (2024e). Future Directions of Digital Twin Architectures for 6G Communication Networks. In Security Issues and Solutions in 6G Communications and Beyond (pp. 197-211). IGI Global.

Pandey, D., Pandey, B. K., Paramashivan, M. A., Mahajan, D. A., Dadheech, P. D., George, A. S., & Hameed, A. S. (2024). Advanced Digital Data Processing Using Cloud Cryptography: Industrial Applications. In Emerging Engineering Technologies and Industrial Applications (pp. 255-268). IGI Global.

Potter, L., Ayala, O., & Palmer, X. L. (2021, February). Biocybersecurity: A converging threat as an auxiliary to war. In *ICCWS 2021 16th international conference on cyber warfare and security* (p. 291).

Rai, P. K., Pandey, D., & Pandey, B. K. (2024). The future of enterprise and innovation is compute as a commodity, or CaaC. *Partners Universal International Research Journal*, *3*(2), 89–94.

Revathi, T. K., Sathiyabhama, B., Sankar, S., Pandey, D., Pandey, B. K., & Dadeech, P. (2022). An intelligent model for coronary heart disease diagnosis. In *Networking Technologies in Smart Healthcare* (pp. 309–327). CRC Press. DOI: 10.1201/9781003239888-15

Sadoughi, F., Behmanesh, A., & Sayfouri, N. (2020). Internet of things in medicine: A systematic mapping study. *Journal of Biomedical Informatics*, *103*, 103383. DOI: 10.1016/j.jbi.2020.103383 PMID: 32044417

Sahani, K., Khadka, S. S., Sahani, S. K., Pandey, B. K., & Pandey, D. (2024b). A possible underground roadway for transportation facilities in Kathmandu Valley: A racking deformation of underground rectangular structures. *Engineering Reports*, *6*(8), e12821. DOI: 10.1002/eng2.12821

Sahani, S. K., Pandey, B. K., & Pandey, D. (2024a). *Single-valued Signals, Multi-valued Signals and Fixed-Point of Contractive Signals*. Mathematics Open. DOI: 10.1142/S2811007224500020

Saravanakumar, R., TamilSelvi, T., Pandey, D., Pandey, B. K., Mahajan, D. A., & Lelisho, M. E. (2024). Big data processing using hybrid Gaussian mixture model with salp swarm algorithm. *Journal of Big Data*, *11*(1), 1–29. DOI: 10.1186/s40537-024-01015-3

Saxena, A., Sharma, N. K., Pandey, D., & Pandey, B. K. (2021). Influence of tourists satisfaction on future behavioral intentions with special reference to desert triangle of Rajasthan. *Augmented Human Research*, *6*(1), 13. DOI: 10.1007/s41133-021-00052-4

Shahul, A., Muniandi, B., Paramashivan, M. A., Pandey, D., Pandey, B. K., Dadheech, P., & George, H. (2024). An Analysis of Algorithms and Methods Based on Image Processing for Medical Applications. In *Emerging Engineering Technologies and Industrial Applications* (pp. 173–186). IGI Global. DOI: 10.4018/979-8-3693-1335-0.ch007

Swapna, H. R., Bigirimana, E., Geetha, R., Paramashivan, M. A., George, A. S., Dadheech, P., & Vyas, V. (2024c). New Insights Into Strategic Consumer Behavior From the Field of Operations Management. In Utilization of AI Technology in Supply Chain Management (pp. 289-298). IGI Global. DOI: 10.4018/979-8-3693-3593-2.ch019

Swapna, H. R., Geetanjali, S., Lakshmi, K. V. N., Paramashivan, M. A., Nikhil, M. S., Dadheech, P., & Vyas, V. (2024b). Navigating the Transformative Journey: AI's Progression in Business Applications. In Utilization of AI Technology in Supply Chain Management (pp. 15-25). IGI Global.

Swapna, H. R., Hukkeri, S. V., Pandey, D., & Paramashivan, M. A. (2024a). Cosmopolitan living during the COVID-19 Era: Navigating Challenges and Uniting Communities-An Impact Analysis. In Impact of Climate Change on Mental Health and Well-Being (pp. 1-10). IGI Global.

Tareke, S. A., Lelisho, M. E., Hassen, S. S., Seid, A. A., Jemal, S. S., Teshale, B. M., & Pandey, B. K. (2022). The prevalence and predictors of depressive, anxiety, and stress symptoms among Tepi town residents during the COVID-19 pandemic lockdown in Ethiopia. *Journal of Racial and Ethnic Health Disparities*, •••, 1–13. PMID: 35028903

Thomasian, N. M., & Adashi, E. Y. (2021). Cybersecurity in the internet of medical things. *Health Policy and Technology*, *10*(3), 100549. DOI: 10.1016/j.hlpt.2021.100549

Chapter 13
Quantum Cryptography for Biomedical Image Security in Next-Generation Telemedicine Networks

L. B. Muralidhar
https://orcid.org/0000-0003-3453-613X
Jain University, India

H. R. Swapna
https://orcid.org/0000-0003-0362-409X
Jain University, India

N. Sathyanarayana
https://orcid.org/0000-0002-4185-7751
Jain University, India

K. Nethravathi
https://orcid.org/0000-0003-4138-0276
Jain University, India

Varanasi Rahul
https://orcid.org/0000-0003-2407-7654
Jain University, India

Digvijay Pandey
https://orcid.org/0000-0003-0353-174X
Department of Technical Education, Government of Uttar Pradesh, India

Pankaj Dadheech
https://orcid.org/0000-0001-5783-1989
Swami Keshvanand Institute of Technology, Management, and Gramothan, India

ABSTRACT

Next-generation telemedicine networks transform healthcare delivery by enabling real-time diagnostics, monitoring, and treatment. However, they face significant cybersecurity challenges, especially in safeguarding sensitive biomedical images. Traditional cryptographic techniques are vulnerable to emerging quantum computing threats, necessitating advanced solutions. Quantum cryptography, leveraging prin-

DOI: 10.4018/979-8-3693-9821-0.ch013

ciples like Quantum Key Distribution (QKD), offers unparalleled security through physical law-based encryption. This chapter explores the integration of quantum cryptography in telemedicine, addressing implementation challenges such as cost, scalability, and infrastructure compatibility. It highlights emerging protocols, like MDI-QKD, and their role in securing biomedical data in applications such as remote surgeries and teleradiology.

INTRODUCTION

Next-generation telemedicine networks epitomise technological innovation in the quest for improved healthcare delivery through enhanced communication systems. These networks are part of the digitisation of healthcare, enabling real-time remote diagnostics, monitoring, and treatment delivery, especially in resource-constrained areas (Sun et al., 2023). An essential aspect of such systems is biomedical image security since the data of patients transmitted over telemedicine networks contains sensitive and confidential information(Kshetri, 2021; Madaan, G., Swapna, H. R., Kumar, A., Singh, A., & David, A., 2021). Considering that these data transmissions have increased in the face of rising cyber threats against health systems worldwide, this chapter reviews the multidimensional dimensions of telemedicine networks, focusing on biomedical image security using theoretical frameworks, comparative perspectives, and the emerging role of quantum cryptography in secure communications.

PROBLEM STATEMENT

In the pace of rapid digital transformation concerning healthcare, telemedicine network architectures have become crucial in both diagnosis and treatment conducted distantly, patient data management, etc.; however, these networks are vulnerable to biomedical image security and protected patient information against rising concerns of cybersecurity threats due to ever-evolving data breaches, ransomware, unauthorised assess, among others. Additionally, conventional cryptographic methods do not have much power to confront the new quantum computers' powers(Pandey, B. K., & Pandey, D., 2025). Quantum cryptography provided some revolutionary solutions to these, including QKD and a variety of other higher-order protocols. On a more macro level, costs, scalability, and possible integrations with existing infrastructure provide barriers to widespread adoption. Resolving these issues is important in ensuring patient privacy and regulatory compliance and opening up global innovation within this sector. The study is conducted to determine how far quantum cryptography would go to meet these challenges, the feasibility of the solution, accessibility, and the ethical plausibility in differing healthcare settings.

OBJECTIVES

1. To evaluate the role of quantum cryptography in enhancing biomedical data security.
2. To examine the feasibility and scalability of quantum cryptographic systems in telemedicine.
3. To propose a strategic roadmap for integrating quantum cryptography into global telemedicine networks

BACKGROUND

Telemedicine networks constantly evolve based on communication and health informatics frameworks like the Technology Acceptance Model, Shannon's Information Theory, and systems theory. Based on TAM, technology adoption by health professionals is predicated upon perceived usefulness and ease of use (Davis, 1989). Shannon's Information Theory states that encryption must be robust so data is not compromised upon transmission, breaching confidentiality (Shannon, 1948). Systems theory considers telemedicine interdependently related entities that must be seamlessly integrated (Von Bertalanffy, 1968). Security frameworks, like the CIA Triad, are fundamental: Confidentiality, Integrity, and Availability(Whitman &Mattord, 2018). Even with regulations like the GDPR, cyberattacks are increasing very fast, including biomedical data(European Commission, 2018).

Consequently, emerging paradigms like ZTA prefer a policy of distrusting internal and external subjects internally, which will be essential in telemedicine networks across organisational boundaries. Additionally, blockchain-based security models introduce data transparency and extra security(Bikis, A. et al.,2025). This has seen workable implementations in Estonia's eHealth system (Zhang et al., 2021). Quantum cryptography enhances security to an advanced level using the process of QKD by sending quantum states to establish tamper-evident keys in QKD (Bennett & Brassard, 1984). Examples of QKD, like the Micius satellite in China, demonstrate a part of its potential, even as high cost and infrastructural needs will limit scalability(Pan et al., 2018).

Critics of quantum cryptography also point out that it is still in its infancy, with ethical considerations regarding unequal access and resource requirements, especially for resource-poor countries(UNESCO, 2022). Blockchain is scalable and cost-effective; however, it does not have the security at a quantum level that QKD does. Hence, vulnerabilities exist(Kumar et al., 2021). Many governments have taken the initiative on telemedicine security through various legislation, such as the U.S. Cybersecurity Act of 2015 and the National Digital Health Mission of India(Government of India, 2020). At the international level, for example, the WHO supports standard cyber security practices and promises support to low- and middle-income countries (ITU, 2023).

Integration of solid security, like multi-factor authentication, encryption, and audits, builds trust with patients, ensures regulatory compliance, and secures financials. Hybrid security mechanisms, such as quantum combined with traditional methods(Sheela, M. S. et al., 2025)

, can effectively deal with various threats. Their practical applications are represented, for example, by such projects as the EU-funded Quantum Internet Alliance and quantum-secured telemedicine platforms of Japan(Yamamoto et al., 2022).

Data breaches still occur. 73% of health organisations experience breaches, while 41% are due to weak encryption(PwC, 2021). The Global Health Security Index also reports that only 10% of countries have strong health cybersecurity(Johns Hopkins University, 2022). This, therefore, means that new innovative security measures in telemedicine networks should be urgently investigated.

Challenges and developments presented in the current section, such as emerging threats to biomedical data security, government initiatives, and innovative strategies, set a foundation for exploring transformative technologies like quantum cryptography(Satheesh, N. et al., 2025). Traditional methods include blockchain and zero-trust architectures, but these are interim solutions, lacking the future-proof security assurances required to handle the vulnerabilities presented by quantum computing advancements (Singh, S., Madaan, G., et.al., 2023). The following section provides an accurate basic overview of quantum cryptography, focusing on its theoretical background, protocols, and uses worldwide. The potential to revolutionise data security: The following section can provide the bridge between addressing cybersecurity challenges and describing the next-generation solutions for the telemedicine network.

FUNDAMENTALS OF QUANTUM CRYPTOGRAPHY

Quantum cryptography is supposed to be a new twist in securing these communication facilities using the principles of quantum mechanics, guaranteeing fundamentally higher security levels than classical cryptography. Technically, there has been key distribution for cryptographic purposes where characteristics of quantum superposition have been used along with its entangled twin to block any access to the vital communication stream(Kumar, M. S. et al., 2025). Analysing and reviewing studies on a multifaceted conceptual framework and different theoretical stances surrounding quantum cryptography, together with the implementation challenges it proposes and actual uses, underline global perspectives with policies on the subject matter with evidence from direct data.

Quantum cryptography sets a whole new basis for quantum mechanics in ensuring information against eavesdropping is secure. Quantum cryptography differs from the usual classical cryptography, in which complex mathematics algorithms are applied. Instead, this cryptography applies the rules of quantum physics to develop the Heisenberg Uncertainty Principle and the No-Cloning Theorem(Konapure, C. G. et al., 2025). These rules make any attempt to intercept the quantum state of particles disturb it, thus alerting the legitimate parties. A forerunner of this idea of cryptography mixed with quantum mechanics first came about in the 1970s but then became in various protocols like BB84 (Bennett & Brassard in 1984).

Principles of Quantum Key Distribution (QKD)

QKD represents one of the first practical applications of quantum cryptography, allowing secure key exchange by transmitting quantum bits over a channel. In the BB84 protocol, the polarisation of photons is used to represent a binary state and their measurements in random bases. Any eavesdropping would alter the qubits' quantum state, producing detectable errors and security(Singh, S. et al., 2025a). Another well-known protocol is E91, based on quantum entanglement proposed by Ekert in 1991, in which the measurement of one particle instantly defines the state of its entangled partner. These protocols represent the shift from computational security to physical security.

Advantages of Quantum Cryptography Over Classical Cryptography

The chief merit of quantum cryptography lies in its resistance to the development of computational power, which covers, among other things, even quantum computers. However, classical encryption, depending on the problem of factorisation of integers or discrete logarithms, will face a real possibility of becoming obsolete with the becoming of quantum computers with Shor's Algorithm. Contrarily, dependence on physical laws means robustness for quantum cryptography(Singh, S. et al., 2025b). Besides this, quantum systems offer unprecedented data integrity and authentication, as is evident from large-scale trials like the Chinese Micius satellite project (Yin et al., 2020). Additionally, quantum cryptography does not require trusted third-party nodes, strengthening the decentralised communication frameworks(Pandey, B. K. et al., 2024a).

So far, two fundamental models have been proposed in quantum cryptography: the BB84 and E91 protocols. While BB84 uses single-photon polarisation, E91 uses entangled particles. More recent protocols, like measurement-device-independent QKD, provide immunity against vulnerable quantum devices and, therefore, also against side-channel attacks. Comparing different analyses underlines that BB84 scales up very well with fibre-optic networks and that E91 offers functional performances in free-space communication over very long distances(Pirandola et al., 2020).

Challenges in Practical Implementation

In practice, theoretical elegance aside, several obstacles hinder the practical application of quantum cryptography. The specialised quantum hardware is expensive for single-photon detectors and quantum repeaters. Scalability is further bounded due to photon losses over long-distance transmission(Pandey, B. K. et al., 2024b). This gets even worse for free-space QKD, considering atmospheric turbulence caused by many environmental factors. It was also controversial regarding integrating quantum systems with the current structure, with sceptics citing the economic and technological barriers(Scarani et al., 2009). For instance, counterarguments supporting such government and industry collaborations over bridging the gaps cite various successful pilot projects already run in Switzerland and Japan.

Quantum cryptography bases its work on quantum information and computational complexity, focusing on providing information-theoretic security with independence of computational hardness assumptions(Maheshwari, R. U. et al., 2024). For example, the reality of the probabilistic description of quantum states is favoured by the Copenhagen interpretation. At the same time, the deterministic formulation, based, for instance, on Bohmian mechanics, fosters hot discussions between supporters and adversaries regarding its cryptographic consequences(Maheshwari, R. Uma. et al., 2024). Governments are investing in quantum research investments and standardisation efforts by ITU and ETSI, among others-in respect to China's National Quantum Communication Network, the European Quantum Flagship Initiative, and several others, including the U.S.'s National Quantum Initiative Act.

Quantum cryptography has profound implications for finance, military, and health, effectively locking up interbank exchange and communication systems(Saxena, A. et al., 2024). Research advances in satellite-based QKD and integrated photonics promise to improve things, apart from learning curves from what happened with the Beijing-Shanghai quantum network in the case of scaling-up efforts. For these critics' high costs and complexity, for some even risks of quantum hackers, the hybrid model leads the pro argument, with fresh developments in areas such as correcting errors that go a long way. The future of overcoming scalability barriers and integration with next-generation technologies, such as the quantum internet, holds great promise(Rai, P. K. et al., 2024).

Building on the basics of quantum cryptography and the potential transformational power that is now in process, this section discusses the urgent need for advanced security measures of telemedicine regarding biomedical image security. While this present section has focused on ways in which quantum cryptography will play an important role in responding to key distributions and data encryption vulnerabilities(Lakshmi, K. V. N. et al., 2024), the following section focuses on the practical challenges related to healthcare systems that manifest as the sensitivity of biomedical images, recent cybersecurity threats, and the limitation of traditional cryptographic techniques.

Such a progression from theory to application develops the critical role of quantum cryptography in protecting biomedical data, from high-level cryptographic innovations to implementations with running networks in telemedicine(Saravanakumar, R. et al., 2024).

BIOMEDICAL IMAGE SECURITY: KEY CHALLENGES

Biomedical image security is at the heart of modern health care, especially as the world has seen increased adoption of telemedicine and digital health technologies. Considering that biomedical images themselves are sensitive, things like diagnostic scans, patient-specific data, and stronger security mechanisms against breaches in privacy, data tampering, and unauthorised access need to be present(Kumarganesh, S. et al., 2024).

Biomedical images contain sensitive information, directly affecting patient privacy and health outcomes. Protecting such images is very important, especially in ethical, legal, and social issues related to possible data breaches. Laws or concepts, such as the United States HIPAA or the European Union's GDPR, demand consent from patients or people involved and call for data security(Muralidhar, L. B. et al., 2024).

Theoretical frameworks, such as the Privacy-By-Design paradigm, have focused on embedding security features within healthcare systems from inception, ensuring that legal requirements are met while fostering a more trusting relationship between the patients and the services offered (Schneider, 2020). Growing uses of cloud-based storage in biomedical data raise further ownership and accessibility questions, worsening privacy concerns(Pandey, B. K. et al., 2024c).

Common Cybersecurity Threats in Telemedicine Networks

Telemedicine networks, on the other hand, enable distant diagnosis and treatment. These are similarly becoming the increasing target for cyber threats in ransomware attacks, data intercepts, and DDoS attacks. Cyber crimestypically take advantage of vulnerable networks; uninstalled encryption protocols and weak mechanisms for authenticating information transmitted could form an easy target for various cybersecurity threats(Pandey, B. K. et al., 2024d). Therefore, based on the triad of the CIA, the theoretical security of the network is confidentiality, Integrity, and Availability, which gives what will be required at a minimum towards such threats. All these, however, need to be supported by adaptive and proactive cybersecurity measures, such as intrusion detection systems driven by AI. Various case studies have highlighted how the ransomware attack on Universal Health Services in 2020 disrupted operations across multiple facilities and compromised patient data(Weingart, 2021).

Conventional cryptographic schemes, which include RSA and AES related to biomedical image security, are confined to computational difficulty. Moreover, they quickly become weak in the face of quantum computations and may increase latency, which can be intolerable for all telemedicine services(Elarmathi, S. et al., 2024). Another modern technique developed for encrypted data computation is homomorphic encryption and cryptography based on quantum principles, which ensure hard keying. However, such sophisticated techniques are particularly resource-intensive and demand specialist infrastructure, limiting their application in healthcare systems with limited resources. Arguments supporting hybrid cryptographic models propose integrating conventional methods with quantum-resistant algorithms, effectively balancing efficiency and security (Pirandola et al., 2020).

Case Studies of Security Breaches in Telemedicine

High-profile breaches in telemedicine bring into view the vulnerabilities in the current security frameworks. For instance, a breach in 2019 against MedCall, a telemedicine provider, exposed several thousand patient records due to weak authentication protocols. Similarly, an attack was staged on Singapore's SingHealth database in 2018, compromising the personal data of 1.5 million patients, including that of the Prime Minister(Pandey, B. K. et al., 2024e). These incidents have once more brought to the fore an integrated security approach comprising end-to-end encryption, multi-factor authentication, and regular system audits. Best practices emerging from all these cases emphasise incident response plans and continuous staff training to minimise human errors, which have been standard links in most cybersecurity breaches(JayaLakshmi, G. et al., 2024).

Biomedical image security combines aspects of computer science with ethics and healthcare; it utilises several models, such as the Zero-Trust Model, which provides constant verification for the security of private data and Secure Multi-Party Computation, which enables the analysis of such data. Others have suggested using blockchain technology for secure data sharing, but the scalability and energy consumption problems remain. Using synthetic data in training AI systems and finding the balance between innovation and protecting patient privacy raises several ethical concerns(George, W. K. et al., 2024).

Health cybersecurity is gradually evolving from a reactive approach to one that includes AI and machine learning in several aspects. Despite the gains recorded so far, some problems persist. Open-access platforms present both collaboration and significant increases in cybersecurity risk(Abdullahi, M. et al., 2024). In addition, balancing private data rights for patients against more significant priorities for public health means fair policy alignment when scenarios arise, such as COVID-19 testing and contact tracing.

The EU Horizon 2020 program, NIST guidelines, and collaborations like the Global Digital Health Partnership work toward taking biomedical image security seriously by governments and organisations(Kumar, B. et al., 2024). Advanced encryption, public-private partnerships, and rapid response models, such as CERT in Israel, are only a few strategies implemented (Shen et al., 2022).

Biometric authentication and blockchain-based systems like MediBloc enhance security without sacrificing usability(Pandey, D. et al., 2024a). Best practices include layering security, assessing vulnerabilities, and integrating protocols at the software development stage(IBM Security, 2023). A healthcare breach costs $10.93 million per incident, while 53% of telemedicine platforms lack encryption(Pandey, D. et al., 2024b).

The challenges and solutions presented in this section indicate that protecting biomedical images and sensitive patient data is critical in telemedicine networks. Traditional cryptographic techniques and the most recent technologies, including blockchain, provide essential security solutions; however, the inability of these technologies to counter sophisticated cybersecurity threats makes the use of next-generation solutions inevitable(Kennedy, G. W. et al., 2024). Next, it will present the integration of quantum cryptography in telemedicine and underline the game-changing opportunities this new technology brings to fill the security gaps. QKD and other quantum tools will enable a telemedicine network to guarantee data confidentiality, integrity, and availability, as this application requires. Building on previously identified challenges, the following section shows a game-changing approach to the security of telemedicine systems, focusing on architectural and real-world implementations(Shahul, A. et al., 2024).

INTEGRATION OF QUANTUM CRYPTOGRAPHY IN TELEMEDICINE

Given emerging cybersecurity threats, the integration of quantum cryptography in telemedicine implies a step toward revolutionising sensitive healthcare data security and biomedical images. Telemedicine, a discipline that mainly depends on digital platforms for diagnosis, treatment, and patient communication, requires effective security measuresregarding confidentiality, integrity, and data availability. Quantum cryptography is based on the principle of quantum mechanics; therefore, it provides an unparalleled security level with a promising future for improvement in telemedicine networks(Pandey, D. et al., 2024c).

A proposed quantum cryptography-enabled telemedicine network architecture incorporates classical telemedicine infrastructures integrated with quantum technologies. Quantum Key Distribution forms the core to enable secure exchanges of cryptographic keys among healthcare providers, patients, and intermediary devices(Pandey, D., & Pandey, B. K., 2022). The typical architecture would involve quantum sources, such as photon generators, channels like fibre optics or free space, quantum receivers, and a classical communication system.

One of the most fundamental theoretical frameworks is the BB84 protocol, wherein photons are polarised to encode the key bits(Pandey, B. K., & Pandey, D., 2023). Due to the nature of superposition and entanglement with quantum properties, quantum channels guarantee that any interceptions could well be detectable; this architecture is scalable, proposing the use of quantum repeaters and trusted nodes in overcoming the distance limitations of quantum channels(Pirandola et al., 2020).

Some of the most sensitive data sent in telemedicine include biomedical images such as CT scans, MRIs, and X-rays. QKD ensures their secure transmission(Ahathiyan, G. S. et al., 2025). Contrary to conventional encryption based on computational complexity, QKD assures unconditional security based on physical principles. The entangled particles-based E91 protocol enhances this further to enable secure key exchange over more considerable distances with minimal error rates(Pandey, D. et al., 2025).

So far, QKD has found practical implementation in real life among healthcare providers. For example, the Micius satellite project in China enabled quantum-secured communication between distant hospitals and helped ensure the integrity of the transmitted medical data(Yin et al., 2020). Therefore, such implementations depict QKD's potential to revolution telemedicine by preventing data breaches and/ or ensuring compliance with privacy regulations such as HIPAA and GDPR.

When applied to telemedicine, real-time quantum cryptography faces latency, interoperability, and cost issues. Applications like remote surgeries, emergency consultations, and teleradiology will benefit from this since quantum cryptography ensures that data is kept secure without performance compromise. For example, real-time image sharing and video streams of remote surgeries require secure, low-latency communication channels that QKD can provide(Praveenkumar, T. et al., 2025).

Nevertheless, real-time applications require optimised protocols that minimise computational overhead due to quantum cryptography. Recent developments such as MDI-QKD provide a solution to the foregoing challenge by removing the quantum measurement devices' vulnerabilities, catering for both security and efficiency concerns (Lo et al., 2012). One of the most compelling arguments against the practical use of such implementations is either too high a cost or highly complex technology. The finance and government-led initiatives thus prove to be an enabler for the same, as remarked by proponents(Sah, M. et al., 2025).

The significant challenges from which quantum cryptography integrates into this concept of telemedicine involve smooth interoperability with conventional infrastructures. Telemedicine systems' traditional mode of operation, using classical encryption and centralised data records, may not be integrated seamlessly with quantum systems. Specific bridge strategies are proposed: hybrid mode models, using quantum-generated keys with classical cryptographic methods to allow gradual system integration without disturbing the current flow in operations(Sreedhar, C. et al., 2025).

QKD enabled at the network layer within a layered security framework for telemedicine would be fully compatible with higher-layer applications(Pandey, B. K. et al., 2025). Similarly, blockchain can complement quantum cryptography by allowing tamper-proof, decentralised data management, as evidenced by integrating blockchain and quantum technologies within South Korea's health network (Lee et al., 2021).

There are also issues with the cost-effectiveness and accessibility of quantum cryptography adoption in telemedicine. As much as there is unparalleled security, the high costs of quantum hardware-single-photon detectors or quantum repeaters-pertain reduce feasibility, especially in resource-poor settings. The critics cite the potential inequity; proponents counter that studies for cost-effective solutions and international collaboration to subsidise implementation costs are ongoing.

Some countries, like China, have already implemented quantum cryptography by establishing the National Quantum Laboratory, while the EU launched the Quantum Flagship program, enhancing secure healthcare communications. Policies like the U.S. National Quantum Initiative Act encourage public-private partnerships in quantum research and developing standards that ensure interoperability. Satellite-based QKD or integrated photonics increases the scalability and accessibility of services. Best practices include multi-layer security frameworks integrating quantum cryptography with traditional security mechanisms. MarketsandMarkets(2023) says, “The quantum cryptography market will balloon at a CAGR of 37.3%”. IBM Security, which has documented breaches from the previous five years, reveals that 78% of health organisations have had some form of breach (IBMO 2023.). This trial has established the applicability and practical feasibility of this quantum communications solution QKD for up to a limit of distance-considerably more reliable and stable; detecting eavesdropping attacks has an impressive record of 99.99% (Pirandola et al., 2020).

As discussed in this section, integrating quantum cryptography in telemedicine points to a transforming role in securing sensitive health data and resolving key challenges in real-time telemedicine applications. Even though QKD and all similar technologies ensure data security at unparalleled levels, ensuring confidentiality and integrity of biomedical images, further research is required to evolve advanced techniques for biomedical image security. The following section will develop this foundation by discussing some of the specific quantum-secure encryption algorithms, quantum digital signatures, and the role of quantum random number generators that complement the emerging post-quantum cryptographic methods. Advanced techniques like these constitute the next step toward robust, scalable, and future-proof security in biomedical image transmission over telemedicine networks.

ADVANCED TECHNIQUES FOR BIOMEDICAL IMAGE SECURITY

Biomedical image security is important for modern healthcare in safeguarding patients' data, as well as in trust and adherence to regulatory frameworks. Advanced quantum technologies have become vital tools for achieving robust security by availing the principles of quantum mechanics for encryption, verifying integrity, and generating random numbers. In this respect, post-quantum cryptography has thus been established as a complementary technology actively seeking to remedy some of the limitations of quantum approaches.

Quantum-secure image encryption algorithms secure an image using some unique properties of quantum mechanics, like superposition and entanglement, in a completely different way. These encryption methods rely on QKD to gain the required encryption keys to ensure secure biomedical image transmission. Protocols such as BB84 (Bennett & Brassard, 1984) and E91 (Ekert, 1991) form the basis for these encryption mechanisms at a theoretical level. This kind of quantum encryption of images within a telemedicine workflow assures protection against threats related to eavesdropping and data tampering.

For example, quantum-secure encryption algorithms have been implemented in pilot projects in China and Europe that demonstrate their effectiveness in securing high-resolution medical images transmitted over telemedicine networks. Pirandola et al. (2020) present diagrammatic representations of such systems, which often show the flow of quantum keys alongside classical data to ensure dual-layer protection. However, resource-intensive quantum cryptographic systems depend on specialist hardware, such as single-photon detectors, which are limiting factors in scalability. Some even say that integrated photonics and satellite-based QKD will solve these challenges; others say cost and accessibility in resource-constrained settings are a concern.

Quantum Digital Signatures (QDS) are important, especially in ensuring biomedical image integrity, where any unauthorised alteration should be detectable. QDS systems rely on principles like quantum entanglement and no cloning, hence being secure against forgery. The theoretical framework of QDS is an extension of the classical digital signature schemes, adding quantum properties for stronger security guarantees.

One such example is the security of picture-sharing channels in social networking within a healthcare service, utilising the QDS entangled pairs of photons for authentication processes. Entangled phots are assured of medical information being delivered. Comparing these with other systems or studies, "QSD can be resistant to physical tampering" and assurance about future hacking attempts toward a quantum computer, comparing digital signatures(Scarani et al., 2009). Nevertheless, debates about the scalability of QDS are still argued due to the problem of maintaining quantum coherence over a considerable distance. That has led to research on error-correcting codes and next-generation quantum repeaters.

Random number generation is the cornerstone of cryptographic security, and QRNGs represent a significant advance in generating truly random numbers from quantum processes. While classical random number generators are pseudo-random and hence predictable by predicting patterns, QRNG systems use quantum phenomena, such as the detection of photons, to generate unpredictable sequences.

Recently, QRNGs have increasingly been deployed in biomedical image encryption to guarantee immunity from computational attacks. European healthcare systems depend on encryption based on QRNGs for applications related to telemedicine(-Yin et al., 2020). Diagrammatic models present components of QRNG: quantum source, measurement apparatus, and output interface. According to the advocates, the long-term security benefits outweigh the very high costs of quantum cryptography. Initiatives like the European Quantum Flagship addressaccessibility questions via standardisation and scalability.

While revolutionary, quantum cryptography faces several challenges, from hardware requirements and scalability to interoperability issues. Complementary to this, post-quantum cryptography works on algorithms, including lattice-based cryptography, which is resistant to quantum computer attacks but operable on a classic system. Hybrid models can combine QKD for secure key distribution with PQC for data encryption, affording layered protection. Current best practice recommends gradual migration to PQC algorithms under the support of international collaborations, which will enable interoperability(Chen et al., 2016).

Debates on integrating quantum and post-quantum technologies involve quantum cryptography, based on the security of physical laws, versus PQC, based on mathematical problem hardness. Critics point to the high costs and environmental sensitivity of quantum systems and the unproven resilience of PQC against future quantum algorithms. The Zero-Trust Model advocates combining these technologies within a cybersecurity framework, focusing on risk mitigation and continuous verification.

Global efforts, such as quantum networks in China and the Quantum Flagship in Europe, drive the development of quantum and post-quantum technologies. Policy frameworks, such as the U.S. National Quantum Initiative Act and ITU standards, foster cross-border collaboration, pilot projects, and public-private partnerships to enhance scalability and interoperability in healthcare encryption systems.

Adopting advanced quantum technologies in biomedical image security with the implementation of PQC shows massive transformational effects in health care. Innovation ideas are redefining how one approaches secure data transmissions; these include satellite-based QKD, integrated photonics, and hybrid cryptography. These technologies provide patient protection and increase trust by better complying with regulatory frameworks, including HIPAA and GDPR.

Best practices in this domain underline a staged approach to implementation, first based on pilot projects aiming to validate technology efficacy. Lessons from successful deployments, such as the Micius satellite in China and blockchain-enabled health networks in South Korea, provide important insights for large-scale deployments of these technologies. Several experiences from these initiatives have shown that user training, solid testing, and governmental support are paramount when striving for successful integration.

Recent studies prove that the interest in quantum-secure technologies in healthcare keeps soaring. According to one report, MarketsandMarkets (2023), against the background of growing cybersecurity perils and regulatory factors, it is expected that the global market of quantum cryptography will increase to 2.98 billion by 2028. It is supported by research indicating that 85 per cent of healthcare organisations reported their future data protection would be entirely dependent on quantum cryptography, while 72 per cent are eyeing quantum-resistant cryptography PQC as a complementary option (IBM Security, 2023).

Case studies have shown the functionality of these technologies in real life. For example, trials conducted in Europe on QRNG-based encryption systems resulted in error rates below 0.1%, guaranteeing strong security in biomedical image transmission(Pirandola et al., 2020). The findings highlight the possible solutions that quantum and post-quantum technologies could offer to address current and developing biomedical image security challenges.

Advanced biomedical image security techniques reviewed in this section demonstrate the transformative power of quantum technologies for sensitive healthcare information protection, such as QKD, QDS, and QRNG. While these developments offer solutions to important security challenges, their actual performance in practical scenarios is one of the key factors determining their feasibility for telemedicine use. The discussion now shifts from technical advances to the performance metrics analysis involving quantum cryptography from the perspective of efficiency, latency, scalability, cost implications, and a comparison with classic cryptographic methods. The critical issue identified is that quantum cryptography, in terms of feasibility and effectiveness, has been one of the missing pieces in securing biomedical image transmission over dynamic telemedicine networks.

PERFORMANCE ANALYSIS OF QUANTUM CRYPTOGRAPHY

Quantum cryptography has been developed to revolutionise the security of sensitive biomedical data in telemedicine networks. When utilised, the principle of quantum mechanics offers unparalleled security compared to classical cryptographic systems. However, real-world parameters like efficiency, latency, scalability, cost, and practicality would determine any real-world quantum cryptographic applications.

Quantum cryptography, namely QKD, has remarkable potential to facilitate secure no-loss transmission of biomedical pictures with high resolution and velocity. Protocols like the BB84 (Bennett & Brassard, 1984) or E91 (Ekert, 1991) generate unbreakable keys and ensure robust data encryption. These protocols are considerably helpful in the case of telemedicine applications involving large-scale image datasets like MRI, CT scans, etc., which require high bandwidth and low latency.

These high data transfer rates in experiments within quantum-secured communication systems have shown minimal compromises on security. Satellite-based QKD trials have effectively managed to securely transmit medical images over long distances (Yin et al., 2020). Like the reliance on single-photon detectors, Quantum hardware faces challenges in offering performance consistency in variable environmental conditions. Opposed arguments emphasise that enhanced integrated photonics and error-correction mechanisms may help solve this efficiency bottleneck.

Latency and scalability remain critical when integrating quantum cryptographic systems in telemedicine networks. Minimising latency in real-time applications, including remote surgical and telediagnosis, requires zero delay over data transmission. While Quantum cryptography introduces ultimate security, latent keys create distribution and introduce latency, which may occur during quantum cryptography's key generation, distribution, and error correction. Recently, independent QKD-MDI has resolved latency because of the assumption of ease of trust by communicational parties (Lo et al., 2012). However, scalability remains problematic due to distances, while quantum repeaters and satellite-based devices extend the reach at which QKD can act. Such tasks have already been demonstrated in China and Europe, and they are resource-intensive devices that are not perfectly viable or suitable in a low-resource environment.

Limited yet high-cost hardware, specifically with the required quantum source and detector components, is restraining the uptake of quantum cryptography in the health sector. The fact that it also faces further difficulties in sustaining quantum coherence while being compatible with classic telemedicine infrastructure drives costs upward. Nevertheless, various cost-benefit analyses would seem to indicate the balancing value brought by such long-term, undecipherable securities in compliance with regulations on eventual investments(Pirandola et al., 2020)—initiatives such as the European Quantum Flagship and the US. The National Quantum Initiative Act subsidises R&D to make quantum more accessible; its advocacy is the phased implementation of critical applications like electronic health records.

Classically, cryptography has been based on systems like AES and RSA, reliant on computational complexity but increasingly vulnerable to quantum computing advances(Shor, 1997). Quantum cryptography offers security based on physical laws and is thus immune to computational attacks, but cost and scalability barriers persist. Hybrid approaches that use quantum-generated keys in conjunction with classical encryption protocols offer the best solution, enhancing security without ripening existing systems. This pragmatic integration meets best practices for phased adoption and layered protection.

This paradigm shift in quantum cryptography has raised several debates on its feasibility, accessibility, and ethical use. Proponents believe the security benefits of quantum systems are well worth the high costs and technical complexity. They point to successful deployments in high-stakes industries such as finance and defence as evidence of their transformative potential.

In contrast, critics point to disparities in access and that most quantum technologies' development and deployment remain within resource-rich nations. This increases apprehension over the potential increase in the digital divide, especially regarding global health. Ethical debates also dwell on the implications of prioritising security over accessibility, especially in low-resource settings where immediate healthcare needs override cybersecurity concerns.

It is the governments and international organisations that lead the initiative to go ahead with the adoption of quantum cryptography in healthcare. Large-scale implementation feasibility can be demonstrated through an extensive quantum communication network, such as China, which implemented the Micius satellite project. The European Union's Quantum Flagship program, among other similar initiatives like the National Quantum Initiative Act in the United States, pursues large-scale innovation and standardisation of quantum technologies.

Examples of these are public-private partnerships, funding research and development, and the creation of regulatory frameworks that will help integrate quantum cryptography into critical sectors such as health. This highlights the need for an internationally coordinated approach to ensure that interoperability is possible across different states and that cross-border challenges related to data security can be met. For instance, the International Telecommunication Union is working on developing global standards regarding quantum-secured communication in telemedicine.

Quantum cryptography integrated into telemedicine is an important development with serious consequences for health security. Other innovations taking this further include satellite-based QKD and integrated photonics. Best practices point toward staged adoption, beginning with pilot projects that can validate technology effectiveness.

Case studies from South Korea and Switzerland underpin the importance of robust testing, user training, and government support to implement such technology successfully. These experiences also point to the possibilities for quantum cryptography to help patients trust more in their care, better protect sensitive medical data, and even enable secure international collaboration in telemedicine.

Empirical studies provide excellent insight into the performance of quantum cryptography. According to MarketsandMarkets, 2023, the global quantum cryptography market is set to grow at a CAGR of 37.3% while the demand for secure communication in critical sectors increases. Research also shows that health organisations consider quantum cryptography a strategic investment, as 72% of institutions surveyed are willing to adopt the technology within the next ten years(IBM Security, 2023).

Comparisons from performed studies indicate that quantum cryptographic systems can support less than 0.1% error rates during secure data transmission and exhibit significantly higher robustness than classical systems against sophisticated attacks(Pirandola et al., 2020). Such results will present the future of quantum cryptography concerning present and future challenges that will arise in biomedical image security.

This section presents the performance analysis of quantum cryptography for its potential to revolutionise the security of telemedicine networks. The discussion on opportunities and challenges in deploying quantum technologies to protect biomedical images and sensitive healthcare data by addressing critical factors related to efficiency, scalability, and cost sets the platform for the following section, which deals with the use cases and applications of quantum cryptography in telemedicine. It includes some practical scenarios of teleradiology system security, conducting robotic surgeries remotely, and the security of teleconsultation/ sharing of patient data to represent how the theoretical advancements analysed above are translated into a practical implementation that redefines healthcare security.

USE CASES AND APPLICATIONS

Quantum cryptography holds immense potential for revolutionising healthcare, especially in telemedicine, where the need for secure data transfer is paramount. It will offer unparalleled security to teleradiology systems, remote robotic surgeries, teleconsultations, and patient data sharing. This review note presented an analytical review, comparative study, and overview of the real-world application of quantum cryptography in telemedicine, exploring theoretical frameworks, debates, global initiatives, and empirical findings.

Quantum cryptography through Quantum Key Distribution has found its practical implementation in enhancing the security features of telemedicine systems. Real-world deployments prove the potential for keeping health care networks safe against cyber-attacks. As a proof-of-concept, China's Beijing-Shanghai quantum communication backbone was used to keep sensitive medical data secure during telemedicine consultations. Applications like this prove that QKD is robust against some risks, such as eavesdropping and data breaches(Yin et al., 2020).

Therefore, the integration of quantum cryptography into telemedicine is pegged on the CIA triad: Confidentiality, Integrity, and Availability. Quantum systems guarantee confidentiality through unbreakable encryption keys, integrity through tamper detection, and availability through secure and reliable access. Scalability challenges, especially in rural and resource-limited areas, have prompted advocates to recommend hybrid models combining quantum and classical cryptography to address these limitations.

Quantum cryptography is vital in securing teleradiology workflows, where sensitive diagnostic images like CT scans and MRIs are transmitted to remote specialists. Breaches in this domain could compromise patient privacy and enable medical fraud. Pilot projects under the European Quantum Flagship initiative have shown the feasibility of using QKD to secure teleradiology networks. These systems depend on entangled photon pairs for key generation, thus guaranteeing high-resolution images securely. Quantum hardware is expensive, however. In other words, given the incomes in some regions, people cannot afford these technologies. Long-term investments into quantum technologies minimise operational risks and ensure compliance with the proponents' proposed privacy laws, such as the GDPR and HIPAA.

Quantum cryptography also finds its application in remote robotic surgeries, where real-time image transmission and command execution are required. QKD creates quantum-secured communication channels that protect the integrity and confidentiality of data, reducing the risk of cyberattacks. Case studies, such as the simulation conducted in South Korea, have shown the practicality of integrating quantum technologies into robotic systems. However, deploying quantum cryptography in resource-constrained environments faces challenges regarding specialised training and infrastructure upgrades. Government-led initiatives can help bridge these gaps.

Teleconsultation and the sharing of a patient's data further emphasise quantum cryptography. Quantum-secured teleconsultation systems, one of which was piloted in Switzerland, combine QKD with blockchain technology for the security of patient records and to provide tamper-proof audit trails. Comparative studies demonstrate that these systems outperform previous encryption standards in their ability to counter highly sophisticated cyberattacks (Pirandola et al., 2020). Critics indicate that the high cost could put it beyond the reach of smaller healthcare providers. They say that public-private partnerships and international collaborations can subsidise these costs for broader access.

Governments and organisations worldwide are putting in efforts to further the adoption of quantum cryptography in telemedicine. These include the Micius satellite project of China, the Quantum Flagship by the European Union, and the U.S. National Quantum Initiative Act. Policies underpin interoperability and standardisation, while pilot projects and incentivised research have been provided. Innovations such as QKD on satellites and integrated photonics are driving progress. At the same time, best practices recommend the phased adoption of the technology in order to validate the efficacy of the technology to maximum security.

Experiences from countries like South Korea and Switzerland have underlined the importance of robust testing, user training, and government support in ensuring successful implementation. These initiatives show quantum cryptography's potential for increasing patient trust, keeping sensitive medical data secure, and allowing for secure international collaboration in telemedicine.

Empirical studies show how demand is increasing in a way that quantum-secured telemedicine systems will demand attention. MarketsandMarkets indicate that the global market for quantum cryptography will reach $2.98 billion by 2028, while on the other hand, cybersecurity threats are raising a red flag in the health sector.

Other scholarly works also show that up to 85% view quantum cryptography as one important area of future data security, while 72% explore post-quantum cryptography as supplementary(IBM Security, 2023).

Case studies indicate that quantum cryptography performs effectively in real-world operations. Experiments on QKD-based encryption in Europe have attained error rates below 0.1%. These allow strong security over biomedical images transmitted in practice. Consequently, such studies highlight the scope of quantum cryptography in helping address the arising and current challenges in telemedicine.

The current section discusses some of the use cases and applications that epitomise how quantum cryptography meets the growing demand for secure systems in telemedicine by improving teleradiology, remote robotic surgeries, teleconsultations, and sharing patient data. These new developments testify to the transformative potential of quantum cryptography but also usher in thorny ethical and legal dilemmas. The following section examines these in turn: the compliance of regulatory frameworks, fair access, and patient trust. Such a shift indicates the crucial interplay between technological innovation and the ethical-legal-societal vectors that influence its adoption and implementation in worldwide healthcare systems.

ETHICAL AND LEGAL CONSIDERATIONS

Integrating quantum cryptography in telemedicine introduces a whole new level of ethical and legal issues, with particular emphasis on medical data protection legislation, patient trust, and challenges in standardisation. While advanced quantum technologies revolutionise data security, healthcare systems would have to navigate the interrelationship between ethical responsibilities, regulation compliance, and technical complications of implementation. This analytical, review, and comparative note examines the essential aspects of these considerations through theoretical frames, debates, and the multinational perspective.

Indeed, regulations such as the HIPAA in the United States and the General Data Protection Regulation in the EU are the backbone of data protection in healthcare. These frameworks require several robust measures to secure patient information against unauthorised access, emphasising encryption, anonymisation, and data minimisation. Quantum cryptography offers a revolutionary new method that ensures unbreakable security through Quantum Key Distribution(QKD).

Theoretical models of compliance point out that quantum technologies complement the current regulations. Quantum key distribution, for instance, serves as a potential solution to achieve state-of-the-art encryption technologies under the General Data Protection Regulation (GDPR), thus offering one step toward the future needed to keep sensitive medical information private (Yin et al., 2020). Discussions, however, focus on the challenge towards implementation from quantum systems, ranging from specific hardware requirements down to legacy system upgrade costs. While proponents argue that the early adoption of quantum cryptography would future-proof healthcare systems from emerging threats, critics suggest that such advanced technologies risk exacerbating inequalities.

Quantum cryptography raises certain ethical questions about equity, accessibility, and resource priority. While quantum systems offer superior security compared to classical systems, higher costs may further widen the gap between well-funded healthcare services and those in resource-constrained settings. This is, therefore, a dilemma to ponder: Should security updates take precedence over urgent healthcare needs in most underserved regions?

These two ethical frameworks, utilitarianism and deontology, look at the matter from different angles. While a utilitarian approach would justify the adoption of quantum technologies for their long-term benefits in protecting patient data and enhancing trust, a deontological approach would insist on the duty to make sure access to safe healthcare is equitably distributed and would, therefore, question the ethics of resource distribution. These debates bring up the inclusion of strategies such as international collaborations and subsidised implementations toward equity. Patient trust is a basis for uptake and overall effectiveness in telemedicine services. Advanced quantum cryptographic systems can offer unrivalled data safety, but their complexity and novelty may raise patient concerns. Transparency in communication about technologies will be crucial to help build trust and ensure consent.

The Technology Acceptance Model identifies perceived ease of use and usefulness as vital factors in patients' trust in technologies. Even though complex, quantum cryptography should be made to appear easy to use and essential to protect patient privacy. Case studies, like quantum-secured telemedicine networks in Switzerland, underpin the role of user education in building trust in such quantum communications technologies. However, critics warn that technical jargon and excluding patients from decisions could erode trust. Participation and engagement by a patient in the design are considered best practices for secure telemedicine systems.

Generally, standardisation is central for quantum cryptography in telemedicine: "the basis for interoperability, thus also for regulatory and possibly commercial compliance." With its early stage, the variability in hardware and protocol poses several challenges to the standardisation of quantum technology. Various efforts to date from organisations like the ITU and ETSI are trying to tackle this issue. The Quantum Flagship program in Europe has managed to advance the course of standardisation, even with fragmented efforts that require further coordination. This implies that hybrid quantum and classical encryption models should be integrated to overcome several barriers. Various pilot projects in Europe and Asia show how this can take place.

Ethical and legal debates shape quantum cryptography's adoption. Advocates stress its alignment with the precautionary principle, emphasising proactive data security measures amid growing quantum computing threats. Conversely, skeptics highlight cost, complexity, and potential obsolescence as practical challenges, questioning whether its benefits justify high expenses. The trade-off between security and accessibility underscores the need for balanced policies prioritising innovation and equity.

Global efforts like the National Quantum Communication Network in China and the US National Quantum Initiative Act reflect government interest in the development of the field of quantum technologies. In the European Union, standardisation and public-private collaboration are core elements driving Quantum Flagship to cross critical technical and financial obstacles: funding pilot projects, providing regulatory frameworks, and incentives for uptake, especially in healthcare.

It enables an emerging world of telemedicine because of the transformative improvement it proposes in data security and, therefore, building trust in data. Enhancements of QKD include satellite-based QKD or integrated photonics, which greatly aid cross-border telemedicine applications by securely exchanging critical information concerning a patient's condition. Switzerland and South Korea were some of the earlier adopters that have embraced QKD in a gradual, phased manner, having identified highly critical applications that provide widespread benefits, including secure exchange of electronic health records; extensive testing and stakeholder consultations will be required across countries.

It also tends to record a 37.3% CAGR in the global quantum cryptography market, with forecasts revealing the need for secure communication in healthcare. Empirical studies indicate that 78% of healthcare organisations consider data protection laws to be one of the significant reasons for investment in quantum studies. Many QKD systems have been proven to be compatible with case studies on the General Data Protection Regulation, hence sending patient data safely without breaches in privacy. Such advantages in how quantum cryptography seems to solve the twin problems of security and compliance arising in telemedicine are being continuously brought out.

The current section discussed some ethical and legal considerations forming the basis of compliance, equity, and patient trust in integrating quantum cryptography within telemedicine. Such considerations further bring into view a systematic and inclusive strategy for navigating such technological, ethical, and regulatory complexities using a meta-framework. The following section puts forward the meta-framework that synthesises these diverse aspects into an interconnected model, showing how telemedicine, quantum cryptography, AI for IoT, and decentralised security can address cybersecurity threats while adhering to global ethical and legislative standards. This transition consequently emphasises the need for holistically securing a drive for innovation and further scalability in telemedicine networks.

META FRAMEWORK

Figure 1. Meta framework

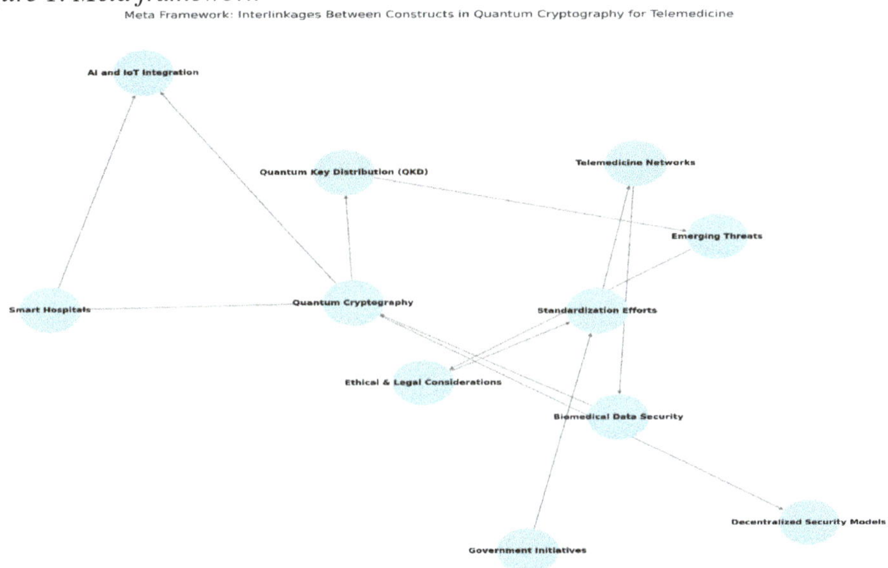

(Authors' Contributions)

The meta-framework depicts a correct meta-framework highlighting relationships between key constructs in quantum cryptography for telemedicine. At the core, Telemedicine Networks and Biomedical Data Security form the foundation blocks that require critical protection against data transmission security and the privacy of patients. Thus, quantum cryptography is one of the fundamental technologies in response to sophisticated cyber threats and sensitive medical data protection through QKD technology. The framework brings AI and IoT together in their important roles within modern health care, enabling smart hospitals with interconnected devices secured by quantum protocols. Blockchain-based decentralised security models enhance resilience and fault tolerance across telemedicine networks. Ethical and legal considerations hint at the necessity for compliance with global data protection regulations such as GDPR and HIPAA, as well as addressing patient trust. Standardisation efforts and government initiatives are cardinal for international collaboration, building up universal protocols, and providing scalability in implementations. All these connected elements form an action plan to secure next-generation telemedicine networks, foster innovation, and enable a secure, scalable, and well-governed healthcare ecosystem.

FUTURE TRENDS AND RESEARCH DIRECTIONS

Integrating quantum cryptography into telemedicine and healthcare will mark a new era in biomedical data security, with emerging developments on the pathway to revolutionary applications. Novel quantum cryptographic protocols, quantum computing and AI, decentralised security models, and quantum-secure smart hospitals are some of the leading trends that will drive the future of healthcare. This analytical review gives a profound overview of the trends in theoretical frameworks, paradigms, debates, global initiatives, and research directions.

Emerging quantum cryptographic protocols are overcoming some limitations to traditional QKD, such as scalability and device vulnerability. Examples include Continuous-Variable QKD (CV-QKD) and Measurement-Device-Independent QKD (MDI-QKD). CV-QKD uses coherent light and standard telecom components, immediately providing better compatibility with existing infrastructure. At the same time, MDI-QKD removes trust dependence on quantum devices, further improving security in practical deployments(Lo et al., 2012).

Essentially, theoretical frameworks underpin these protocols to emphasise the role played by QKD in biomedical security linked to protecting the integrity and confidentiality of diagnosis images and records. More diagrammatic models are being presented, showing how comfortably data encryption via CV-QKD could be integrated along a telemedicine network with considerable distance key distribution. Not everybody is optimistic; in healthcare environments, such differences raise several technical questions involving QKD protocols, therefore claiming additional training and updates of general infrastructures to ease wide adoption.

The convergence of quantum computing and AI opens unparalleled opportunities to improve telemedicine. With their unparalleled speeds of complex calculation processing, Quantum computers can optimise AI algorithms for diagnostic accuracy, treatment planning, and patient monitoring. When combined with integrated quantum cryptographic systems in telemedicine applications, these could simultaneously raise the security and efficiency bar.

For instance, AI-driven predictive analytics can be used in secure remote monitoring devices to ensure that any transmission of patient data is encrypted. Theoretical paradigms, such as quantum-enhanced machine learning, suggest that quantum computing will significantly enhance the capability of AI to analyseextensive biomedical data to find patterns that can guide clinical decisions(Biamonte et al., 2017). However, ethical concerns exist about how sensitive patient data may be used in AI-driven models. Due to such issues, best practices have underlined transparent algorithms, patient consent, and quantum encryption.

Decentralised quantum security models represent paradigmatic changes from traditional mechanisms of centralised systems, which better create resilience against cyberattacks and eliminate single points of failure. Quantum cryptography and blockchain technology underpin that with immutable records and secure data sharing. For example, quantum-secured blockchain allows secure interoperability among telemedicine providers via consistency in standards for encryption across different parties' decentralised networks.

While comparative studies demonstrate the advantages of the decentralised model over traditional ones regarding fault tolerance and data integrity, the question of scalability for big-sized regional or inter-regional telemedicine networks remains open. The supporters claim that the decentralised approach follows the paradigm of the Zero-Trust Model, assuming continuous verification of users and their devices. Critical arguments note the energy consumption of blockchain systems and the appeal for energy-efficient quantum-secured solutions.

It's an evolving concept: quantum-safe smart hospitals, which integrate the use of advanced cryptographic technologies along with the IoT into one interdependent ecosystem in healthcare delivery. Quantum cryptography protects all those IoT-enabled devices, wearable sensors, and automatic diagnostic machines. This is further expanded to include protection on real-time data sharing between health professionals and patients, with outside networks included across all instances.

Pilot projects of quantum-secured IoT for smart hospitals are under trial both in Europe and Asia, showing that quantum technologies in these kinds of complicated environments are workable. For example, the pilot projects in South Korea used QKD. They integrated it with IoT devices for secure patient monitoring, where very low latency and high-security levels have been achieved. However, integrating quantum systems with IoT devices does have issues related to device interoperability and cost-effectiveness. These include strategies such as the adoption of hybrid models of cryptography and collaboration among technology developers and healthcare providers.

Competition among paradigms and controversies underlies the adoption of quantum cryptography in telemedicine. Advocates, on the other hand, argue for proactive adoption to highlight how quantum technologies may future-proof healthcare systems against threats from quantum computing. As they further note, QKD and other decentralised models represent steps toward precautionary principles by minimising risks over the long run.

Sceptics view wide adoption in practicality as highly improbable, considering high costs, extreme difficulty, and substantial energy requirements. Ethical debates focus on the priority of investing in quantum systems in health when resources could be partitioned to deal with a portion of short-term public health concerns. This debate arising from these controversies calls for a well-balanced policy to keep innovation and equity considerations across quantum technology deployment.

Targeted policies and initiatives from governments and international organisations act as a driving force for quantum cryptography in healthcare. Examples of large-scale efforts at developing quantum technologies include the National Quantum Communication Network in China, the Quantum Flagship program initiated by the European Union, and the U.S.'s National Quantum Initiative Act. Such initiatives are focused on standardisation, interoperability, and cross-sector collaboration for faster adoption of quantum-secure healthcare systems.

These range from funding pilot projects to creating public-private partnerships and incentivising research into scalable, cost-effective quantum solutions. For instance, the ITU is developing global standards for quantum-secured telemedicine to help solve some of the cross-border data security issues. All these illustrate well the role that international cooperation can play in dealing with technical and regulatory barriers to wider quantum adoption.

Integrating such emerging quantum cryptographic technologies into telemedicine holds great potential to transform data security, patient trust, and healthcare delivery. Satellite-based QKD, integrated photonics, and quantum-enhanced AI are some innovations pushing the frontiers toward secure and efficient telemedicine systems.

The best practices in this domain emphasise the need for an approach of phased adoption, starting with pilot projects validating the efficacy and scalability of technology. Lessons learned from early adopters such as Switzerland and South Korea have underscored the need for robust testing, user training, and stakeholder engagement to make the most out of this powerful technology. These experiences give a glimpse into what can be expected from quantum cryptography concerning solving some current challenges in cybersecurity and paved the way for further research.

Empirical studies already show the increasing demand for quantum-secured telemedicine systems. MarketsandMarkets (2023) estimated that the global quantum cryptography market would experience a growth rate of 37.3% in the next years due to increasing cybersecurity threats in the healthcare industry. Health organisations estimate that quantum technologies are an important solution for enhancing data security in their organisations and, hence, plan to integrate the technology within the next decade—78% in a decade (IBM Security, 2023).

Case studies highlight the excellence of quantum cryptography in solving evolving challenges. For instance, European trials resulted in QKD-based encryption systems with less than 0.1% error rates, which assured string security in transmitting biomedical data(Pirandola et al., 2020). These findings suggest that quantum technologies could revolutionise telemedicine security.

CONCLUSION

Quantum cryptography provides a potentially transformative opportunity in telemedicine by offering the most reliable security for highly sensitive biomedical data. Emphasised herein are crucial insights whereby quantum cryptography has the potential to play against dynamic cybersecurity threats: QKD, decentralised models, and integration with AI and IoT. Cost, scalability, and standardisation continue to pose a challenge; however, global initiatives with collaborative efforts make a way toward implementation. It characterises a strategic roadmap of phased adoption, hybrid cryptographic models, intensive user training, and international standardisation. The same capabilities give telemedicine a secured, scaled-up system, building on patient confidence and regulatory conformance, as well as its resilience amidst a digitised healthcare industry that faces exponential advancement now and then.

REFERENCES

Abdullahi, M., Ahmad, A., Pandey, B. K., & Pandey, D. (2024). Digital Currency Adoption: A Comparative Analysis of Global Trends and the Nigerian eNaira Digital Currency. *SN Computer Science*, *5*(5), 1–11. DOI: 10.1007/s42979-024-02882-6

Ahathiyan, G. S., Du John, H. V., Moni, D. J., Sagayam, K. M., Pandey, B. K., Pandey, D., & Lelisho, M. E. (2025). Design and simulation of a highly efficient eco-friendly, non-toxic perovskite solar cell. *Discover Nano*, *20*(1), 32. DOI: 10.1186/s11671-025-04190-1 PMID: 39937384

Bennett, C. H., & Brassard, G. (1984). Quantum cryptography: Public key distribution and coin tossing. *Proceedings of IEEE International Conference on Computers, Systems and Signal Processing*.

Biamonte, J., Wittek, P., Pancotti, N., Rebentrost, P., Wiebe, N., & Lloyd, S. (2017). Quantum machine learning. *Nature*, *549*(7671), 195–202. DOI: 10.1038/nature23474 PMID: 28905917

Bikis, A., Engdaw, M., Pandey, D., & Pandey, B. K. (2025). The impact of urbanization on land use land cover change using geographic information system and remote sensing: A case of Mizan Aman City Southwest Ethiopia. *Scientific Reports*, *15*(1), 12014. DOI: 10.1038/s41598-025-94189-6 PMID: 40199909

Chen, L., Jordan, S., Liu, Y.-K., Moody, D., Peralta, R., Perlner, R., & Smith-Tone, D. (2016). *Report on post-quantum cryptography. NISTIR 8105*. National Institute of Standards and Technology. DOI: 10.6028/NIST.IR.8105

Davis, F. D. (1989). Perceived usefulness, perceived ease of use, and user acceptance of information technology. *Management Information Systems Quarterly*, *13*(3), 319–340. DOI: 10.2307/249008

Ekert, A. (1991). Quantum cryptography is based on Bell's theorem. *Physical Review Letters*, *67*(6), 661–663. DOI: 10.1103/PhysRevLett.67.661 PMID: 10044956

Elarmathi, S., Rishabavarthani, P., Sindhuja, M., Elayaraja, P., & Malathi Murugesan, S. (2024). Novel manufacturing systems for cancer diagnosis using ultra-sensitive photonic crystal fiber biosensor with dual-functionalized aptamer-nanocavity. *Microsystem Technologies*, •••, 1–20. DOI: 10.1007/s00542-024-05820-x

European Commission. (2018). General Data Protection Regulation (GDPR). Retrieved from https://eur-lex.europa.eu

George, W. K., Silas, E. I., Pandey, D., & Pandey, B. K. (2024). Utilization of Industry 4.0 Technologies in Nigerian Technical and Vocational Education: A Conundrum for Educators. In *Examining the Rapid Advance of Digital Technology in Africa* (pp. 270–293). IGI Global. DOI: 10.4018/978-1-6684-9962-7.ch014

Government of India. (2020). National Digital Health Mission: Data privacy policy. Retrieved from https://www.ndhm.gov.in

JayaLakshmi. G., Pandey, D., Pandey, B. K., Kaur, P., Mahajan, D. A., & Dari, S. S. (2024). Smart big data collection for intelligent supply chain improvement. In AI and Machine Learning Impacts in Intelligent Supply Chain (pp. 180-195). IGI Global.

Johns Hopkins University. (2022). Global Health Security Index. Retrieved from https://www.ghsindex.org

Kennedy, G. W., Sunday, S. E., Pandey, D., Kabari, A. D., Pandey, B. K., George, A. S., & Dadheech, P. (2024). Building Information Modeling: Harnessing Innovations for Professional Proficiency. In Emerging Engineering Technologies and Industrial Applications (pp. 305-331). IGI Global.

Konapure, C. G., Pandey, D., Shete, H., Thakar, C. M., Pandey, B. K., & George, A. S. (2025). Artificial Intelligence in Automated Concrete Mix Design Using Computerized Grading Curves. Interdisciplinary Approaches to AI, Internet of Everything, and Machine Learning, 567-586.

Kshetri, N. (2021). Cybersecurity management for healthcare organisations. *Journal of Business Research*, *124*, 749–756.

Kumar, B., Pandey, D., Pandey, B. K., & George, A. S. (2024). Higher Education in the Last Four Decades: A Review of Paradigm Shifts in Policy Frameworks. Design and Implementation of Higher Education Learners' Learning Outcomes (HELLO), 333-348.

Kumar, M. S., Prasanna, P. L., Lalitha, M., Joy, M., Jha, S. S., & Pandey, B. K. (2025). Utilizing the Internet of Everything and Artificial Intelligence for Real-Time Workforce Management. In Role of Internet of Everything (IOE), VLSI Architecture, and AI in Real-Time Systems (pp. 153-168). IGI Global Scientific Publishing.

Kumarganesh, S., & Malathi Murugesan, C. (2024). Hybrid plasmonic biosensors with deep learning for colorectal cancer detection. *Plasmonics*, •••, 1–15. DOI: 10.1007/s11468-024-02568-y

Lakshmi, K. V. N., Rajan, R., Pandey, D., & Pandey, B. K. (2024). Circular economy: A catalyst for economic growth-an empirical study. *Circular Economy and Sustainability*, •••, 1–22.

Lee, S., Kim, H., & Park, J. (2021). Enhancing healthcare security using blockchain and quantum cryptography. *Journal of Medical Internet Research, 23*(6), e27682.

Lo, H.-K., Curty, M., & Qi, B. (2012). Measurement-device-independent quantum key distribution. *Physical Review Letters, 108*(13), 130503. DOI: 10.1103/PhysRevLett.108.130503 PMID: 22540686

Madaan, G., Swapna, H. R., Kumar, A., Singh, A., & David, A. (2021). Enactment of sustainable technovations on healthcare sectors. *Asia Pacific Journal of Health Management, 16*(3), 184–192. DOI: 10.24083/apjhm.v16i3.989

Maheshwari, R., Kumarganesh, S., K v M, S., Gopalakrishnan, A., Selvi, K., Paulchamy, B., Rishabavarthani, P., Sagayam, K. M., Pandey, B. K., & Pandey, D. (2024). Advanced plasmonic resonance-enhanced biosensor for comprehensive real-time detection and analysis of deepfake content. *Plasmonics*, •••, 1–18. DOI: 10.1007/s11468-024-02407-0

Maheshwari, R. U., Paulchamy, B., Pandey, B. K., & Pandey, D. (2024). Enhancing sensing and imaging capabilities through surface plasmon resonance for deepfake image detection. *Plasmonics*, •••, 1–20. DOI: 10.1007/s11468-024-02492-1

Mosca, M. (2018). Cybersecurity in an era with quantum computers. *Communications of the ACM, 61*(10), 62–71.

Muralidhar, L. B., Lakshmi, K. V. N., Swapna, H. R., Rupani, J., Nethravathi, K., Pandey, B. K., & Pandey, D. (2024). Impact of Organizational Culture on The Level of Corporate Social Responsibility Investments: An Exploratory Study. *Circular Economy and Sustainability, 4*(3), 1–19. DOI: 10.1007/s43615-024-00371-9

Pan, J. W.. (2018). Long-distance quantum key distribution using entangled photons. *Nature, 549*, 43–47.

Pandey, B. K., Kanike, U. K., George, A. S., & Pandey, D. (Eds.). (2024d). *AI and machine learning impacts in intelligent supply chain*. IGI Global. DOI: 10.4018/979-8-3693-1347-3

Pandey, B. K., Nassa, V. K., Mukundan, A. P., Mahajan, D. A., Pandey, D., George, A. S., & Dadheech, P. (2024c). An Industry-Focused Traffic System Utilising Internet of Things. In *Emerging Engineering Technologies and Industrial Applications* (pp. 200–213). IGI Global. DOI: 10.4018/979-8-3693-1335-0.ch009

Pandey, B. K., & Pandey, D. (2023). Parametric optimization and prediction of enhanced thermoelectric performance in co-doped CaMnO3 using response surface methodology and neural network. *Journal of Materials Science Materials in Electronics, 34*(21), 1589. DOI: 10.1007/s10854-023-10954-1

Pandey, B. K., & Pandey, D. (2025). Securing healthcare medical image information using advance morphological component analysis, information hiding systems, and hybrid convolutional neural networks on IoMT. *Computers in Biology and Medicine*, *185*, 109499. DOI: 10.1016/j.compbiomed.2024.109499 PMID: 39642698

Pandey, B. K., Pandey, D., & Lelisho, M. E. (2024a). Face mask identification with enhanced cuckoo optimization and deep learning-based faster regional neural network. *Scientific Reports*, *14*(1), 29719. DOI: 10.1038/s41598-024-78746-z PMID: 39613761

Pandey, B. K., Pandey, D., & Sahani, S. K. (2024b). Autopilot control unmanned aerial vehicle system for sewage defect detection using deep learning. *Engineering Reports*, •••, 12852.

Pandey, B. K., Pandey, D., & Sahani, S. K. (2025). Autopilot control unmanned aerial vehicle system for sewage defect detection using deep learning. *Engineering Reports*, *7*(1), e12852. DOI: 10.1002/eng2.12852

Pandey, B. K., Paramashivan, M. A., Pandey, D., George, A. S., Agarwal, A., Mahajan, D. A., . . . Pramanik, S. (2024e). Future Directions of Digital Twin Architectures for 6G Communication Networks. In Security Issues and Solutions in 6G Communications and Beyond (pp. 197-211). IGI Global.

Pandey, D., Nassa, V. K., Pandey, B. K., Thankachan, B., Dadheech, P., Mahajan, D. A., & George, A. S. (2024a). Artificial Intelligence and Machine Learning and Its Application in the Field of Computational Visual Analysis. In Emerging Engineering Technologies and Industrial Applications (pp. 36-57). IGI Global. DOI: 10.4018/979-8-3693-1335-0.ch003

Pandey, D., & Pandey, B. K. (2022). An efficient deep neural network with adaptive galactic swarm optimization for complex image text extraction. In *Process Mining Techniques for Pattern Recognition* (pp. 121–137). CRC Press. DOI: 10.1201/9781003169550-10

Pandey, D., Pandey, B. K., Nassa, V. K., Mahajan, D. A., George, A. S., & Dadheech, P. (2024c). Optimized Throughput-Based Broadcasting for Next Generation Wireless Networks. In Emerging Engineering Technologies and Industrial Applications (pp. 355-368). IGI Global. DOI: 10.4018/979-8-3693-1335-0.ch018

Pandey, D., Pandey, B. K., Paramashivan, M. A., Mahajan, D. A., Dadheech, P. D., George, A. S., & Hameed, A. S. (2024b). Advanced Digital Data Processing Using Cloud Cryptography: Industrial Applications. In Emerging Engineering Technologies and Industrial Applications (pp. 255-268). IGI Global.

Pandey, D., Sharma, M., Talwar, R., & Pandey, B. K. (2025). A compact quintuple band miniaturized elliptical planar monopole antenna for 5G/6G wireless systems. *Analog Integrated Circuits and Signal Processing*, *122*(3), 1–16. DOI: 10.1007/s10470-025-02310-6

Pirandola, S., Andersen, U. L., Banchi, L., Berta, M., Bunandar, D., Colbeck, R., & Wehner, S. (2020). Advances in quantum cryptography. *Advances in Optics and Photonics*, *12*(4), 1012–1236. DOI: 10.1364/AOP.361502

Praveenkumar, T., Anthoniraj, S., Kumarganesh, S., Somaskandan, M., Martin Sagayam, K., Pandey, B. K., Pandey, D., & Sahani, S. K. (2025). Enhanced Circuit Board Analysis: Infrared Image Segmentation Utilizing Markov Random Field (MRF) and Level Set Techniques. *Engineering Reports*, *7*(3), e70029. DOI: 10.1002/eng2.70029

PwC. (2021). Healthcare Cybersecurity: A rising priority. Retrieved from https://www.pwc.com

Rai, P. K., Pandey, D., & Pandey, B. K. (2024). The future of enterprise and innovation is compute as a commodity, or CaaC. *Partners Universal International Research Journal*, *3*(2), 89–94.

Sah, M., Chaudhary, R., Sahani, S. K., Sahani, K., Pandey, B. K., Pandey, D., & Lelisho, M. E. (2025). Quantum physical analysis of caffeine and nicotine in CCL4 and DMSO solvent using density functional theory. *Scientific Reports*, *15*(1), 10372. DOI: 10.1038/s41598-025-91211-9 PMID: 40140665

Saravanakumar, R., TamilSelvi, T., Pandey, D., Pandey, B. K., Mahajan, D. A., & Lelisho, M. E. (2024). Big data processing using hybrid Gaussian mixture model with salp swarm algorithm. *Journal of Big Data*, *11*(1), 167. DOI: 10.1186/s40537-024-01015-3

Satheesh, N., Gopisankar, N., Kumarganesh, S., Anthoniraj, S., Saravanakumar, S., & Martin Sagayam, K. (2025). Advanced AI-driven emergency response systems for enhanced vehicle and human safety. *Iran Journal of Computer Science*, •••, 1–16. DOI: 10.1007/s42044-025-00228-w

Saxena, A., Agarwal, A., Pandey, B. K., & Pandey, D. (2024). Examination of the Criticality of Customer Segmentation Using Unsupervised Learning Methods. *Circular Economy and Sustainability*, *4*(2), 1–14. DOI: 10.1007/s43615-023-00336-4

Scarani, V., Bechmann-Pasquinucci, H., Cerf, N. J., Dušek, M., Lütkenhaus, N., & Peev, M. (2009). The security of practical quantum key distribution. *Reviews of Modern Physics*, *81*(3), 1301–1350. DOI: 10.1103/RevModPhys.81.1301

Schneider, F. B. (2020). Cybersecurity and the protection of privacy in telehealth. *Journal of Medical Internet Research, 22*(6), e20257.

IBM Security. (2023). *Cost of a Data Breach Report 2023.*

Shahul, A., Muniandi, B., Paramashivan, M. A., Pandey, D., Pandey, B. K., Dadheech, P., & George, H. (2024). An Analysis of Algorithms and Methods Based on Image Processing for Medical Applications. In *Emerging Engineering Technologies and Industrial Applications* (pp. 173–186). IGI Global. DOI: 10.4018/979-8-3693-1335-0.ch007

Sheela, M. S., Kumarganesh, S., Pandey, B. K., & Lelisho, M. E. (2025). Integration of silver nanostructures in wireless sensor networks for enhanced biochemical sensing. *Discover Nano, 20*(1), 7. DOI: 10.1186/s11671-024-04159-6 PMID: 39804434

Shen, W., Xu, Z., & Li, Z. (2022). Blockchain technology in biomedical imaging: Opportunities and challenges. *IEEE Transactions on Biomedical Engineering, 69*(4), 1123–1135.

Singh, S., Madaan, G., Kaur, J., Swapna, H. R., Pandey, D., Singh, A., & Pandey, B. K. (2023). Bibliometric Review on Healthcare Sustainability. *Handbook of Research on Safe Disposal Methods of Municipal Solid Wastes for a Sustainable Environment*, 142-161.

Singh, S., Madaan, G., Swapna, H. R., Singh, A., Pandey, B. K., George, A. S., & Pandey, D. (2025b). Unleashing the Power of AI and Data Analysis: Transforming Insights into Action. In Interdisciplinary Approaches to AI, Internet of Everything, and Machine Learning (pp. 1-24). IGI Global Scientific Publishing.

Singh, S., Madaan, G., Swapna, H. R., Singh, A., Pandey, D., George, A. S., & Pandey, B. K. (2025a). Empowering Connectivity: Exploring the Internet of Things. In Interdisciplinary Approaches to AI, Internet of Everything, and Machine Learning (pp. 89-116). IGI Global Scientific Publishing.

Sreedhar, C., Kallam, S., Ghantasala, G. P., Anthoniraj, S., Kumarganesh, S., Sagayam, K. M., & Pandey, D. (2025). Enhancing healthcare data security using RFE and CRHSM for big data. *Computers in Biology and Medicine, 190*, 110063. DOI: 10.1016/j.compbiomed.2025.110063 PMID: 40154199

Weingart, S. N. (2021). Ransomware in healthcare: An emerging threat. *The New England Journal of Medicine, 384*(9), 843–845.

Whitman, M. E., & Mattord, H. J. (2018). *Principles of information security.* Cengage Learning.

Yamamoto, K.. (2022). Quantum-secured telemedicine for remote surgery: A pilot study. *Journal of Medical Internet Research, 24*(6), e32743.

Yin, J., Cao, Y., Li, Y.-H., Ren, J.-G., Liao, S.-K., Zhang, L., & Pan, J.-W. (2020). Entanglement-based secure quantum cryptography over 1,120 kilometres. *Nature, 582*(7813), 501–505. DOI: 10.1038/s41586-020-2401-y PMID: 32541968

Zhang, P., Schmidt, D. C., & White, J. (2021). Blockchain applications in healthcare: Strengths and weaknesses. *Health Informatics Journal, 27*(1), 0039–52.

Compilation of References

Abdulkarim, Y. I., Awl, H. N., Muhammadsharif, F. F., Saeed, S. R., Sidiq, K. R., Khasraw, S. S., Dong, J., Pandey, B. K., & Pandey, D. (2024). Metamaterial-based sensors loaded corona-shaped resonator for COVID-19 detection by using microwave techniques. *Plasmonics, 19*(2), 595–610. DOI: 10.1007/s11468-023-02007-4

Abdullahi, M., Ahmad, A., Pandey, B. K., & Pandey, D. (2024). Digital Currency Adoption: A Comparative Analysis of Global Trends and the Nigerian eNaira Digital Currency. *SN Computer Science*, *5*(5), 1–11. DOI: 10.1007/s42979-024-02882-6

Aceto, G., Persico, V., & Pescapé, A. (2020). Industry 4.0 and health: Internet of things, big data, and cloud computing for healthcare 4.0. *Journal of Industrial Information Integration*, *18*, 100129. DOI: 10.1016/j.jii.2020.100129

Agbo, C. C., Mahmoud, Q. H., & Eklund, J. M. (2019, April). Blockchain technology in healthcare: A systematic review. [). MDPI.]. *Health Care*, *7*(2), 56. PMID: 30987333

Ahathiyan, G. S., Du John, H. V., Moni, D. J., Sagayam, K. M., Pandey, B. K., Pandey, D., & Lelisho, M. E. (2025). Design and simulation of a highly efficient eco-friendly, non-toxic perovskite solar cell. *Discover Nano*, *20*(1), 32. DOI: 10.1186/s11671-025-04190-1 PMID: 39937384

Al Kuwaiti, A., Nazer, K., Al-Reedy, A., Al-Shehri, S., Al-Muhanna, A., Subbarayalu, A. V., Al Muhanna, D., & Al-Muhanna, F. A. (2023). A review of the role of artificial intelligence in healthcare. *Journal of Personalized Medicine*, *13*(6), 951. DOI: 10.3390/jpm13060951 PMID: 37373940

Alenoghena, C. O., Onumanyi, A. J., Ohize, H. O., Adejo, A. O., Oligbi, M., Ali, S. I., & Okoh, S. A. (2022). eHealth: A survey of architectures, developments in mHealth, security concerns and solutions. *International Journal of Environmental Research and Public Health*, *19*(20), 13071. DOI: 10.3390/ijerph192013071 PMID: 36293656

Ali, A., Rahim, H. A., Pasha, M. F., Dowsley, R., Masud, M., Ali, J., & Baz, M. (2021). Security, privacy, and reliability in digital healthcare systems using blockchain. *Electronics (Basel)*, *10*(16), 2034. DOI: 10.3390/electronics10162034

Alsubaei, F., Abuhussein, A., Shandilya, V., & Shiva, S. (2019). IoMT-SAF: Internet of medical things security assessment framework. *Internet of Things : Engineering Cyber Physical Human Systems*, *8*, 100123. DOI: 10.1016/j.iot.2019.100123

Annamalai, M., & Jesintha, D. X. M. (2021). Smart iot system based patient monitoring and medicine reminder based on registry service selection scheme. *European Journal of Molecular and Clinical Medicine*, *7*, 2710–2721.

Asghari, P., Rahmani, A. M., & Javadi, H. H. S. (2019). Internet of Things applications: A systematic review. *Computer Networks*, *148*, 241–261. DOI: 10.1016/j.comnet.2018.12.008

Atkinson, A., Ellenberger, B., Piezzi, V., Kaspar, T., Salazar-Vizcaya, L., Endrich, O., Leichtle, A. B., & Marschall, J. (2023). Extending outbreak investigation with machine learning and graph theory: Benefits of new tools with application to a nosocomial outbreak of a multidrug-resistant organism. *Infection Control and Hospital Epidemiology*, *44*(2), 246–252. DOI: 10.1017/ice.2022.66 PMID: 36111457

Bajwa, J., Munir, U., Nori, A., & Williams, B. (2021). Artificial intelligence in healthcare: Transforming the practice of medicine. *Future Healthcare Journal*, *8*(2), e188–e194. DOI: 10.7861/fhj.2021-0095 PMID: 34286183

Basha, A. J., Maheshwari, R. U., Pandey, B. K., & Pandey, D. (2024). Ultra-sensitive photonic crystal fiber–based SPR sensor for cancer detection utilizing hybrid nanocomposite layers. *Plasmonics*, •••, 1–15. DOI: 10.1007/s11468-024-02584-y

Bennett, C. H., & Brassard, G. (1984). Quantum cryptography: Public key distribution and coin tossing. *Proceedings of IEEE International Conference on Computers, Systems and Signal Processing*.

Bhatt, D., Swapna, H. R., Madaan, G., Gayathri, D. K., Mahajan, D. A., Mahajan, R. D., & Paramashivan, M. A. (2024). From Theory to Practice: The Evolution of Artificial Intelligence in Business. In Utilization of AI Technology in Supply Chain Management (pp. 1-14). IGI Global.

Bhattacharya, S., Reddy Maddikunta, P. K., Pham, Q. V., Gadekallu, T. R., & Krishnan, S. (2020, November). S. R., Chowdhary, C. L., Alazab, M., &JalilPiran, M. (2021). Deep learning and medical image processing for coronavirus (COVID-19) pandemic: A survey. *Sustainable Cities and Society*, *65*, 102589. DOI: 10.1016/j.scs.2020.102589 PMID: 33169099

Biamonte, J., Wittek, P., Pancotti, N., Rebentrost, P., Wiebe, N., & Lloyd, S. (2017). Quantum machine learning. *Nature, 549*(7671), 195–202. DOI: 10.1038/nature23474 PMID: 28905917

Bikis, A., Engdaw, M., Pandey, D., & Pandey, B. K. (2025). The impact of urbanization on land use land cover change using geographic information system and remote sensing: A case of Mizan Aman City Southwest Ethiopia. *Scientific Reports, 15*(1), 12014. DOI: 10.1038/s41598-025-94189-6 PMID: 40199909

Brian Brenner, M. D., Scott Brancolini, M. D., Yashar Eshraghi, M. D., Maged Guirguis, M. D., Shravani Durbhakula, M. D., David Provenzano, M. D., & Kevin Vorenkamp, M. D. (2022). Telemedicine implementation in pain medicine: A survey evaluation of pain medicine practices in spring 2020. *Pain Physician, 25*, 387–390. PMID: 35901479

Calegari, L. P., & Fettermann, D. C. (2022). A review of e-health technologies applications. *International Journal of Bioinformatics Research and Applications, 18*(4), 318–357. DOI: 10.1504/IJBRA.2022.126742

Campbell, I. M., Crowley, T. B., Keena, B., Donoghue, S., McManus, M. L., & Zackai, E. H. (2022). The experience of one pediatric geneticist with telemedicine-based clinical diagnosis. *American Journal of Medical Genetics. Part A, 188*(12), 3416–3422. DOI: 10.1002/ajmg.a.62920 PMID: 35906847

Chakraborty, C., Gupta, B., & Ghosh, S. K. (2013). A review on telemedicine-based WBAN framework for patient monitoring. *Telemedicine Journal and e-Health, 19*(8), 619–626. DOI: 10.1089/tmj.2012.0215 PMID: 23841489

Chen, L., Jordan, S., Liu, Y.-K., Moody, D., Peralta, R., Perlner, R., & Smith-Tone, D. (2016). *Report on post-quantum cryptography. NISTIR 8105*. National Institute of Standards and Technology. DOI: 10.6028/NIST.IR.8105

Davis, F. D. (1989). Perceived usefulness, perceived ease of use, and user acceptance of information technology. *Management Information Systems Quarterly, 13*(3), 319–340. DOI: 10.2307/249008

Devaraj, S. J., & Ezra, K. (2011, April). Current trends and future challenges in wireless telemedicine system. In *2011 3rd International Conference on Electronics Computer Technology* (Vol. 4, pp. 417-421). IEEE. DOI: 10.1109/ICECTECH.2011.5941933

Devasenapathy, D., Madhumathy, P., Umamaheshwari, R., Pandey, B. K., & Pandey, D. (2023). Transmission-efficient grid-based synchronized model for routing in wireless sensor networks using Bayesian compressive sensing. *SN Computer Science, 5*(1), 128. DOI: 10.1007/s42979-023-02410-y

Dhanasekar, S., Martin Sagayam, K., Pandey, B. K., & Pandey, D. (2023). Refractive index sensing using metamaterial absorbing augmentation in elliptical graphene arrays. *Plasmonics*, •••, 1–11.

Dhanvijay, M. M., & Patil, S. C. (2019). Internet of Things: A survey of enabling technologies in healthcare and its applications. *Computer Networks*, *153*, 113–131. DOI: 10.1016/j.comnet.2019.03.006

Du John, H. V., Jose, T., Jone, A. A. A., Sagayam, K. M., Pandey, B. K., & Pandey, D. (2022). Polarization insensitive circular ring resonator based perfect metamaterial absorber design and simulation on a silicon substrate. *Silicon*, *14*(14), 9009–9020. DOI: 10.1007/s12633-021-01645-9

Dwivedi, R., Mehrotra, D., & Chandra, S. (2022). Potential of Internet of Medical Things (IoMT) applications in building a smart healthcare system: A systematic review. *Journal of Oral Biology and Craniofacial Research*, *12*(2), 302–318. DOI: 10.1016/j.jobcr.2021.11.010 PMID: 34926140

Ekert, A. (1991). Quantum cryptography is based on Bell's theorem. *Physical Review Letters*, *67*(6), 661–663. DOI: 10.1103/PhysRevLett.67.661 PMID: 10044956

Elarmathi, S., Rishabavarthani, P., Sindhuja, M., Elayaraja, P., & Malathi Murugesan, S. (2024). Novel manufacturing systems for cancer diagnosis using ultra-sensitive photonic crystal fiber biosensor with dual-functionalized aptamer-nanocavity. *Microsystem Technologies*, •••, 1–20. DOI: 10.1007/s00542-024-05820-x

European Commission. (2018). General Data Protection Regulation (GDPR). Retrieved from https://eur-lex.europa.eu

Filonenko, A., & Jo, K. H. (2016). Unattended object identification for intelligent surveillance systems using sequence of dual background difference. *IEEE Transactions on Industrial Informatics*, *12*(6), 2247–2255. DOI: 10.1109/TII.2016.2605582

Ge, H., Li, L., Zhang, D., & Ma, F. (2022). Applications of digital Medicine in oncology: Prospects and challenges. *Cancer Innovation*, *1*(4), 285–292. DOI: 10.1002/cai2.37 PMID: 38089082

George, W. K., Silas, E. I., Pandey, D., & Pandey, B. K. (2024). Utilization of Industry 4.0 Technologies in Nigerian Technical and Vocational Education: A Conundrum for Educators. In *Examining the Rapid Advance of Digital Technology in Africa* (pp. 270–293). IGI Global. DOI: 10.4018/978-1-6684-9962-7.ch014

Ghannam, R. B., & Techtmann, S. M. (2021). Machine learning applications in microbial ecology, human microbiome studies, and environmental monitoring. *Computational and Structural Biotechnology Journal, 19*, 1092–1107. DOI: 10.1016/j.csbj.2021.01.028 PMID: 33680353

Government of India. (2020). National Digital Health Mission: Data privacy policy. Retrieved from https://www.ndhm.gov.in

Guidance, W. H. O. (2021). *Ethics and governance of artificial intelligence for health.* World Health Organization.

Hameed, K., Ali, A., Naqvi, M. H., Jabbar, M., Junaid, M., & Haider, A. (2016, August). Resource management in operating systems-a survey of scheduling algorithms. In *Proceedings of the International Conference on Innovative Computing (ICIC)*, Lanzhou, China (pp. 2-5).

Hester, R. J. (2020). Bioveillance: A techno-security infrastructure to preempt the dangers of informationalised biology. *Science as Culture, 29*(1), 153–176. DOI: 10.1080/09505431.2019.1705270

IBM Security. (2023). *Cost of a Data Breach Report 2023.*

Islam, S. R., Kwak, D., Kabir, M. H., Hossain, M., & Kwak, K. S. (2015). The internet of things for health care: A comprehensive survey. *IEEE Access : Practical Innovations, Open Solutions, 3*, 678–708. DOI: 10.1109/ACCESS.2015.2437951

Istiaque Ahmed, K., Tahir, M., Hadi Habaebi, M., Lun Lau, S., & Ahad, A. (2021). Machine learning for authentication and authorization in iot: Taxonomy, challenges and future research direction. *Sensors (Basel), 21*(15), 5122. DOI: 10.3390/s21155122 PMID: 34372360

JayaLakshmi. G., Pandey, D., Pandey, B. K., Kaur, P., Mahajan, D. A., & Dari, S. S. (2024). Smart big data collection for intelligent supply chain improvement. In AI and Machine Learning Impacts in Intelligent Supply Chain (pp. 180-195). IGI Global Scientific Publishing.

JayaLakshmi. G., Pandey, D., Pandey, B. K., Kaur, P., Mahajan, D. A., & Dari, S. S. (2024). Smart big data collection for intelligent supply chain improvement. In AI and Machine Learning Impacts in Intelligent Supply Chain (pp. 180-195). IGI Global.

Johns Hopkins University. (2022). Global Health Security Index. Retrieved from https://www.ghsindex.org

Kamilaris, A., & Prenafeta-Boldú, F. X. (2018). Deep learning in agriculture: A survey. *Computers and Electronics in Agriculture, 147*, 70–90. DOI: 10.1016/j.compag.2018.02.016

Kennedy, G. W., Sunday, S. E., Pandey, D., Kabari, A. D., Pandey, B. K., George, A. S., & Dadheech, P. (2024). Building Information Modeling: Harnessing Innovations for Professional Proficiency. In *Emerging Engineering Technologies and Industrial Applications* (pp. 305-331). IGI Global.

Khadka, M., Sah, M., Chaudhary, R., Sahani, S. K., Sahani, K., Pandey, B. K., & Pandey, D. (2025). Spectroscopic, quantum chemical, and topological calculations of the phenylephrine molecule using density functional theory. *Scientific Reports, 15*(1), 208. DOI: 10.1038/s41598-024-81633-2 PMID: 39747169

Khan, B., Hasan, A., Pandey, D., Ventayen, R. J. M., Pandey, B. K., & Gowwrii, G. (2021). Fusion of datamining and artificial intelligence in prediction of hazardous road accidents. In *Machine learning and iot for intelligent systems and smart applications* (pp. 201–223). CRC Press. DOI: 10.1201/9781003194415-12

Kim, B., Psannis, K., & Bhaskar, H. (2017). Special section on emerging multimedia technology for smart surveillance system with IoT environment. *The Journal of Supercomputing, 73*(3), 923–925. DOI: 10.1007/s11227-016-1939-9

Kim, H., Kim, S. H., Hwang, J. Y., & Seo, C. (2019). Efficient privacy-preserving machine learning for blockchain network. *IEEE Access : Practical Innovations, Open Solutions, 7*, 136481–136495. DOI: 10.1109/ACCESS.2019.2940052

Kim, I. C., Kim, Y. J., & Chin, S. Y. (2022). Sound localization framework for construction site monitoring. *Applied Sciences (Basel, Switzerland), 12*(21), 10783. DOI: 10.3390/app122110783

Kokkonis, G., Psannis, K. E., Roumeliotis, M., & Schonfeld, D. (2017). Real-time wireless multisensory smart surveillance with 3D-HEVC streams for internet-of-things (IoT). *The Journal of Supercomputing, 73*(3), 1044–1062. DOI: 10.1007/s11227-016-1769-9

Konapure, C. G., Pandey, D., Shete, H., Thakar, C. M., Pandey, B. K., & George, A. S. (2025). Artificial Intelligence in Automated Concrete Mix Design Using Computerized Grading Curves. Interdisciplinary Approaches to AI, Internet of Everything, and Machine Learning, 567-586.

Kshetri, N. (2021). Cybersecurity management for healthcare organisations. *Journal of Business Research, 124*, 749–756.

Kumar Pandey, B., Pandey, D., Nassa, V. K., Ahmad, T., Singh, C., George, A. S., & Wakchaure, M. A. (2021). Encryption and steganography-based text extraction in IoT using the EWCTS optimizer. *Imaging Science Journal*, *69*(1-4), 38–56. DOI: 10.1080/13682199.2022.2146885

Kumar, B., Pandey, D., Pandey, B. K., & George, A. S. (2024). Higher Education in the Last Four Decades: A Review of Paradigm Shifts in Policy Frameworks. Design and Implementation of Higher Education Learners' Learning Outcomes (HELLO), 333-348.

Kumar, M. S., Prasanna, P. L., Lalitha, M., Joy, M., Jha, S. S., & Pandey, B. K. (2025). Utilizing the Internet of Everything and Artificial Intelligence for Real-Time Workforce Management. In Role of Internet of Everything (IOE), VLSI Architecture, and AI in Real-Time Systems (pp. 153-168). IGI Global Scientific Publishing.

Kumarganesh, S., & Malathi Murugesan, C. (2024). Hybrid plasmonic biosensors with deep learning for colorectal cancer detection. *Plasmonics*, •••, 1–15. DOI: 10.1007/s11468-024-02568-y

KVM, S., Pandey, B. K., & Pandey, D. (2024). Design of Surface Plasmon Resonance (SPR) Sensors for Highly Sensitive Biomolecular Detection in Cancer Diagnostics. *Plasmonics*, •••, 1–13.

Lakshmi, K. V. N., Rajan, R., Pandey, D., & Pandey, B. K. (2024). Circular economy: A catalyst for economic growth-an empirical study. *Circular Economy and Sustainability*, •••, 1–22.

Lakshmi, K. V. N., Rajan, R., Pandey, D., & Pandey, B. K. (2024). Circular Economy: A Catalyst for Economic Growth-An Empirical Study. *Circular Economy and Sustainability*, •••, 1–22.

Lee, D., & Yoon, S. N. (2021). Application of artificial intelligence-based technologies in the healthcare industry: Opportunities and challenges. *International Journal of Environmental Research and Public Health*, *18*(1), 271. DOI: 10.3390/ijerph18010271 PMID: 33401373

Lee, S., Kim, H., & Park, J. (2021). Enhancing healthcare security using blockchain and quantum cryptography. *Journal of Medical Internet Research*, *23*(6), e27682.

Lin, Z., Ding, G., Han, J., & Wang, J. (2016). Cross-view retrieval via probability-based semantics-preserving hashing. *IEEE Transactions on Cybernetics*, *47*(12), 4342–4355. DOI: 10.1109/TCYB.2016.2608906 PMID: 28113531

Liu, J., Li, X., Ye, L., Zhang, H., Du, X., & Guizani, M. (2018, December). BPDS: A blockchain based privacy-preserving data sharing for electronic medical records. In *2018 IEEE Global Communications Conference (GLOBECOM)* (pp. 1-6). IEEE. DOI: 10.1109/GLOCOM.2018.8647713

Lo, H.-K., Curty, M., & Qi, B. (2012). Measurement-device-independent quantum key distribution. *Physical Review Letters, 108*(13), 130503. DOI: 10.1103/PhysRevLett.108.130503 PMID: 22540686

Lütkepohl, H. (2010). *Impulse response function.* DOI: 10.1057/9780230280830_16

Madaan, G., Swapna, H. R., Kumar, A., Singh, A., & David, A. (2021). Enactment of sustainable technovations on healthcare sectors. *Asia Pacific Journal of Health Management, 16*(3), 184–192. DOI: 10.24083/apjhm.v16i3.989

Maglietta, R., Carlucci, R., Fanizza, C., & Dimauro, G. (2022). Machine Learning and Image Processing Methods for Cetacean Photo Identification: A Systematic Review. *IEEE Access : Practical Innovations, Open Solutions, 10*(July), 80195–80207. DOI: 10.1109/ACCESS.2022.3195218

Maheshwari, R. U., Paulchamy, B., Pandey, B. K., & Pandey, D. (2024). Enhancing sensing and imaging capabilities through surface plasmon resonance for deepfake image detection. *Plasmonics*, •••, 1–20. DOI: 10.1007/s11468-024-02492-1

Maheshwari, R., Kumarganesh, S., K v M, S., Gopalakrishnan, A., Selvi, K., Paulchamy, B., Rishabavarthani, P., Sagayam, K. M., Pandey, B. K., & Pandey, D. (2024). Advanced plasmonic resonance-enhanced biosensor for comprehensive real-time detection and analysis of deepfake content. *Plasmonics*, •••, 1–18. DOI: 10.1007/s11468-024-02407-0

Martin, R. (2015). The internet of things (iot)–removing the human element. *Infosec Writers, 28*, 12.

Mbonihankuye, S., Nkunzimana, A., & Ndagijimana, A. (2019). Healthcare data security technology: HIPAA compliance. *Wireless Communications and Mobile Computing, 2019*(1), 1927495.

Mekala, M. S., & Viswanathan, P. (2017, August). A Survey: Smart agriculture IoT with cloud computing. In 2017 international conference on microelectronic devices, circuits and systems (ICMDCS) (pp. 1-7). IEEE.

Mohammed, M. A., Mohammed, V. A., & Mohammed, V. A. (2022). Impact of Artificial Intelligence on the Automation of Digital Health System. [IJSEA]. *International Journal of Software Engineering and Its Applications*, •••, 13.

Moore, M. (1999). The evolution of telemedicine. *Future Generation Computer Systems*, *15*(2), 245–254. DOI: 10.1016/S0167-739X(98)00067-3

Mosca, M. (2018). Cybersecurity in an era with quantum computers. *Communications of the ACM*, *61*(10), 62–71.

Muniandi, B., Nassa, V. K., Pandey, D., Pandey, B. K., Dadheech, P., & George, A. S. (2024). Pattern Analysis for Feature Extraction in Complex Images. In Using Machine Learning to Detect Emotions and Predict Human Psychology (pp. 145-167). IGI Global. DOI: 10.4018/979-8-3693-1910-9.ch007

Muralidhar, L. B., Lakshmi, K. V. N., Swapna, H. R., Rupani, J., Nethravathi, K., Pandey, B. K., & Pandey, D. (2024). Impact of Organizational Culture on The Level of Corporate Social Responsibility Investments: An Exploratory Study. *Circular Economy and Sustainability*, *4*(3), 1–19. DOI: 10.1007/s43615-024-00371-9

Niu, K., Chen, Y., & Shen, J. (2021). Dual-channel night vision image restoration method based on deep learning. *Computer Applications (Nottingham)*, *41*(6), 10.

Oh, J. G., & Hong, M. C. (2022). Low-Light Image Enhancement Using Hybrid Deep-Learning and Mixed-Norm Loss Functions. *Sensors (Basel)*, *22*(18), 6904. Advance online publication. DOI: 10.3390/s22186904 PMID: 36146252

Palaniappan, S. V. R., & David, B. (2022). Prediction of epidemic disease dynamics on the infection risk using machine learning algorithms. *SN Computer Science*, *3*(1), 47. DOI: 10.1007/s42979-021-00902-3 PMID: 34755116

Palmer, X., Potter, L. N., & Karahan, S. (2021). COVID-19 and biocybersecurity's increasing role on defending forward. [IJCWT]. *International Journal of Cyber Warfare & Terrorism*, *11*(3), 15–29. DOI: 10.4018/IJCWT.2021070102

Pandey, B. K., Mukundan, A. P., Nassa, V. K., Pandey, D., George, A. S., Hameed, A. S., & Dadheech, P. (2024f). Deployment of Load Balancing in Cloud Computing: Industrial Application and Benefits. In Emerging Engineering Technologies and Industrial Applications (pp. 342-354). IGI Global.

Pandey, B. K., Paramashivan, M. A., Hasan, A., Pramanik, S., Dadheech, P., Manaktala, S. S., & George, A. S. (2024a). Social Psychological Obstacles to the Implementation of Artificial Intelligence in Supply Chain Management. In AI and Machine Learning Impacts in Intelligent Supply Chain (pp. 17-24). IGI Global. DOI: 10.4018/979-8-3693-1347-3.ch002

Pandey, B. K., Paramashivan, M. A., Nassa, V. K., Mahajan, D. A., Dadheech, P., George, A. H., & George, A. S. (2024h). Blockchain's Potential Effect on the Healthcare Industry. In Emerging Engineering Technologies and Industrial Applications (pp. 214-232). IGI Global. DOI: 10.4018/979-8-3693-1335-0.ch010

Pandey, B. K., Paramashivan, M. A., Pandey, D., George, A. S., Agarwal, A., Mahajan, D. A., . . . Pramanik, S. (2024d). Future Directions of Digital Twin Architectures for 6G Communication Networks. In Security Issues and Solutions in 6G Communications and Beyond (pp. 197-211). IGI Global.

Pandey, B. K., Paramashivan, M. A., Pandey, D., George, A. S., Agarwal, A., Mahajan, D. A., . . . Pramanik, S. (2024e). Future Directions of Digital Twin Architectures for 6G Communication Networks. In Security Issues and Solutions in 6G Communications and Beyond (pp. 197-211). IGI Global.

Pandey, D., Nassa, V. K., Pandey, B. K., Thankachan, B., Dadheech, P., Mahajan, D. A., & George, A. S. (2024a). Artificial Intelligence and Machine Learning and Its Application in the Field of Computational Visual Analysis. In Emerging Engineering Technologies and Industrial Applications (pp. 36-57). IGI Global. DOI: 10.4018/979-8-3693-1335-0.ch003

Pandey, D., Pandey, B. K., Nassa, V. K., Mahajan, D. A., George, A. S., & Dadheech, P. (2024c). Optimized Throughput-Based Broadcasting for Next Generation Wireless Networks. In Emerging Engineering Technologies and Industrial Applications (pp. 355-368). IGI Global. DOI: 10.4018/979-8-3693-1335-0.ch018

Pandey, D., Pandey, B. K., Paramashivan, M. A., Mahajan, D. A., Dadheech, P. D., George, A. S., & Hameed, A. S. (2024). Advanced Digital Data Processing Using Cloud Cryptography: Industrial Applications. In Emerging Engineering Technologies and Industrial Applications (pp. 255-268). IGI Global.

Pandey, D., Pandey, B. K., Paramashivan, M. A., Mahajan, D. A., Dadheech, P. D., George, A. S., & Hameed, A. S. (2024b). Advanced Digital Data Processing Using Cloud Cryptography: Industrial Applications. In Emerging Engineering Technologies and Industrial Applications (pp. 255-268). IGI Global.

Pandey, B. K., Kanike, U. K., George, A. S., & Pandey, D. (Eds.). (2024d). *AI and machine learning impacts in intelligent supply chain*. IGI Global. DOI: 10.4018/979-8-3693-1347-3

Pandey, B. K., Nassa, V. K., Mukundan, A. P., Mahajan, D. A., Pandey, D., George, A. S., & Dadheech, P. (2024c). An Industry-Focused Traffic System Utilising Internet of Things. In *Emerging Engineering Technologies and Industrial Applications* (pp. 200–213). IGI Global. DOI: 10.4018/979-8-3693-1335-0.ch009

Pandey, B. K., & Pandey, D. (2023). Parametric optimization and prediction of enhanced thermoelectric performance in co-doped CaMnO3 using response surface methodology and neural network. *Journal of Materials Science Materials in Electronics*, *34*(21), 1589. DOI: 10.1007/s10854-023-10954-1

Pandey, B. K., & Pandey, D. (2025). Securing healthcare medical image information using advance morphological component analysis, information hiding systems, and hybrid convolutional neural networks on IoMT. *Computers in Biology and Medicine*, *185*, 109499. DOI: 10.1016/j.compbiomed.2024.109499 PMID: 39642698

Pandey, B. K., Pandey, D., & Agarwal, A. (2022). Encrypted information transmission by enhanced steganography and image transformation. [IJDAI]. *International Journal of Distributed Artificial Intelligence*, *14*(1), 1–14. DOI: 10.4018/IJDAI.297110

Pandey, B. K., Pandey, D., Dadheech, P., Mahajan, D. A., George, A. S., & Hameed, A. S. (2023). Review on Smart Sewage Cleaning UAV Assistance for Sustainable Development. In *Handbook of Research on Safe Disposal Methods of Municipal Solid Wastes for a Sustainable Environment* (pp. 69–79). IGI Global. DOI: 10.4018/978-1-6684-8117-2.ch005

Pandey, B. K., Pandey, D., & Lelisho, M. E. (2024a). Face mask identification with enhanced cuckoo optimization and deep learning-based faster regional neural network. *Scientific Reports*, *14*(1), 29719. DOI: 10.1038/s41598-024-78746-z PMID: 39613761

Pandey, B. K., Pandey, D., & Sahani, S. K. (2024b). Autopilot control unmanned aerial vehicle system for sewage defect detection using deep learning. *Engineering Reports*, •••, 12852.

Pandey, B. K., Paramashivan, M. A., Kanike, U. K., Mahajan, D. A., Mahajan, R., George, A. S., & Hameed, A. S. H. (2024b). Impacts of Artificial Intelligence and Machine Learning on Intelligent Supply Chains. In *AI and Machine Learning Impacts in Intelligent Supply Chain* (pp. 57–73). IGI Global. DOI: 10.4018/979-8-3693-1347-3.ch005

Pandey, D., & Pandey, B. K. (2022). An efficient deep neural network with adaptive galactic swarm optimization for complex image text extraction. In *Process Mining Techniques for Pattern Recognition* (pp. 121–137). CRC Press. DOI: 10.1201/9781003169550-10

Pandey, D., Sharma, M., Talwar, R., & Pandey, B. K. (2025). A compact quintuple band miniaturized elliptical planar monopole antenna for 5G/6G wireless systems. *Analog Integrated Circuits and Signal Processing*, *122*(3), 1–16. DOI: 10.1007/s10470-025-02310-6

Pandian, P. S., Safeer, K. P., Shakunthala, D. T. I., Gopal, P., & Padaki, V. C. (2007). Store and Forward Applications in Telemedicine for Wireless IP Based Networks. *J. Networks*, *2*(6), 58–65. DOI: 10.4304/jnw.2.6.58-65

Pan, J. W.. (2018). Long-distance quantum key distribution using entangled photons. *Nature*, *549*, 43–47.

Pirandola, S., Andersen, U. L., Banchi, L., Berta, M., Bunandar, D., Colbeck, R., & Wehner, S. (2020). Advances in quantum cryptography. *Advances in Optics and Photonics*, *12*(4), 1012–1236. DOI: 10.1364/AOP.361502

Plageras, A. P., Psannis, K. E., Ishibashi, Y., & Kim, B. G. (2016, October). IoT-based surveillance system for ubiquitous healthcare. In *IECON 2016-42nd Annual Conference of the IEEE Industrial Electronics Society* (pp. 6226-6230). IEEE. DOI: 10.1109/IECON.2016.7793281

Potter, L., Ayala, O., & Palmer, X. L. (2021, February). Biocybersecurity: A converging threat as an auxiliary to war. In *ICCWS 2021 16th international conference on cyber warfare and security* (p. 291).

Praveenkumar, T., Anthoniraj, S., Kumarganesh, S., Somaskandan, M., Martin Sagayam, K., Pandey, B. K., Pandey, D., & Sahani, S. K. (2025). Enhanced Circuit Board Analysis: Infrared Image Segmentation Utilizing Markov Random Field (MRF) and Level Set Techniques. *Engineering Reports*, *7*(3), e70029. DOI: 10.1002/eng2.70029

Provenzano, S., Santangelo, O. E., Giordano, D., Alagna, E., Piazza, D., Genovese, D., & Firenze, A. (2019). Predicting disease outbreaks: Evaluating measles infection with Wikipedia Trends. *Recenti Progressi in Medicina*, *110*(6), 292–296. PMID: 31282485

Pryor, L., Dave, R., Seliya, J., & Boone, E. S. (2021, December). Machine learning algorithms in user authentication schemes. In *2021 International Conference on Electrical, Computer and Energy Technologies (ICECET)* (pp. 1-6). IEEE. DOI: 10.1109/ICECET52533.2021.9698440

Puvvadi, U. L., Di Benedetto, K., Patil, A., Kang, K. D., & Park, Y. (2015). Cost-effective security support in real-time video surveillance. *IEEE Transactions on Industrial Informatics*, *11*(6), 1457–1465. DOI: 10.1109/TII.2015.2491259

PwC. (2021). Healthcare Cybersecurity: A rising priority. Retrieved from https://www.pwc.com

Qayyum, A., Qadir, J., Bilal, M., & Al-Fuqaha, A. (2020). Secure and robust machine learning for healthcare: A survey. *IEEE Reviews in Biomedical Engineering*, *14*, 156–180. DOI: 10.1109/RBME.2020.3013489 PMID: 32746371

Rai, P. K., Pandey, D., & Pandey, B. K. (2024). The future of enterprise and innovation is compute as a commodity, or CaaC. *Partners Universal International Research Journal*, *3*(2), 89–94.

Ray, P. P. (2018). A survey on Internet of Things architectures. *Journal of King Saud University. Computer and Information Sciences*, *30*(3), 291–319. DOI: 10.1016/j.jksuci.2016.10.003

Revathi, T. K., Sathiyabhama, B., Sankar, S., Pandey, D., Pandey, B. K., & Dadeech, P. (2022). An intelligent model for coronary heart disease diagnosis. In *Networking Technologies in Smart Healthcare* (pp. 309–327). CRC Press. DOI: 10.1201/9781003239888-15

Roth, J. A., Battegay, M., Juchler, F., Vogt, J. E., & Widmer, A. F. (2018). Introduction to machine learning in digital healthcare epidemiology. *Infection Control and Hospital Epidemiology*, *39*(12), 1457–1462. DOI: 10.1017/ice.2018.265 PMID: 30394238

Roy, S., Biswas, P., & Ghosh, P. (2021). Spatiotemporal tracing of pandemic spread from infection data. *Scientific Reports*, *11*(1), 17689.

Sadoughi, F., Behmanesh, A., & Sayfouri, N. (2020). Internet of things in medicine: A systematic mapping study. *Journal of Biomedical Informatics*, *103*, 103383. DOI: 10.1016/j.jbi.2020.103383 PMID: 32044417

Sahani, K., Khadka, S. S., Sahani, S. K., Pandey, B. K., & Pandey, D. (2024b). A possible underground roadway for transportation facilities in Kathmandu Valley: A racking deformation of underground rectangular structures. *Engineering Reports*, *6*(8), e12821. DOI: 10.1002/eng2.12821

Sahani, S. K., Pandey, B. K., & Pandey, D. (2024a). *Single-valued Signals, Multi-valued Signals and Fixed-Point of Contractive Signals*. Mathematics Open. DOI: 10.1142/S2811007224500020

Sah, M., Chaudhary, R., Sahani, S. K., Sahani, K., Pandey, B. K., Pandey, D., & Lelisho, M. E. (2025). Quantum physical analysis of caffeine and nicotine in CCL4 and DMSO solvent using density functional theory. *Scientific Reports*, *15*(1), 10372. DOI: 10.1038/s41598-025-91211-9 PMID: 40140665

Saravanakumar, R., TamilSelvi, T., Pandey, D., Pandey, B. K., Mahajan, D. A., & Lelisho, M. E. (2024). Big data processing using hybrid Gaussian mixture model with salp swarm algorithm. *Journal of Big Data*, *11*(1), 167. DOI: 10.1186/s40537-024-01015-3

Satheesh, N., Gopisankar, N., Kumarganesh, S., Anthoniraj, S., Saravanakumar, S., & Martin Sagayam, K. (2025). Advanced AI-driven emergency response systems for enhanced vehicle and human safety. *Iran Journal of Computer Science*, ●●●, 1–16. DOI: 10.1007/s42044-025-00228-w

Saxena, A., Agarwal, A., Pandey, B. K., & Pandey, D. (2024). Examination of the Criticality of Customer Segmentation Using Unsupervised Learning Methods. *Circular Economy and Sustainability*, *4*(2), 1–14. DOI: 10.1007/s43615-023-00336-4

Saxena, A., Sharma, N. K., Pandey, D., & Pandey, B. K. (2021). Influence of tourists satisfaction on future behavioral intentions with special reference to desert triangle of Rajasthan. *Augmented Human Research*, *6*(1), 13. DOI: 10.1007/s41133-021-00052-4

Scarani, V., Bechmann-Pasquinucci, H., Cerf, N. J., Dušek, M., Lütkenhaus, N., & Peev, M. (2009). The security of practical quantum key distribution. *Reviews of Modern Physics*, *81*(3), 1301–1350. DOI: 10.1103/RevModPhys.81.1301

Schneider, F. B. (2020). Cybersecurity and the protection of privacy in telehealth. *Journal of Medical Internet Research*, *22*(6), e20257.

Shamshad, F., Khan, S., Zamir, S. W., Khan, M. H., Hayat, M., Khan, F. S., & Fu, H. (2023). Transformers in medical imaging: A survey. *Medical Image Analysis*, *88*, 102802. DOI: 10.1016/j.media.2023.102802 PMID: 37315483

Sharma, M., Talwar, R., Nassa, V. K., Binay, K., & Pandey, D. (2025). Design and performance analysis of a multiband vivaldi antenna for wireless broadband communication in 3-5.6 GHz spectrum. In *Artificial Intelligence and Information Technologies* (pp. 86–91). CRC Press.

Sheela, M. S., Kumarganesh, S., Pandey, B. K., & Lelisho, M. E. (2025). Integration of silver nanostructures in wireless sensor networks for enhanced biochemical sensing. *Discover Nano*, *20*(1), 7. DOI: 10.1186/s11671-024-04159-6 PMID: 39804434

Shelton, J., Rice, C., Singh, J., Jenkins, J., Dave, R., Roy, K., & Chakraborty, S. (2018, August). Palm print authentication on a cloud platform. In 2018 International Conference on Advances in Big Data, Computing and Data Communication Systems (icABCD) (pp. 1-6). IEEE. DOI: 10.1109/ICABCD.2018.8465479

Shen, W., Xu, Z., & Li, Z. (2022). Blockchain technology in biomedical imaging: Opportunities and challenges. *IEEE Transactions on Biomedical Engineering*, *69*(4), 1123–1135.

Shreyas, K. K., Rajeev, S., Panetta, K., & Agaian, S. S. (2017, April). Fingerprint authentication using geometric features. In *2017 IEEE International Symposium on Technologies for Homeland Security (HST)* (pp. 1-7). IEEE.

Siddiqui, N., Pryor, L., & Dave, R. (2021). User authentication schemes using machine learning methods—a review. In Proceedings of International Conference on Communication and Computational Technologies: ICCCT 2021 (pp. 703-723). Springer Singapore. DOI: 10.1007/978-981-16-3246-4_54

Singh, S., Madaan, G., Kaur, J., Swapna, H. R., Pandey, D., Singh, A., & Pandey, B. K. (2023). Bibliometric Review on Healthcare Sustainability. *Handbook of Research on Safe Disposal Methods of Municipal Solid Wastes for a Sustainable Environment*, 142-161.

Singh, S., Madaan, G., Swapna, H. R., Singh, A., Pandey, B. K., George, A. S., & Pandey, D. (2025b). Unleashing the Power of AI and Data Analysis: Transforming Insights into Action. In Interdisciplinary Approaches to AI, Internet of Everything, and Machine Learning (pp. 1-24). IGI Global Scientific Publishing.

Singh, S., Madaan, G., Swapna, H. R., Singh, A., Pandey, D., George, A. S., & Pandey, B. K. (2025). Empowering Connectivity: Exploring the Internet of Things. In Interdisciplinary Approaches to AI, Internet of Everything, and Machine Learning (pp. 89-116). IGI Global Scientific Publishing.

Singh, S., Madaan, G., Swapna, H. R., Singh, A., Pandey, D., George, A. S., & Pandey, B. K. (2025a). Empowering Connectivity: Exploring the Internet of Things. In Interdisciplinary Approaches to AI, Internet of Everything, and Machine Learning (pp. 89-116). IGI Global Scientific Publishing.

Sreedhar, C., Kallam, S., Ghantasala, G. P., Anthoniraj, S., Kumarganesh, S., Sagayam, K. M., & Pandey, D. (2025). Enhancing healthcare data security using RFE and CRHSM for big data. *Computers in Biology and Medicine*, *190*, 110063. DOI: 10.1016/j.compbiomed.2025.110063 PMID: 40154199

Stergiou, C., Psannis, K. E., Plageras, A. P., Kokkonis, G., & Ishibashi, Y. (2017, June). Architecture for security monitoring in IoT environments. In *2017 IEEE 26th international symposium on industrial electronics (ISIE)* (pp. 1382-1385). IEEE. DOI: 10.1109/ISIE.2017.8001447

Stergiou, C., Psannis, K. E., Kim, B. G., & Gupta, B. (2018). Secure integration of IoT and cloud computing. *Future Generation Computer Systems*, *78*, 964–975. DOI: 10.1016/j.future.2016.11.031

Stewart, L. A., Clarke, M., Rovers, M., Riley, R. D., Simmonds, M., Stewart, G., & Tierney, J. F. (2015). Preferred reporting items for a systematic review and meta-analysis of individual participant data: The PRISMA-IPD statement. *Journal of the American Medical Association*, *313*(16), 1657–1665. DOI: 10.1001/jama.2015.3656 PMID: 25919529

Swapna, H. R., Bigirimana, E., Geetha, R., Paramashivan, M. A., George, A. S., Dadheech, P., & Vyas, V. (2024c). New Insights Into Strategic Consumer Behavior From the Field of Operations Management. In Utilization of AI Technology in Supply Chain Management (pp. 289-298). IGI Global. DOI: 10.4018/979-8-3693-3593-2.ch019

Swapna, H. R., Geetanjali, S., Lakshmi, K. V. N., Paramashivan, M. A., Nikhil, M. S., Dadheech, P., & Vyas, V. (2024b). Navigating the Transformative Journey: AI's Progression in Business Applications. In Utilization of AI Technology in Supply Chain Management (pp. 15-25). IGI Global.

Swapna, H. R., Hukkeri, S. V., Pandey, D., & Paramashivan, M. A. (2024a). Cosmopolitan living during the COVID-19 Era: Navigating Challenges and Uniting Communities-An Impact Analysis. In Impact of Climate Change on Mental Health and Well-Being (pp. 1-10). IGI Global.

Tareke, S. A., Lelisho, M. E., Hassen, S. S., Seid, A. A., Jemal, S. S., Teshale, B. M., & Pandey, B. K. (2022). The prevalence and predictors of depressive, anxiety, and stress symptoms among Tepi town residents during the COVID-19 pandemic lockdown in Ethiopia. *Journal of Racial and Ethnic Health Disparities*, •••, 1–13. PMID: 35028903

Thomasian, N. M., & Adashi, E. Y. (2021). Cybersecurity in the internet of medical things. *Health Policy and Technology*, *10*(3), 100549. DOI: 10.1016/j.hlpt.2021.100549

Tortorella, G. L., Saurin, T. A., Fogliatto, F. S., Rosa, V. M., Tonetto, L. M., & Magrabi, F. (2021). Impacts of Healthcare 4.0 digital technologies on the resilience of hospitals. *Technological Forecasting and Social Change*, *166*, 120666. DOI: 10.1016/j.techfore.2021.120666

Usak, M., Kubiatko, M., Shabbir, M. S., Viktorovna Dudnik, O., Jermsittiparsert, K., & Rajabion, L. (2020). Health care service delivery based on the Internet of things: A systematic and comprehensive study. *International Journal of Communication Systems*, *33*(2), e4179. DOI: 10.1002/dac.4179

Vinodhini, V., Kumar, M. S., Sankar, S., Pandey, D., Pandey, B. K., & Nassa, V. K. (2022). IoT-based early forest fire detection using MLP and AROC method. *International Journal of Global Warming*, *27*(1), 55–70. DOI: 10.1504/IJGW.2022.122794

Vinod, S. K., Jameson, M. G., Min, M., & Holloway, L. C. (2016). Uncertainties in volume delineation in radiation oncology: A systematic review and recommendations for future studies. *Radiotherapy and Oncology : Journal of the European Society for Therapeutic Radiology and Oncology*, *121*(2), 169–179. DOI: 10.1016/j.radonc.2016.09.009 PMID: 27729166

Vora, J., Italiya, P., Tanwar, S., Tyagi, S., Kumar, N., Obaidat, M. S., & Hsiao, K. F. (2018, July). Ensuring privacy and security in e-health records. In *2018 International conference on computer, information and telecommunication systems (CITS)* (pp. 1-5). IEEE. DOI: 10.1109/CITS.2018.8440164

Vyas, S., Bhargava, D., & Khan, S. (2023). Healthcare 4.0: A systematic review and its impact over conventional healthcare system. Artificial Intelligence for Health 4.0: Challenges and Applications, 1-17.

Wang, S., Cao, G., Wang, Y., Liao, S., Wang, Q., Shi, J., Li, C., & Shen, D. (2021). Review and prospect: Artificial intelligence in advanced medical imaging. *Frontiers in Radiology*, *1*, 781868. DOI: 10.3389/fradi.2021.781868 PMID: 37492170

Weingart, S. N. (2021). Ransomware in healthcare: An emerging threat. *The New England Journal of Medicine*, *384*(9), 843–845.

Whitman, M. E., & Mattord, H. J. (2018). *Principles of information security*. Cengage Learning.

Yamamoto, K.. (2022). Quantum-secured telemedicine for remote surgery: A pilot study. *Journal of Medical Internet Research*, *24*(6), e32743.

Yang, X., Qian, X., & Mei, T. (2015). Learning salient visual word for scalable mobile image retrieval. *Pattern Recognition*, *48*(10), 3093–3101. DOI: 10.1016/j.patcog.2014.12.017

Yan, L., Fu, J., Wang, C., Ye, Z., Chen, H., & Ling, H. (2021). Enhanced network optimized generative adversarial network for image enhancement. *Multimedia Tools and Applications*, *80*(9), 14363–14381. DOI: 10.1007/s11042-020-10310-z

Yin, J., Cao, Y., Li, Y.-H., Ren, J.-G., Liao, S.-K., Zhang, L., & Pan, J.-W. (2020). Entanglement-based secure quantum cryptography over 1,120 kilometres. *Nature*, *582*(7813), 501–505. DOI: 10.1038/s41586-020-2401-y PMID: 32541968

Yusof, M. M., Papazafeiropoulou, A., Paul, R. J., & Stergioulas, L. K. (2008). Investigating evaluation frameworks for health information systems. *International Journal of Medical Informatics*, *77*(6), 377–385. DOI: 10.1016/j.ijmedinf.2007.08.004 PMID: 17904898

Zarei, M., Mohammadian, A., & Ghasemi, R. (2016). Internet of things in industries: A survey for sustainable development. *International Journal of Innovation and Sustainable Development, 10*(4), 419–442. DOI: 10.1504/IJISD.2016.079586

Zhang, P., Schmidt, D. C., & White, J. (2021). Blockchain applications in healthcare: Strengths and weaknesses. *Health Informatics Journal, 27*(1), 0039–52.

Zhang, P. (2022). Image Enhancement Method Based on Deep Learning. *Mathematical Problems in Engineering, 2022*, 1–9. Advance online publication. DOI: 10.1155/2022/6797367 PMID: 35781947

Zhang, R., Guo, L., Huang, S., & Wen, B. (2021). ReLLIE: Deep reinforcement learning for customized low-light image enhancement.In *Proceedings of the 29th ACM international conference on multimedia*, pp. 2429-2437. DOI: 10.1145/3474085.3475410

About the Contributors

Binay Kumar Pandey is an Assistant Professor at Govind Ballabh Pant University of Agriculture and Technology in Pantnagar, Uttarakhand, India. He obtained his education qualification in the field of Information Technology, with a focus on Bioinformatics, image processing, and high-performance computing. In 2005, he received his first degree in B. Tech. from IET Lucknow (Uttar Pradesh Technical University, Uttar Pradesh, Lucknow), India. He started working as an assistant professor in the department of information technology at Govind Ballabh Pant University of Agriculture and Technology in Pantnagar in 2010 and has since worked on a wide range of UG and PG projects. He has over a decade of experience in the fields of teaching and research. He has over 70 publications in prestigious journals, including those from renowned publishers Springer, Inderscience, Taylor & Francis (SCIE/Scopus Indexed Journals, and others), as well as three patents published in the Indian official journal of patents and two patents published in the Australian official journal of patents. He is also an editor of scientific books published by international publishers such as NOVA International. He has received numerous awards, including the PM Scholarship, among others. He chaired a session at the IEEE International Conference on Advent Trends in Multidisciplinary Research and Innovation (ICATMRI-2020) on December 30, 2020, hosted by Pankaj Laddhad Institute of Technology and Management Studies in Buldhana, Maharashtra, India, and is a reviewer for SCI/Scopus indexed journals published by Springer, Wiley, Inder Science, Tech Science Publishers, Elsevier, and several others. He is an associate editor of SN Social Sciences, a multidisciplinary journal published by Springer Nature and Partners Universal International Research Journal (PUIRJ).

A. Shaji George Cooperate advisory board of trustees as a Deputy Vice President (Administration) West Coast University International, Nigeria, West Africa. Trainer and Counsellor of the National Human Rights and Humanitarian Federation -NHRF, Kerala India. A recognized technical expert in ICT Systems,

Network & Telecommunication, designed and deployed large scale ICT projects. Having published more than sixty research papers in National and International Journals with impact factors, his research interests include Wireless, Networking, Cloud Computing, Image Processing Big Data, IoT and industrial automation systems.

Sameer Tiwari is a highly dedicated and established biological scientist with 16 years of research experience in diverse areas relevant to infectious diseases, and gastrointestinal disorders. After his master's in microbiology, he learned molecular techniques, research skills, and drug testing from nationally importance research institutions. He started his research career with a doctoral study focused on the role of mycobacterial kinases in pathogenicity. His postdoctoral work involves the role of autophagy in maintaining homeostasis in intestinal goblet cells, investigating virulence factors of mycoplasma infection in mammary glands, serving several prestigious institutions around the globe, such as CSIR-Central Drug Research Institute, India; PGIMER Chandigarh, India; University of Calgary, Canada, and Hebrew University of Jerusalem, Israel. Moreover, during the COVID-19 pandemic, he served as a scientist and founding member of a BSL2 laboratory and played a significant role in the SARS-Cov2 diagnosis from patient samples by RT-PCR. Currently, he is associated with George Mason University, Virginia, USA as a postdoctoral scientist focused on investigating the antiviral mechanisms that prevent HIV from invading target cells. He has accomplishments include presenting at several national and international conferences and publishing several manuscripts as author and co-author in reputed journals.

Salah A Albermany is working as senior Professor in Department of Computer Science, Faculty of Computer Science and Mathematics, Kufa University, Iraq. In expert in field of Algorithms Computer Communications (Networks) Computer Security and Reliability. Skills and expertise Authentication Cryptography Network Security Computer Networks Security Applied Cryptography Algorithm Analysis Wireless Security Algorithms Encryption Digital Signature Number Theory Algebraic Number Theory Algebraic Cryptography

Ho Sy Hung is currently a lecturer at Hong Duc University, Vietnam. His position is the head of the department of pre-school education of Hong Duc University. He has been teaching in the education field for more than 10 years. He has a PhD in educational science from Hanoi National University of Education in 2020. This is the best quality pedagogical school in Vietnam. He spends most of my time teaching and researching education, especially early childhood education

***

Mukundan A P is a seasoned data professional with over 20 years of experience in driving strategic growth and innovation through data-driven strategies. Currently serving as the Director & Chief Growth Officer at Champions Group, Singapore, Mukundan excels in leveraging advanced analytics, machine learning, and data governance to optimize business operations and expand global markets. His technical expertise spans SQL, Hadoop, Python, R, and cloud platforms like AWS and Google Cloud. Mukundan is also proficient in data mining, machine learning, and data visualization tools such as Tableau and Power BI. He has a strong background in Statistical Analysis and Big Data technologies, making him a well-rounded leader in the data science field. Mukundan's leadership style is holistic and collaborative, focusing on nurturing talent and fostering high-performing teams. He is known for his ability to translate complex data insights into actionable growth strategies, aligning them with business goals. His work has been recognized with several awards. As a mentor and public speaker, Mukundan shares his knowledge with the next generation of data professionals, emphasizing the importance of data ethics and responsible technology use. His visionary yet pragmatic approach ensures that his strategies are not only innovative but also ethically sound. Mukundan's extensive experience in data management and strategic leadership makes him a valuable asset in any organization looking to drive growth through data-driven decision-making.

Joshuva Arockia Dhanraj is currently an Associate Professor in Computer Science and Engineering (AI & ML) at the School of Engineering, Dayananda Sagar University. Previously, he worked at the Centre for Automation and Robotics (ANRO), Department of Mechatronics Engineering, Hindustan University, Chennai, Tamil Nadu, India. He also served as a Post-Doctoral Researcher in Environmental Assessment and Technology for Hazardous Waste Management Research Center at the Faculty of Environmental Management, Prince of Songkla University, Thailand. He is associated as Adjunct Faculty at the University Centre for Research & Development (UCRD), Chandigarh University, Mohali, Punjab, India and also as an Adjunct Faculty at the Research and Development Cell, Lovely Professional University, Jalandhar-Delhi Grand Trunk Road, Phagwara, Punjab, India and the Chief Research Manager and Advisor of Smart Green Grid Solutions, India. He earned his Bachelor of Engineering in Electronics and Communication Engineering from Anna University, Chennai, Tamil Nadu, India, in 2012, his Master of Technology in Mechatronics from VIT University, Chennai Campus, Tamil Nadu, India, and his Master of Business Administration in Human Resource Management from the University of Madras, Chennai, Tamil Nadu, India, in 2015. He completed his doctoral degree in Mechanical Engineering (Mechatronics specialization) from

VIT University, Chennai Campus, Tamil Nadu, India, in 2018. With 6+ years of teaching experience, 3 years of research experience, and 1 year of post-doctoral experience, he has published over 190+ papers in peer-reviewed SCI/Scopus-indexed international journals and has filed nearly 11 national and 10 international patents. His research interests include Artificial Intelligence and Machine Learning, Mechatronics, Machine Fault Diagnosis and Prognosis, Robotics and Automation, Structural Health and Condition Monitoring, and Renewable Energy Applications towards Sustainable Development Goals (SDG).

Joshuva Arockia Dhanraj is currently an Associate Professor in Computer Science and Engineering (AI & ML) at the School of Engineering, Dayananda Sagar University. Previously, he worked at the Centre for Automation and Robotics (ANRO), Department of Mechatronics Engineering, Hindustan University, Chennai, Tamil Nadu, India. He also served as a Post-Doctoral Researcher in Environmental Assessment and Technology for Hazardous Waste Management Research Center at the Faculty of Environmental Management, Prince of Songkla University, Thailand. He is associated as Adjunct Faculty at the University Centre for Research & Development (UCRD), Chandigarh University, Mohali, Punjab, India and also as an Adjunct Faculty at the Research and Development Cell, Lovely Professional University, Jalandhar-Delhi Grand Trunk Road, Phagwara, Punjab, India and the Chief Research Manager and Advisor of Smart Green Grid Solutions, India. He earned his Bachelor of Engineering in Electronics and Communication Engineering from Anna University, Chennai, Tamil Nadu, India, in 2012, his Master of Technology in Mechatronics from VIT University, Chennai Campus, Tamil Nadu, India, and his Master of Business Administration in Human Resource Management from the University of Madras, Chennai, Tamil Nadu, India, in 2015. He completed his doctoral degree in Mechanical Engineering (Mechatronics specialization) from VIT University, Chennai Campus, Tamil Nadu, India, in 2018. With 5.5 years of teaching experience, 3 years of research experience, and 1 year of post-doctoral experience, he has published over 190+ papers in peer-reviewed SCI/Scopus-indexed international journals and has filed nearly 11 national and 7 international patents. His research interests include Artificial Intelligence and Machine Learning, Mechatronics, Machine Fault Diagnosis and Prognosis, Robotics and Automation, Structural Health and Condition Monitoring, and Renewable Energy Applications towards Sustainable Development Goals (SDG).

Muralidhar L B is a professionally qualified dental surgeon. He holds a Ph.D. from Canara Bank School of Management Studies, Bangalore University, after his MBA from Christ University. He is qualified in management at UGC - NET and KSET. He has 18 years of total teaching experience spanning across dental education, healthcare management and general management and 4 years of corporate experience. He has worked as a research associate in the Institute for Social and Economic Change, Bangalore in a project entitled as "Management By and For Common Man: An Exploration of the Concept and Direction for Future"post Ph.D. He had secured 28th rank in the S.S.L.C. examination for Karnataka State in 1993. His 25 patents have been published, and 2 design patents have been granted. He has 36 research publications to his credit, of which 13 are Scopus-indexed and 5 are ABDC indexed. He has co-authored 11 books and 6 book chapters.. He is supervising Ph.D. research of 3 research scholars at JAIN (Deemed to be University). He works as an assistant professor in the Department of Business Management Studies, School of Commerce, Jain Deemed to be a University student in Bangalore.

Prince Chelladurai S is an Assistant Professor in the Department of Computational Intelligence at SRM University Chennai. He received his Ph.D. in Information and Communication Engineering from Anna University Chennai. His research interests span both Cryptography and Network Security. Much of his work has been on improving the understanding, design, and performance of cloud, IOT and networked computer systems, mainly through the application of Cryptography and Network Security.

Pankaj Dadheech is currently working as a Professor & Deputy Head in the Department of Computer Science & Engineering (NBA Accredited), Swami Keshvanand Institute of Technology, Management & Gramothan (SKIT), Jaipur, Rajasthan, India (Accredited by NAAC A++ Grade). He has more than 18 years of experience in teaching. He is currently working a Professor & Dy. HOD in the Department of Computer Science & Engineering (NBA Accredited), Swami Keshvanand Institute of Technology, Management & Gramothan (SKIT), Jaipur, Rajasthan, India. He has published 25 Patents at Intellectual Property India, Office of the Controller General of Patents, Design and Trade Marks, Department of Industrial Policy and Promotion, Ministry of Commerce and Industry, Government of India. He has published 8 International Patents (USA, South African, Australian, Germany) & 2 Copyrights. He has 73 publications in various International & National Journals, 63 papers in various National & International conferences. He has published 9 Books & 45 Book Chapters.

Sonia Duggal With 28 years of extensive experience in both education and corporate sectors, Dr. Sonia Duggal brings a wealth of knowledge and expertise. Her domain expertise spans Cloud Computing and the Internet of Things (IoT), areas in which she has made significant contributions through numerous publications, edited books, published chapters, and patents. Her work is well-recognized in the academic community, with several publications indexed in Scopus. She is known for her unwavering commitment and dedication to her roles and responsibilities, consistently demonstrating high levels of professionalism and excellence. Professional Experience • Education and Corporate Experience: Over 28 years of experience in various roles, including teaching, research, and corporate positions, providing a unique blend of practical and theoretical knowledge. • Domain Expertise: Specialized in Cloud Computing and IoT, with a strong track record of research and innovation in these fields. Publications and Contributions • Scopus-Indexed Publications: Authored numerous research papers published in high-impact journals indexed in Scopus. • Edited Books and Published Chapters: Edited several books and contributed chapters to various academic publications, showcasing a broad range of expertise and thought leadership. • Patents: Holder of multiple patents, reflecting a strong emphasis on innovation and practical applications of research. Commitment and Dedication • Professionalism: Known for a high level of commitment and dedication in all roles, consistently delivering quality work and contributing to the advancement of knowledge in the field. • Leadership and Collaboration: Demonstrated ability to lead research projects and collaborate with peers, fostering a productive and innovative research environment. Skills and Competencies • Research and Analysis: Strong analytical skills with a proven ability to conduct thorough research and present findings effectively. • Editorial Skills: Experienced in editing and reviewing academic manuscripts, ensuring the highest standards of quality and integrity. • Communication: Excellent written and verbal communication skills, capable of conveying complex ideas clearly and concisely. Professional Affiliations • Memberships: Active member of various professional organizations related to Cloud Computing and IoT, staying updated with the latest trends and developments in the field. • Editorial Boards: Served on the editorial boards of several reputed journals, contributing to the peer-review process and editorial decision-making.

Ashish Jolly is an Assistant Professor in the Department of Computer Science at the Govt PG College Ambala Cantt Haryana.

K Nethravathi is a program coordinator and assistant professor at SOC, JAIN (Deemed-to-be University) Bangalore, Karnataka, India.

G.Kalaiarasi has received her B.Tech., degree in Information Technology from Srinivasa Institute of Engineering & Technology affiliated to Madras University. She has completed M.E., in Computer Science & Engineering Dhanalakshmi Srinivasan Engineering College which is affiliated to Anna University. She obtained her Ph.D., degree in Information & Communication Engineering, Anna University, Chennai.

She has published papers in National & International Journals and Conferences. Her research areas are Computer Vision, Image Processing, Image Retrieval, Content Based Multimedia Retrieval and Data Mining. She has served at various Educational Institutions. She has more than twelve years of teaching experience. Currently she is working in Sathyabama Institute of Science and Technology.

Lakshmi Chandrakanth Kasireddy holds a Master of Computer Applications (MCA) degree from Jawaharlal Nehru Technological University, Kakinada, and a Bachelor of Science (B.Sc.) degree from Andhra University. He is currently based in the United States, working as a Cloud Architect, leveraging his expertise in Cloud Architecture to design and implement robust cloud solutions. With over 14 years of experience in the computer science industry, Chandra has developed a deep specialization in Cloud Architecture. He is also pursuing a Ph.D. with a focus on AI-Driven Cybersecurity, contributing to cutting-edge research in the intersection of artificial intelligence and cybersecurity. Chandra has published several research papers in prestigious journals and conferences, particularly in the fields of Cybersecurity, Artificial Intelligence, and Machine Learning. His work has been featured in renowned platforms such as Web of Science, Scopus-indexed journals, and IEEE conferences, reflecting his significant contributions to both industry and academia.

Krishna Murthy Inumula holds the position of Associate Professor at Symbiosis Institute of International Business (SIIB), Pune. He possesses 20 years of experience in the field of management education. His research interests encompass Data-Driven Models, Predictive Modeling, Simulation, and Benchmarking. He has authored and contributed to management topics, with over 50 papers and articles published in national and international journals and presented at conferences.

Devanga Dharani Lakshmi Working as Assistant Professor(T&C), Department of Computer science in Central University of Andhra Pradesh. I have completed my Ph.D. from JNTUA in the year of 2023 with specialization in Power Electronics, Artificial Intelligence and Data science. I completed my masters and Bachelors from Anantha Lakshmi Institute of Technology and sciences in the year of 2017 and 2014. I have total 6.5 years of Experience in both Teaching and Industrial Experience

Niladri Maiti is serving as the Founding Dean of School of Dentistry, Central Asian University, Tashkent, Uzbekistan.

Anantha Murthy is an accomplished academic and researcher in the field of Artificial Intelligence, with a special focus on Machine Learning, Deep Learning, Computer Vision, Natural Language Processing, and Cultural Informatics. Currently serving as an Assistant Professor (III) at NMAM Institute of Technology, Nitte, he brings over 17 years of teaching and research experience, complemented by a recent Ph.D. in Artificial Intelligence from Srinivas University, Mangalore. Dr. Murthy's work spans a diverse range of applications, including predictive analytics in agriculture and healthcare, and the innovative use of AI in cultural contexts like Yakshagana imagery.

Digvijay Pandey is a Lecturer in the Department of technical Education and a Research Scholar at IET Lucknow, India.

Shailendra Pardeshi is an Assistant Professor in the Computer Engineering Department at the R C Patel Institute of Technology, Shirpur, MH, India.

R Yogitha graduated from Anna University with Bachelor's Degree in Computer Science and Engineering and from Sathyabama Institute of Science and Technology with Master's Degree in Computer Science and Engineering in 2018. She has more than five years of teaching experience in Department of Computer Science and Engineering at Sathyabama Institute of Science and Technology. Her area of research is Deep Learning Machine Learning and Artificial Intelligence. She has presented her paper work conferences and published her research works in some reputed journals.

Varanasi Rahul is an Assistant Professor at JAIN University (Bangalore), Semi qualified Cost Accountant, holding three Post graduations M. Com (Acct & Tax), M .Com(Mgt.) and MA (History). He has cleared UGC NET in Commerce Twice, cleared AP SET in Commerce, History and Management and TS SET in Commerce. He has 5 years of experience as Ass. Professor and 6 months of experience as Corporate Tax Associate for Australian Taxation in PWC (Big 4). He is a Freelance Archaeologist, Epigraphist in Brahmi (Practicing), and Numismatist. More than 30 newspaper articles have been published in Deccan Chronical, Times of India and other Local new papers. He presented and participated in 29 National and International Seminars and published 3 research article in SCOPUS, 2 in Web of science, 2 in ABDC (C), 4 research articles in Peer reviewed Journals. He is a story writer and 5 of his stories has been published in top magazines of AP. He authored 3 books, 2 in the field of History and Epigraphy and 1 book about Extradition of fugitive offenders. He published 11 Patents, received design grant for 2 Indian designs and 2 UK designs

M. Rajkumar is in the Department of Smart Computing at the School of computer science Engineering and Information Systems at Vellore Institute of Technology, VIT University, Vellore.

Bhawna Janghel Rajput, Assistant Professor Department of Computer Science & Engineering, Rungta College of Engineering and Technology, Bhilai, durg.(C.G.) She has 12 years of teaching experince. She has Guided 6 Ph.d Scholars undergoing. she has published 25 papaers in reputed National and International Journals.she has published 2 Patents. She is a reviewer of IEEE and member of Inence –Innovation and Science as well as Reviewer .She is a chairman Board of studies in bharti Vishwavidyalaya,durg, She is also guiding Ph.D. Scholars in various area of research includes Computer Networking, Sensor Networks, Data Mining, information systems and security and Cloud Computing etc.

N Sathyanarayana has over 15 years of teaching experience at the UG and PG levels. He holds a Master's in Business Administration and Commerce and is pursuing a Ph.D. He currently holds the position of Assistant Professor in the School of Commerce at Jain (Deemed-to-be University), Bangalore. He has published 22 research papers in international journals, 7 research papers in national journals, and presented 14 research papers at international conferences and 11 research papers at national conferences. He has co-authored 2 books at national level and 8 book chapters (Scopus indexed).

M. Selvi has received her B.E., degree in Computer Science & Engineering from Sri Sairam Engineering College affiliated to Anna University. She has completed M. Tech., in Information Technology from Sathyabama University. She obtained her Ph.D., degree in Computer Science and Engineering at Sathyabama Institute of Science and Technology, Chennai. She has published papers in National & International Journals and Conferences. Her research areas are Wireless Sensor Network(WSN), Data Mining, Network Security, Machine Learning, Image Processing and Web Mining. She has more than Seventeen years of teaching experience. Currently she is working in Sathyabama Institute of Science and Technology.

Mukta Sharma presently working as Professor and Director Research, IIMT University, Meerut, Uttar Pradesh, India. Previously she was working as Professor and head, Department of Microbiology at Shree Bankey Bihari Dental College, Ghaziabad. She has been teaching Microbiology for the last twenty four years. Her research work is focused on Bacteriocin (Nisin) production and probiotics. She has published a number of scientific research papers in national and international journals. She has been published twelve books and has conducted many research programmes on Microbiology. She has five granted patents and 14 awards. She was also invited as keynoter speaker to present her scientific research work in many international and national conferences. She has been awarded with many academic awards. She has successfully completed a course of Medical Microbiology conducted by University of Goettingen, Germany. She is an Editorial Board Member of Journal of Pure and Applied Science & Technology and Academic Journals Online and lifetime member of Indian Journal of Microbiology.

Kawerinder Singh Sidhu has a total work experience of more than 24 years. His experience includes more than 14 years in the industry and 10 years in the Academics. He worked in domains like HRM, Training, MIS, Finance, Operations and Research. His industrisal experience includes working with organizations like Indian Military Academy, Grenada e-Services, Exl Services Ltd and HCL Technologies Ltd. Besides that, he worked in an ICSSR sponsored research project assigned to Doon University, Dehradun. He is UGC NET/SLET qualified in Management and currently working as Assistant Professor in Uttaranchal University, Dehradun. He has many publications on his name which are featured in Scopus database.

T. Illakiya is working as an Assistant professor in the Department of Computational Intelligence, SRM Institute of Science and Technology, Chennai, India. She has completed Ph.D. from the School of Computer Science and Engineering, Vellore Institute of Technology, Chennai, India. She received the M.Tech. degree in Information Technology from Anna University, India. She has published more than 20 research papers in journals and conferences. Her research interests include deep learning, computer vision, and medical image analysis.

Shikha Verma, an Associate Professor at MMICTBM (MCA), is a distinguished academic and resource person in the domains of Artificial Intelligence, Machine Learning, Sentiment Analysis, and their application in the stock market. With over a decade of teaching experience and prior contributions to Santan Dharma College, Ambala Cantt (affiliated with Kurukshetra University), Dr. Verma has delivered insightful lectures and workshops as a resource person. Her expertise, reflected in her numerous research papers published in reputable journals and conferences, underscores her commitment to advancing knowledge and innovation in these evolving fields. Dr. Verma's lectures as a resource person have been instrumental in shaping the academic landscape and fostering learning excellence. She has taught many Certificate courses online during Covid Like Python for Beginners, LaTeX, Open-Source Research Tools, Web Development, Design Hassle Free Websites Using Word press. She has done Ph.D. in Computer Applications, CT University. Experienced educator and researcher specializing in applying machine learning techniques to the stock market. Holds an MCA from Kurukshetra University and a BCA from the same institution. Proficient in teaching a diverse range of subjects

Index

www.ingramcontent.com/pod-product-compliance
Ingram Content Group UK Ltd.
Pitfield, Milton Keynes, MK11 3LW, UK
UKHW051038091026
15624UKWH00011B/523

9 798369 398210